In the Face of Death

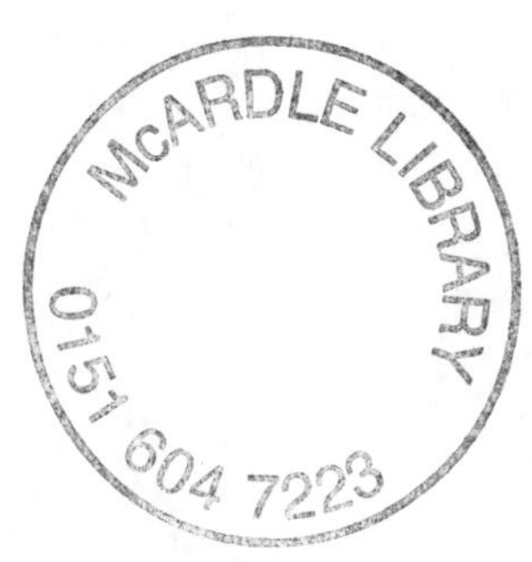

Danai Papadatou, PhD, is a professor of clinical psychology at the Faculty of Nursing of the University of Athens. Her clinical experience, research interests, and publications focus mostly on issues related to pediatric palliative care, bereavement support, and health care providers' responses to the death of their patients. Her work is known internationally through her publications, presentations at scientific meetings, and active involvement in international work groups and societies. She has organized several conferences and symposia and, along with her father Costas Papadatos, organized in 1989 the First International Conference on Children and Death and subsequently edited the book *Children and Death* (1991). She has received an award from Children's Hospice International (1989), and the Death Educator Award from the Association for Death Education and Counseling (2001). She had the honor to serve from 1999 to 2004 as chair of the International Work Group on Death, Dying, and Bereavement, an organization of leaders in the field of thanatology.

Dr. Papadatou is also the founder and president of a Greek nonprofit organization ("Merimna"), which provides services to children and families who are coping with illness and death experiences, offers training to professionals who support seriously ill and bereaved children and adolescents, organizes psychosocial interventions in disaster situations, and sensitizes the Greek public on issues related to death and dying.

In the Face of Death

Professionals Who Care for the Dying and the Bereaved

DANAI PAPADATOU, PhD

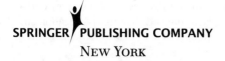

Springer Publishing Company, LLC
11 West 42nd Street
New York, NY 10036
www.springerpub.com

Acquisitions Editor: Sheri W. Sussman
Production Editor: Julia Rosen
Cover design: Mimi Flow
Composition: Apex CoVantage

09 10 11 / 5 4 3 2 1

Library of Congress Cataloging-in-Publication Data

Papadatou, Danai.
In the face of death: professionals who care for the dying and the bereaved/ Danai Papadatou.
p. cm.
Includes bibliographical references and index.
ISBN 978-0-8261-0256-0 (alk. paper)
1. Terminal care. 2. Bereavement. 3. Grief therapy. I. Title.
R726.8.P35 2009
616'.029—dc22 2008050933

Printed in the United States of America by Hamilton Printing Company.

To Costas, my father,
and
Clea, my mother,
who gave me the roots
and wings of confidence
to explore the challenges of life.

Contents

Foreword *xi*
Preface *xiii*
Acknowledgments *xix*

SECTION I: THE CARING RELATIONSHIP 1

1 Society, Science, and Death 3

The Medical Model of Care 5
The Biopsychosocial and Holistic Model of Care 6
The Relationship-Centered Approach to Care 9

2 A Relationship of Care 21

Partners in Care 22
The Attachment Bond 24
Request for Services in Death Situations 25
The Person's Attachment Behaviors 28
The Professional's Caregiving Behaviors 32
Bond Affirmation Through Belonging 35

3 Distinct Features of the Helping Relationship 39

Exposure to Death and Mortality Awareness 40
Inevitability of Suffering Versus Potential for Growth 47
Experience of an Altered Sense of Time 50
Involvement in the Caregiving Relationship 54

4 The Accompanying Process 61

The Myth 61
From Myth to Reality: Assuming a Companioning Role 67
Condition 1: Establishing an Appropriate Frame 70

Condition 2: Being Fully Present 79
Condition 3: Being Vulnerable Enough 92
Condition 4: Developing a Holding Environment for Ourselves and Co-Workers 103
Working in Private Practice 105
When the Care Provider Is Seriously Ill or Dying 108
The End of Accompaniment 110

SECTION II: THE CARE PROVIDER IN DEATH SITUATIONS 113

5 The Wounded Healer 115

From Myth to Reality: The Suffering of the Care Provider 117
Aspects of Care Providers' Suffering 120
Grief: A Healthy Response to Death Situations 128

6 A Model for Professionals' Grieving Process 131

Proposition 1: Professionals Who Experience the Death of a Person as a Personal Loss Are Likely to Grieve 134
Proposition 2: Grieving Involves a Fluctuation Between Experiencing and Avoiding Loss and Grief 139
Proposition 3: Through Grieving, Meanings Are Attributed to Death, Dying, and Caregiving 146
Proposition 4: Personal Meanings Are Affected by Meanings That Are Shared by Co-workers, and Vice Versa 155
Proposition 5: Grief Overload and Grief Complications Occur When There Is No Fluctuation Between Experiencing and Avoiding Loss and Grief 159
Proposition 6: Grief Offers Opportunities for Personal Growth 163
Proposition 7: The Professional's Grieving Process is Affected by Several Interacting Variables 167

7 The Rewards of Caregiving 175

Obstacles to Rewarding Experiences 178
Conditions That Promote Rewarding Experiences 179
The Wisdom of the Wounded Healer 186

SECTION III: THE TEAM IN THE FACE OF DEATH 189

8 Caregiving Organizations and Death 191

Suffering in the Workplace 193

The Organization's Myths and Ideals 196
The Organization's Primary Tasks and Mode of Functioning 198

9 Team Functioning in Death Situations 203

Principle 1: Team Functioning Is Affected by the Organization's Culture 206
Principle 2: Team Rules Determine How Professionals Should Care for Dying and Bereaved People and Cope With Suffering 209
Principle 3: There Are No Functional or Dysfunctional Teams—Only Teams That Use Functional and Dysfunctional Patterns to Cope With Loss, Death, and Suffering 217
Principle 4: The Chronic Use of Dysfunctional Patterns Renders a Team Vulnerable to Various Types of Disorganization 230
Principle 5: Crises Are Inevitable; They Hold the Potential for Team Disorganization as Well as Team Growth 236
Principle 6: All Teams Have the Potential to Function With Competence 242
Principle 7: Interprofessional Collaboration Is an Unfolding Process That Is Reflective of a Team's Development and Growth 256
Principle 8: Resilience Is Enhanced by the Team's Ability to Cope Effectively With Suffering, and to Creatively Use Its Resources to Foster Change and Growth 260

10 The Good-Enough Team 269

Team Narratives of Traumas and Achievements 271
Leaders in Good-Enough Teams 275
Supervisors and Consultants 278
Toward a Community of Support 281

11 The Challenges of Educating Health Care Professionals 285

Challenge 1: Develop a Philosophy of Teaching That Promotes Relational Learning and Reflective Practice 287
Challenge 2: Develop Curricula That Include Goals, Learning Objectives, and Methods of Teaching That Focus on Relationships With the Dying, the Bereaved, and Co-Workers 288
Challenge 3: Integrate Current Knowledge Into Educational Programs and Supervised Clinical Applications 290
Challenge 4: Evaluate Training Outcomes as Well as the Context and Process by Which Learning Occurs 291
Challenge 5: Integrate Formal and Informal Learning Activities Into the Work Context 293

Epilogue 297
Appendix: Brief Description of Bowlby's Theory on Attachment 301
References 305
Index 321

Foreword

Doctor, Doctor, shall I die?
Yes, my child, and so shall I.

Skipping Rhyme, circa 1894

This old rhyme encapsulates the painful reality that underlies this remarkable book. We are all in the same boat, and the main difference between the dying patient and the doctor is that the patient will probably die before the doctor.

Life-threatening illnesses, such as cancer, invade families and societies as well as patients. We are all changed by them. "Send not to learn for whom the bell tolls/it tolls for thee (John Donne)." The implication is that, if we are to be of help, we must include death's influence on all of the relationships that surround and are affected by it.

Much of the literature in recent years about palliative care (the care of the dying) and bereavement care (the care of the bereaved) has the patient and the bereaved individual as the objects of study. In this book, Danai Papadatou does something quite different. She draws on her considerable experience of working with nurses, doctors, and other members of the caring professions along with wide reading and her own systematic research to explain how death affects the caregivers, both as individuals and teams, and how this then affects their care of people facing death or the death of those they love. From this analysis she draws out an approach of relational care—care based on an understanding of relationships—that should be essential reading for these professions.

Although she makes use of sophisticated educational, psychological, and sociological knowledge, Papadatou writes in an engaging and nontechnical language, managing to convey complex ideas in a manner that is accessible to all.

As a psychiatrist with a special interest in people's attachments to each other and the consequences when those attachments are severed by death, I found Papadatou's extension of this field of study to include the caring team both enlightening and personally challenging. I suspect that I am not the only reader who will realize that our own needs sometimes conflict with those of our patients. But we are never too old to learn, and it is reassuring to find that we do not have to be 'perfect' but simply 'good enough.' As an author, teacher, psychologist, and friend, Danai Papadatou is certainly good enough for me.

Colin Murray Parkes OBE, MD, FRCPsych

Preface

Thousands of years ago, during the fifth century B.C., Hippocrates described medicine as a practice and an art. The Hippocratic Corpus, his collected writings as well as those of his students, states that the healer who exercises his skill and knowledge for the benefit of the sick may experience suffering in the process. Hippocrates perceived and described the healer's suffering as integral to the care of the ill person:

> There are some arts which to those that possess them are painful, but to those that use them are helpful, a common good to laymen, but to those that practice them grievous. Of such arts there is one which the Greeks call medicine. For the medical man sees terrible sights, touches unpleasant things, and the misfortunes of others bring a harvest of sorrows that are peculiarly his; yet the sick—of means of this art—get rid themselves of the worst of evils: disease, suffering, pain and death. (Jones, 1923, p. 227)

Twenty-five centuries later, even with advances in medicine and nursing, suffering among health care professionals is largely disenfranchised and neglected despite its integral role in their work. There is a widespread belief that suffering is not supposed to happen to experts. It happens only to people who are ill, dying, or bereaved and these are the people who receive help to enable them to cope with and alleviate it. The suffering of care providers has been ignored, mostly because they prefer to suppress it or keep it private. The privatization of their pain prevents them from openly acknowledging their anxiety, anger, sadness, guilt, fear, disgust, and grief, which remains hidden, along with the sense of helplessness, hopelessness, meaninglessness, or confusion that is experienced at times. However, by dismissing and denying suffering, they concurrently close their eyes, shut their ears, and turn their back on any person, family, or situation that triggers disturbing thoughts, feelings, or responses.

Most studies on burnout suggest that one of the most stressful situations that health care providers experience on the job is death. Recent studies of trauma workers who are empathically engaged with people who are traumatized by death, abuse, and disasters suggest that professionals are vulnerable to vicarious traumatization and compassion fatigue. This may be true. But are compassion stress, traumatic disorders, and burnout all we experience in the face of death, or is there a wider and more complex process that occurs in illness, dying, and bereavement situations? Should we focus on understanding our intrapsychic and idiosyncratic responses, or should we expand our perspective and explore how we develop relationships with dying and bereaved people, what we bring into these relationships, how we affect them, and how we are affected in return? Do we suffer? Can suffering be totally eliminated in the face of human loss and death? Can it be changed or transformed?

"You will get used to death," the medical director of a pediatric oncology unit told me compassionately when he saw me crying over the death of my first young patient. I realized over the years that one can never get used to death. Nor can one ever become immune to human pain and suffering without paying a high price. Occasionally, we get used to the sight of death or to listening to stories of trauma. It is natural. Unfortunately, some get used to a sense of futility ("What's the point?"), hopelessness ("There is nothing we can offer"), or despair and learn to avoid relationships with dying and bereaved people in order to protect themselves.

When our personal suffering remains untapped, unexplored, and hidden, our relationships with individuals, families, and colleagues are deeply affected. This happens because suffering does not occur in a vacuum. It stems from relationships; it develops within relationships and affects them in positive or negative ways. Yet it is within relationships that suffering can also be alleviated and/or transformed. By shedding light upon our own responses in the face of serious illness, dying, and death, we bring them out of the darkness, understand them, and seek alternative ways to accept them, own them, cope, and occasionally change them. It is with such a goal that this book was written. It aims to explore the experiences of care providers who care for seriously ill, dying, or bereaved children, adolescents, or adults, and to offer a framework in which their responses can be understood, addressed, and transformed. Based upon theory, research findings, and clinical illustrations, this book intends to trigger readers' thinking and hopefully elicit reflection and debate among colleagues.

The first section of the book, "The Caring Relationship," adopts a primarily interpersonal perspective by focusing on the relationship between the person who is dying or grieving and the care provider. Its main purpose is to describe the nature of services that are provided at the end of life and through bereavement according to the medical and biopsychosocial model of care, and propose as an alternative *a relationship-centered approach to care*. This approach acknowledges the reciprocal influence between care seekers and care providers, each of whom brings his or her own unique set of experiences, values, and perspectives to the caring relationship. Special emphasis is placed on the dynamics involved, and on the characteristics that render this relationship distinct from other helping relationships. The Greek myth of the labyrinth and the ferocious minotaur that Theseus succeeded in killing with the help of Ariadne's love and wisdom is used to illustrate the unique aspects and conditions that facilitate an accompanying process through the dark and unfamiliar paths of dying and bereavement.

The second section, "The Care Provider in Death Situations," adopts an intrapsychic approach and addresses our personal responses to death. Another Greek myth, that of the wounded healer, is used to illustrate how the ability to care is enhanced when we learn to recognize and accept our suffering as part of being human and empathic in our relations with others. Suffering is discussed in relation to the concepts of burnout, compassion fatigue, and vicarious traumatization, while a new framework is offered for understanding some of our healthy responses in the face of death. A model for the grieving process of health professionals based on the findings of studies that I conducted with my colleagues in Greece and Hong Kong is presented, and its seven basic propositions are analyzed. Physicians' and nurses' accounts illustrate aspects of their grief that are affected by personal, interpersonal, and social variables. Special consideration is given to the difficulties and grief complications that some professionals experience, as well as to conditions that promote rewarding experiences and enhance personal growth.

Finally, the third section, "The Team in the Face of Death," adopts a systemic perspective and focuses on the organizational context within which care services are offered. Attention is given to how a team organizes itself and develops functional and/or dysfunctional patterns in order to cope with loss and death. Eight principles illuminate how teams cope with death encounters at a systemic level. Special consideration is given to dysfunctional patterns as well as to the risk of team disorganization when such patterns are perpetuated over time. Three key conditions that enhance team functioning and resilience in death situations are analyzed: (1) commitment to goals, tasks, and co-workers, (2) establishment of a holding environment that allows team members to contain, reflect on, and transform suffering, and (3) open teamwork that enables professionals to move beyond the team's boundaries and—through meaningful collaborations—offer interdisciplinary services that benefit dying and bereaved people as well as themselves. This section ends with an invitation to review our philosophy, goals, and methods of teaching palliative and bereavement care in order to adopt a relational approach that promotes learning through relationships among students, instructors, patients, families, and practitioners. Five challenges are discussed, innovative approaches as to the methods of teaching are presented, and special emphasis is placed on how best to prepare students and young practitioners to accompany dying and bereaved people and cope with loss and death issues in their professional and personal lives.

I have tried to avoid using the impersonal word *patient* as much as possible, because I believe that we care primarily for *people* in death situations, who are assigned the role of patients. Whenever the word is used, it is not with the intent of undermining my respect for each individual's uniqueness.

My thinking and writing have been influenced by several theoretical approaches, rather than by a single psychological school of thought. My European studies in psychodynamic theories and my American postgraduate education in humanistic psychology and a systemic approach to care have been integrated in my clinical practice, which was enriched by the recent contributions of phenomenology to the health care field. Influential in my work with dying and bereaved people have been the works of John Bowlby on human bonds and separation; of Alfred Adler on self-determination and social belonging; of my teacher and mentor Oscar Christensen on families; of Eric Cassell, Kay Toombs, and Arthur Frank on the phenomenology of illness; and of René Kaës on institutions. A source of incredible learning has also been my relationships with individuals, families, and colleagues with whom I have shared death experiences. They enabled me to explore unknown territories and expand my horizons of understanding. The content of this book derives from three major sources: my clinical experience in pediatric palliative and bereavement care, my academic experience in the education of health care professionals, and my research on care providers who are repeatedly exposed to death encounters.

The book is addressed to professionals who work in caregiving organizations (e.g., hospitals, hospices, home care programs, bereavement centers) or in private practice. This includes nurses, physicians, psychologists, social workers, chaplains, palliative care specialists, bereavement counselors, and other health care specialists who provide services to seriously ill people and support families through the illness, dying, and bereavement process. It is also intended for trainees as well as for educators who design courses or seminars on death and dying, on health psychology, on communication skills, and on stress management and staff support. Health managers can also benefit from understanding the complexity of employees' and teams' responses and of the necessity of building appropriate structures to support care providers in their caregiving role. In addition, the book can be of value to researchers who wish to design qualitative studies and advance our knowledge of a critical topic that deserves deeper exploration and consideration. Even though it is written for professionals, I believe that it can also apply to volunteers who accompany families through dying and bereavement.

Over the past decades, clinicians, researchers, and educators have emphasized the importance of humanizing the care of sick and dying people who are institutionalized and of bereaved individuals, who have been negatively affected by the growth of a grief industry that pathologizes bereavement. It is my belief that in order to ensure the humanization of care, we need to humanize the role we assume in death situations instead of idealizing it or projecting onto it powers and qualities we do not possess. Of all living experiences, death reminds us that we are all finite and mortal. But death also invites us to value life, invest it with meaning, and honor it.

The process of writing this book has been filled with emotional, cognitive, and spiritual challenges as well as with personal transformations. I relived the deaths of several children I have accompanied through the end of life, as well as the bereavements of many families. I reflected on the quality of services we provide and read and reread the transcripts of colleagues who confided in me their most intimate thoughts and work-related experiences in the context of my research studies.

This book is a small token of my deep gratitude to all the children, adolescents, and adults whom I have been privileged to accompany in death situations. Through their suffering and personal growth, they taught me about living and valuing the present moment while striving to contribute to the creation of a better and more human world for all.

Acknowledgments

Throughout the journey of writing this book several people have been very supportive, and I am indebted to them. Robert Kastenbaum was most encouraging of my decision to undertake and commit myself to this challenging endeavor. Barbara Sourkes, my dearest colleague and friend, was always available to read the manuscript at critical stages of its development, discuss key issues, and offer constructive feedback. She has been a valuable companion and an excellent critic. I am also deeply thankful to Colin Parkes, Chuck Corr, and Scott Long, who read a few chapters, offered constructive feedback, and enabled me to clarify some of my thinking. My appreciation also extends to Kelly Moraiti and Eleni Kotrozou for their assistance with the organizational details of the manuscript, as well as to Thanassis Goudzivelakis and Eleni Kotsani, two nurses, who gave me permission to use their drawings in this book. Some of the content in chapters four and six also appear in the Oxford Textbook of Palliative Care of Children (2006) with permission from the author.

I wish to express my gratitude to Sheri W. Sussman, editorial vice president at Springer Publishing Company, who played a key role as the acquisitions editor of this book, and who has supported me with her encouragement, understanding, and persistence. Finally, I offer my heartfelt thanks and endless love to my daughter Alexia for being so understanding of my desire to write this book and so eager to celebrate its completion.

Acknowledgments

The Caring Relationship

SECTION I

1 Society, Science, and Death

It is widely assumed that Western societies are death denying. This assumption has been reinforced by the seminal work of the French historian Ariès (1974, 1981), who studied the representations and management of death in Europe from the early Middle Ages through modern times. Ariès described how death, which was initially "tamed" and perceived as a familiar event in the lives of people who were frequently exposed to it, progressively came to be an alien experience, cut off from the rest of life, and denied as a result of historical and social developments. He argued that modern society's denial of death is reflected in the prevailing attitudes toward dying individuals, who are put away in health care institutions, and toward bereaved people, whose grief is expected to occur in private. Perceived as a threat to social order, death became a taboo topic that is excluded from social discourse.

Ariès' thesis on the denial of death is questioned by some sociologists, who offer an alternative interpretation. They claim that modern secular societies "face up" to the reality of death by organizing themselves in order to actively cope with the irreversible disruption of social bonds caused by death (Albery, Elliot, & Elliot, 1993; Parsons, 1978; Seale, 1998). According to Kastenbaum (1977), each society develops a death system that more or less formally and explicitly comprises a system of symbols, meanings, and practices assigned to specific people with defined roles (e.g., health care providers, funeral directors, lawyers) and designated locations (e.g., health care institutions, cemeteries, funeral homes). Academic, legal, religious, and health care institutions define which death is "acceptable" and which is "unacceptable" and hide certain aspects of dying and bereavement while rendering others public (Seale, 1998). In most Western societies, for example, academic institutions propose a scientific body of knowledge that guides professionals in how to perceive, control, and manage death and how to care for the dying and the bereaved; legal institutions create laws that specify which deaths are socially acceptable (e.g., war-related deaths, death by capital punishment, or euthanasia) and which are not and should be controlled or sanctioned (e.g., death by murder, suicide); religious institutions offer systems of beliefs that explain death and create rituals to help people cope with mortality and suffering; and the media shapes representations of death through the display of certain images (e.g., of violent deaths caused by accidents, disasters, terrorist attacks), the avoidance of others (e.g., slow, lingering deaths), the use of specific words and phrases (e.g., "war casualties"), or the creation of narratives about death events. Thus, every society has its own unique death system that shapes and affects death-related experiences.

Western secular societies, which have attempted to hide—rather than deny—death during the last century, are currently confronted with a new reality. Disasters, terrorist acts and threats, and war events are introduced directly or indirectly—through the media—into our daily lives. They do not happen only to others living in foreign lands. These out-of-the-ordinary experiences can happen to anybody. We are repeatedly reminded that we live in a world that is not safe. Tight controls and warnings about our safety in airports, at big gatherings, even in schools; alerts about hurricanes, floods, and fires; or the practice of safety procedures in the case of earthquakes and human-induced disasters are a few examples that highlight the uncertainty of our existence. Concurrently, extraordinary achievements by the biomedical sciences create new hopes. Cloning, stem cell research, organ transplantation, and spectacular pharmaceutical developments that prolong or attempt to create life raise new ethical dilemmas and concerns regarding the limits of our living existence.

In this era, life-and-death issues are increasingly brought out in the open. Attracted and threatened by them, secular societies are challenged to address these issues. People who are sick, dying, and bereaved are affected by these conflicting pulls as well as by the new ethical dilemmas that determine their trajectory through dying and bereavement.

Concurrently, we, the care providers, are challenged to offer services in ways that are acceptable and meaningful to them as well as to us, and to society. We are incited to review the models of care that guide our actions and orient our clinical practice and eventually revise, expand, and/or change them. With this goal in view, I will briefly examine two prevailing models that affect our approach to the care of dying and bereaved people: the medical model of care and the biopsychosocial or holistic model of care. Each offers a context that defines caregiving and consequently affects death experiences for those who seek services and those who provide them.

THE MEDICAL MODEL OF CARE

The medical model is concerned with the assessment and treatment of sick bodies, diseases, and mental health conditions. These are perceived as independent of the person who suffers. They are assessed, objectively measured, classified, labeled, and treated. Dying and bereavement, which are natural processes, are perceived as dysfunctional conditions to be controlled by science. More precisely, dying is medicalized through the management of physical symptoms located in a dysfunctional body that hosts a life-threatening disease, while bereavement is pathologized and viewed as atypical. In both situations, care aims to restore health and resolve grief through a return to "normalcy," which was disrupted by illness or the loss of a loved person.

The medical model of care sets as its primary goal the "solution of a riddle" rather than the care of a person (Nuland, 1994). The riddle in dying is posed by the life-threatening nature of the disease, and in bereavement, by the intensity and duration of grief symptoms. Solving the riddle comprises the identification of a correct assessment or diagnosis, an appropriate treatment or intervention, and an accurate prognosis as to the possibility of health recovery or grief resolution.

The care provider assumes a role of "expert" in the solution of the riddle, while the dying or bereaved person is turned into a case to be solved. A relationship between the professional and the person is developed via a body that hosts the disease or via a psyche that hosts an atypical mental health condition. Their relationship is governed by strict rules and expectations that protect both participants from becoming emotionally involved. They cooperate against a *dis-ease* or *dis-order* caused by illness, death, and suffering and become adversaries when their goals are not achieved.

A heroic script is assigned to "experts," who assume the responsibility of all decisions and treatments, while a victim script is assigned to dying and bereaved people, who conform to orders, rules, and regulations. These heroic versus victimizing scripts are perpetuated with the consent of both individuals seeking services and practitioners who abide by the values of a medical model that promotes an illusion of control over death and over suffering. When interventions fail to control death and suffering, dying and bereaved people are either subjected to futile treatments and therapies that compromise the quality of life or abandoned by clinicians, who, in turn, are rejected and accused by those who showed trust in their "expertise." Care providers who are not successful in restoring health or resolving grief are left to cope with a sense of failure, helplessness, and despair over the pursuit of unrealistic goals.

While the medical model has never been able to fully control death, it has succeeded in *owning* death by defining it in scientific and biological terms. Consider death certificates. All define death as a bodily event that is measurable, objective, and located in a dysfunctional body. It is never recorded as a natural event due to old age, or as a psychological event caused by the decision to end one's life, or as a social event triggered by the suffering of a broken heart or bereavement. Death is presented and understood *only* in biological terms, and it is presented as such to the dying as well as to bereaved people.

Over the past few decades, the dramatic increase of scientific knowledge of life-threatening illnesses as well as of bereavement has contributed to spectacular advances in the care of dying and bereaved people. As a side effect, however, it has also contributed to the pathologization of normal processes such as dying and grieving. Dying and bereavement are therefore de-normalized and often de-humanized as they are transformed into scientific riddles. This pathologization and medicalization have increased the marginalization of people and have served as a form of social control over death and suffering. Care seekers and care providers are, therefore, deprived of the meaningful and personal relationships that often develop in death situations.

THE BIOPSYCHOSOCIAL AND HOLISTIC MODEL OF CARE

In protest of the over-medicalization and dehumanization of care, an alternative model, the biopsychosocial model of care, made its appearance by the end of the 20th century. Charts on the rights of sick people forced professionals to redefine their goals and values, and George Engel (1977, 1980, 1997) set the foundation of a model that took into account their psychosocial needs. This model adopts a patient-centered approach that deals with individuals rather than diseases and clinical cases. It advocates that each individual be treated as a unique human being and understood in his or her wholeness (Balint, 1969). The concept of wholeness refers to the undivided unity of a person's body and mind, which is in reciprocal interaction with the physical and social environment.

The principles of this holistic model were implemented and further developed by some inspirational health professionals who cared for people at the end of life. Cicely Saunders, Elisabeth Kübler-Ross, Jeanne Quint Benoliel, Florence Wald, Balfour Mount, Ida Martinson, and Colin Murray Parkes were some of the charismatic leaders who contributed to the development of the palliative care approach. This approach was based on a new set of values that humanized the care of dying individuals, who were invited to actively participate in their care, and of families who were supported before and after the patient's death. The message of these pioneers was loud and clear: individuals have the right to have a say in their experiences and the care they receive in the face of death. Dying and bereavement are experiences that belong to *them,* not to professionals.

Thus, focus shifted from professionals, who know what is "best" for others, to individuals and families, who identify what is important to them when life comes to an end (Egan, 1998; Egan & Labyak, 2001). Care providers with different scientific backgrounds and experience adopt an interdisciplinary team approach that addresses physical, psychological, social, and spiritual needs and ensures a dignified death that corresponds to each person's and family's values, desires, and preferences. This approach turned into a social movement that spread around the world. The response was so impressive that within only 30 years, approximately 5,000 hospice, palliative, and bereavement care services were developed in several countries across all the continents (Clark, 2002).

There are four distinct ways in which palliative care differs from the biomedical model and offers an alternative approach to the care of dying and bereaved people:

1 Death is defined as a natural, unavoidable life event that causes increased suffering due to the final and irreversible rupture of human bonds. Interventions aim not to fight death when it is imminent, but to ensure dignified conditions for the dying person and to offer support for the bereaved. Focus is shifted from the

prevention and control of death to the experience of living with the awareness and reality of death. Palliative care is introduced when life-threatening disease is diagnosed, and grief counseling is made available to facilitate the family's acceptance and adjustment to loss.

2. The person's lived experience and, by extension, his or her biopsychosocial and spiritual needs become the main focus of care. This patient-centered approach is expanded to include significant others. Thus, holism is ensured through a family-centered approach that addresses the needs of family members, who participate in shaping experiences at the end of life and through bereavement. This approach acknowledges the impact of death upon networks of people who are changed forever as a result of loss.
3. Teamwork is redefined so as to promote interdisciplinary collaboration among professionals with different expertise, who cooperate with each other instead of compartmentalizing their services. The team's goal is to integrate various services into a comprehensive plan of care that addresses the needs, preferences, and desires of each person and family who is faced with death and bereavement.
4. Care providers are encouraged to develop personal relationships with dying and bereaved people and to accompany them in their trajectories. The hazards of caregiving are recognized, and the importance of professionals' support is acknowledged.

The palliative care approach assigns an active role both to professionals, and to dying and grieving individuals, who are expected to develop a partnership toward the achievement of a good death or recovery from loss. In this partnership, a heroic script is usually assigned to terminally ill people, who are expected to display courage by being aware of their dying; by being expressive of their innermost feelings, thoughts, and needs; and by being autonomous in their decisions. In a similar way, the bereaved are expected to openly express their feelings and thoughts, work through their grief, and move toward "restoration," or "resolution."

Open awareness, self-expression, and self-determination are Western values reinforced by the practice of palliative and bereavement care in contemporary secular societies. Studies undertaken in North America, the United Kingdom, and other European countries confirm a shift in physicians' attitudes toward truth telling and the use of advance directives in the face of death. The person seeking services is expected to lead the journey through dying or grief, while the professional assumes the role of a companion who offers information, guidance, and support. This role is believed to require expertise and involves helping people to come to terms with their mortality; live meaningfully in the face of death; address physical, psychosocial, and spiritual needs; share farewells with loved ones; prepare for the funeral; and be supported through bereavement (Seale, 1998). These activities function as rituals that prepare the dying for death, orient bereaved families toward living, and guide professionals in their interventions. They bring a sentiment of order that enhances control over death, dying, and bereavement.

The palliative care approach reflects modern society's active attempt to face up to the reality of death by introducing dying and bereavement into the midstream of life. It personalizes care by addressing individualized needs and attempts to humanize it by rendering it social. People receive support from the caring communities of home care programs, hospices, and bereavement centers rather than being marginalized or alienated.

THE RELATIONSHIP-CENTERED APPROACH TO CARE

Where do we stand at the dawn of the 21st century? I believe we are at a crossroads. Much has been accomplished within a short period of time, and a great deal remains to be learned. We are challenged to critically review our models of care and evaluate our practices, raise critical questions, and seek answers that will help us to move forward. This process has just begun in both end-of-life and bereavement care (e.g., Fins, Miller, Acres, Bacchett, Huzzard, & Rapkin, 1999; Larson & Hoyt, 2007; Randall & Downie, 2006; Stroebe, Hansson, Stroebe, & Schut, 2007; SUPPORT Investigators, 1995).

Studies conducted in North America with large populations of terminally ill patients indicate that the biomedical model of care is still widely prevalent, while serious obstacles compromise the application of palliative care. In spite of people's preference for a humanized death that occurs at home, the majority continue to die in hospitals and nursing homes, where they are treated as diseases or "cases" to be managed.

The use of life-sustaining interventions remains excessive, and physical pain is largely mismanaged, causing increased suffering among dying patients and their relatives (e.g., Fins et al., 1999; SUPPORT Investigators, 1995). Evidence indicates that palliative services are offered only to limited populations, particularly patients with life-threatening diseases that have a predictable course and outcome, such as cancer and AIDS. Elderly people and patients with chronic conditions for which death cannot be predicted (e.g., chronic heart failure, chronic obstructive airways disease, diabetes) are deprived of psychosocial and spiritual care. Even though they suffer from a terminal condition, they are not viewed as dying, and consequently, their needs are totally neglected. They come in and out of health care institutions until one day they "suddenly" succumb and die as a result of health complications (Field, 1996; Seale, 1996). Finally, limited access to end-of-life care is common among people with minority ethnic backgrounds. The care they do receive is often compromised by professionals' insensitivity to their cultural beliefs and practices regarding life-and-death issues. As a result, they grow to mistrust the health care system, which they perceive as inconsiderate of their values, needs, and preferences (Krakauer, Crenner, & Fox, 2002).

Similar findings reflect the status of pediatric palliative care (for a review, see Liben, Papadatou, & Wolfe, 2008). Most children in Western countries die in hospitals, and some in intensive care units. Despite the fact that home care has been repeatedly found to have beneficial effects upon parents' and siblings' adjustment to loss, professionals are reluctant to refer children and adolescents to home care programs or hospice facilities because of their insistence on the use of disease-directed therapy (Fowler, Poehling, Billheimer, Hamilton, Wu, Mulder, & Frangould, 2006). Pain and symptoms are mismanaged, causing unnecessary suffering in children (Goldman, Hewitt, Collins, Childs, & Hain, 2006; Wolfe et al., 2000) and in parents, who remain dissatisfied with the quality of care that they and the sick child receive (Contro, Larson, Scofield, Sourkes, & Cohen, 2002, 2004; Meyer, Burns, Griffith, & Truog, 2002).

What about bereavement care? Outcomes regarding the efficacy of bereavement services have been more confusing. Meta-analytic reviews have led to erroneous claims that grief counseling is at best mildly effective, and at worst harmful to the bereaved. This unwarranted pessimism, which is reflected in some literature reviews and in the popular media, has caused some damage to the reputation of grief counseling. A critical review of all available meta-analyses on grief counseling undertaken by Larson and Hoyt (2007) has recently brought to light statistical limitations that contribute to these erroneous conclusions. Their investigation led them to conclude that there is no empirical evidence that bereaved people are harmed by counseling or that individuals who are "normally" bereaved are at any special risk. It is, therefore, prudent to maintain a cautious optimism as to the empirical findings and conduct more rigorous research on individual and group counseling, which will determine who among the bereaved benefits from what kind of professional help, and when.

Another major issue of concern in the field of bereavement is related to the identification and classification of pathological forms of bereavement. Professionals have been involved in heated debates about the pros and cons of introducing a diagnostic category of pathological grief (potentially to be referred to as traumatic grief or protracted grief) into the *Diagnostic Statistical Manual of Mental Disorders.* The question remains as to who will benefit from such a classification: The bereaved, whose difficulties will be recognized and treated? The professionals, who will use a shared code of communication with regard to grief complications or who will negotiate reimbursement for services? Pharmaceutical industries, which will produce and promote new drugs for profit? Or society, which will find a new way to control undesirable behavior?

There is no doubt that at the dawn of the 21st century, we are faced not only with new challenges with regard to the care of the dying and bereaved, but also with new concerns that affect every person on this planet. Nowadays, we all have to live with the uncertainty that is evoked by natural disasters, by terrorism and nuclear threats, and by the consequences of contemporary biotechnology (e.g., excessive prolongation of life, proliferation of genetically modified organisms in the food chain, genetic manipulation, human cloning). Death is not something that happens only to *others,* but a reality that affects us all. As a result, it cannot be ignored.

Both as individuals and as care providers, we must begin by staring death in the face and confronting our mortality. In so doing, we may realize that such a confrontation is also an awakening experience that can help to not only temper our fear of death but also enrich our lives (Yalom, 2008). Such a realization can assist us in supporting seriously ill and bereaved people to engage in a similar process and come to terms with the reality of death. While some benefit from direct confrontation and open discussions about death, dying, and grief, others do not. Confronting death does not preclude an unverbalized awareness of dying and grieving that helps some individuals to continue viewing life as "normal" in order to protect their bonds from any threat or impending separation, and to avoid the anxiety that is associated with existential concerns or a narrative reconstruction (Seale, 1998). In our multicultural society, the needs, values, priorities, and preferences of the dying and bereaved vary to such a degree that those of us who provide services to them must possess—besides specialized knowledge and skills—an ability to relate with sensitivity and to create caring communities in which bonds are affirmed and belonging is enhanced in the face of death, loss, and separation.

Recent evidence shows that people's relationships to care providers constitute a key factor that determines satisfaction with end-of-life and bereavement care (e.g., Contro et al., 2002; Heller & Solomon, 2005; Hickey, 1990; Malacrida et al., 1998; Meyer et al., 2002; Solomon & Browning, 2005; Steinhauser, Christakis, Clipp, McNeilley, McIntyre, & Tulsky, 2000; Steinhauser, Clipp, McNeilly, Christakis, McIntyre, & Tulsky, 2000). Dying and bereaved people report that the primary source of satisfaction regarding the care they receive is related to their relationships with care providers who are caring, humane, and sensitive to their needs. Interestingly, the major source of their distress is associated with unsatisfying relationships with professionals who provide inadequate pain relief, fragmented care, insensitive support, and unclear or no information. It therefore becomes evident that individuals and families expect something from caregiving relationships that is qualitatively distinct from what they actually receive. They ask for more understanding of what they are going through, more genuine concern, more compassion for their suffering, and more humanness.

How do we respond to such requests? Usually by striving to operationalize understanding, compassion, and genuine concern in measurable skills that will permit us to address the psychosocial and spiritual dimensions of a person's illness or loss experience. These skills are taught in workshops and seminars that offer specific guidelines about how to communicate bad news, how to cope with difficult patients, how to use active listening skills, how to assess spiritual needs or deal with unfinished business, how to use interview guides, and how to provide grief support. The problem with most of these educational approaches is that they train care providers to apply specific skills with people who are expected to fit prescribed guidelines or interventions. Moreover, they create the expectation that if the acquired skills are implemented according to the guidelines (e.g., the SPIKES model of the breaking of bad news[1]), then care providers will relate effectively with people in death situations.

Ironically, this educational approach, although holistic in theory, creates a reductionism that objectifies both the individual and his or her dying and bereavement condition that is managed by the use of protocols or a prescribed set of guidelines.

What we, as care providers, tend to forget is that we are an integral aspect of the care process and that we bring into relationships something personal that transcends knowledge and skills. Our goals, needs, and motives for providing services in this field are mistakenly perceived as unimportant and independent of the way we relate to others, while our personal responses to death situations are viewed as subjective and obstructive to caregiving. We act as if quality of care is independent of who we are. In our striving to understand or assist another person, we often times remain dissociated and estranged from ourselves. While this protects us from realizing how we are being affected by the illness or grief experience of others, it also deprives us of the opportunity to be human in our encounters with dying and bereaved people.

It is my firm belief that our holistic approaches to the care of dying and bereaved individuals should expand their scope and pay closer attention to care providers, who affect and are being affected by the people they accompany through dying and bereavement, by the practitioners they collaborate with, and by the community in which they provide their services. A relationship-centered approach, rather than a patient-centered or family-centered approach, may serve as a first step toward a new understanding of care.

The basic idea of the relationship-centered approach is that care cannot be perceived or understood independently of the relationships in which it occurs. In these relationships the reciprocal influence between care seekers and care providers—each of whom brings his or her own unique set of experiences, values, and perspectives—is recognized (Beach, Inui, & Relationship-Centered Care Research Network, 2006). Such an approach invites professionals to understand not only the other person, but also the selves they bring to their encounters, as well as the relationship that results from such meetings. We can no longer offer solely specialized knowledge and skills. Expertise in palliative and bereavement care, although important, is not enough. No matter how "expert" we become—or strive to appear—dying and bereaved people remind us that we are human and equal in the face of death. We all die—some sooner, others later. In this field of work, we are all affected by the transience of life, the irreversibility of death, the suffering that loss engenders, and an existential quest for meaning.

To this day, phenomenological and narrative approaches have contributed significantly to our understanding of the dying or grieving person's subjective world. Unfortunately, these approaches have not had the same impact on the exploration of the private worlds of health care professionals. It is only recently that studies began to shed light on the subjective experiences of health care professionals in death-related situations (see chapter 5). Preliminary evidence shows that behind the facade of a false professionalism that promotes rational thinking, objectivity, and detached concern, care providers are affected by death encounters. Their accounts reveal aspects of the professional as a person who suffers but seldom acknowledges it or does something about it. Focusing on oneself (both as a person and a care provider) is imperative, according to the relationship-centered approach. Knowing oneself becomes equally important as knowing the person one is invited to help. Both are necessary for the building of a relationship in which care is offered and received.

To illustrate the reciprocal influence of the person and of the professional, take a moment to look carefully at Escher's 1938 drawing titled *Two Birds* (Illustration 1.1).

In order to see the figures, one must first focus on the white birds, which appear on a shaded background, and then focus on the shaded birds, which appear on a white background. The beauty of the image is neither in the white birds nor in the shaded birds alone, but in their combination.

The relationship-centered approach poses a similar challenge. It requires that we learn to shift the focus of our attention from the person's subjective world (the white bird) to our own subjective world (the shaded bird), and from ourselves back to the person in order to understand what unfolds in an intersubjective space that is shared and is unique to our relationship.

Notice that in Escher's picture, the perfect fit between two birds becomes evident only if these are perceived within a larger context that comprises several birds. In a parallel way, relationship-centered care also requires that we pay attention to significant others who are brought—directly or indirectly—into our dyadic interaction. A dying or bereaved person, for example, brings into the relationship with the care provider his or her personal story, along with a world of family and significant other relations (the white birds). These relationships form the context in which both he or she and significant others experience dying or bereavement, and grow in the face of multiple changes that

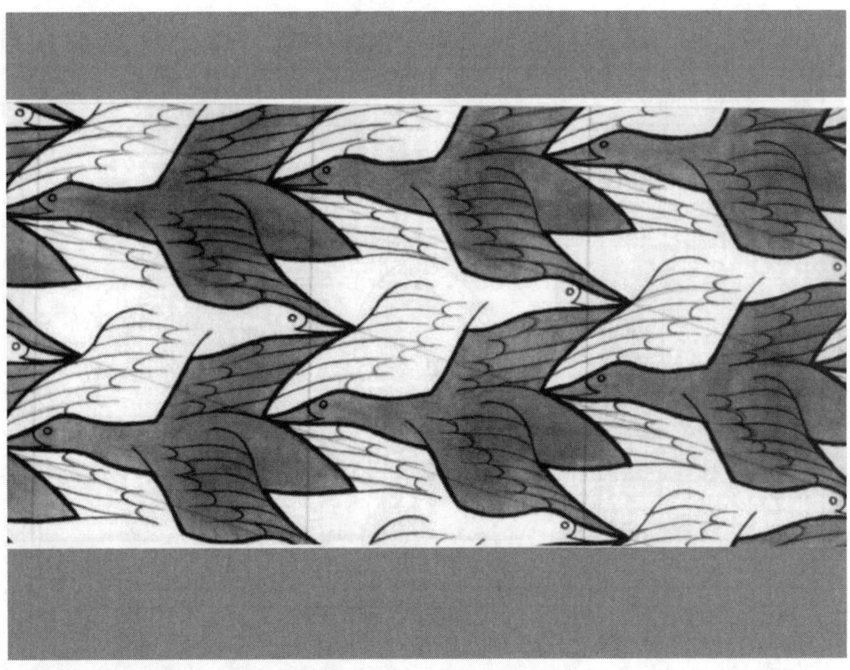

Illustration 1.1. M. C. Escher, 1938

occur within themselves and in their environment. We, on the other hand, bring into our relationship with each person our personal and family histories as well as a network of team and other professional relations that are shaped by the organization's goals, values, and ideals (the shaded birds). These relationships affect the quality of care we provide and determine the stresses and rewards we reap from the process of caregiving. Although each set of birds is facing in a different direction, the observer has the impression that they move together as a result of a perfect fit. Quality care results from a similar fit, which requires a collaboration between people who face a life that is uncertain or dramatically changed as a result of impending death or the death of a loved person, and care providers who face in the direction of a more or less stable life with an anticipated future. The space in which they meet, interact, and coexist is enlarged and enriched as a result of their collaboration.

A relationship-centered approach focuses on whatever transpires when the world of care seekers and the world of care providers meet and interact in a setting of care and community context (Figure 1.1). To

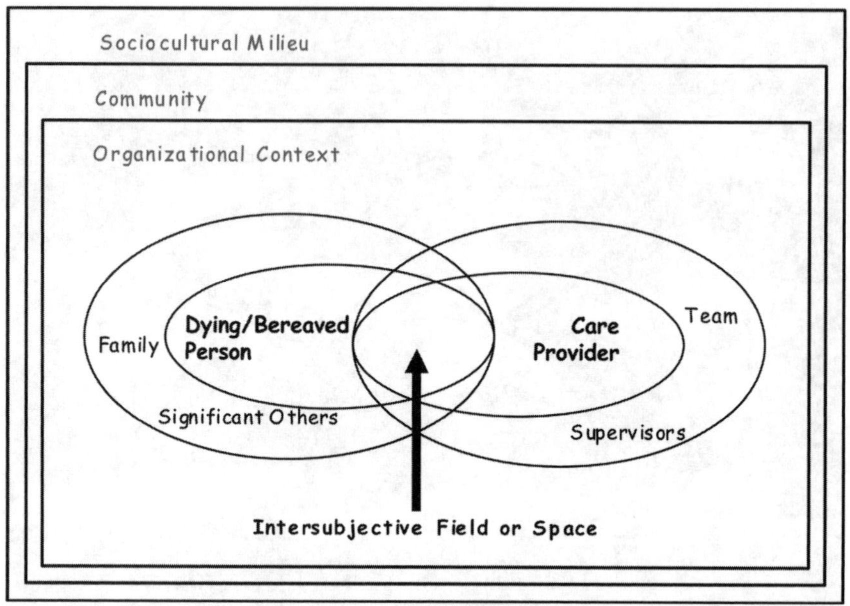

Figure 1.1 The context of the caregiving relationship

better understand the outcomes of such encounters, it is important to consider its basic components. These involve:

1. The acknowledgment of the subjective world of the dying or bereaved individual who seeks care
2. The acknowledgement of the subjective world of the care provider
3. The influence of other key persons (i.e., family members, team members, other colleagues) who are—directly or indirectly—involved in the caregiving or care-receiving process
4. The intersubjective space or field that is formed as a result of their encounter
5. The organizational or work context in which care is offered and received at the end of life and through bereavement
6. The community and sociocultural milieu in which care in life and death situations unfolds

It becomes evident that not only the relationship between a person and a care provider, but their respective relations with family members, significant others, colleagues, co-workers, and supervisors, is important.

These are further affected by the work, community, and sociocultural context in which care is being offered.

When these worlds meet, an *intersubjective field* is developed that belongs neither to the person nor to the professional, but to their relationship, which is embedded and affected by a wider network of relationships. Whatever unfolds in this intersubjective field is brought by the person back to the members of his or her family, who are subsequently affected; in a parallel way, whatever transpires in this intersubjective space is brought by the professional back to the team and organization, whose goals, values, and practices are reinforced, disconfirmed, challenged, or changed.

What is the intersubjective field or space? Stern (2004) defines it as "the domain of feelings, thoughts, knowledge that two (or more) people share about the nature of their current relationship" (p. 243). When the professional and the patient enact prescribed scripts and roles, they remain oblivious to their own and the other's subjective experiences. In contrast, when they are open to each other, and in touch with themselves, the intersubjective field is enlarged and offers opportunities for change and growth as a result of their interaction. For example, in the presence of an empathic professional, the dying or bereaved person may view and experience him- or herself in a new light. Similarly, in the presence of a grieving individual, the professional may discover aspects of him- or herself that were unknown to him or her but emerge as he or she revisits past experiences of loss. Insights and changes that occur in the intersubjective field are often subtle, implicit, and unverbalized, but nonetheless significant. They provide opportunities for new explorations, new experiences, and new narratives that are co-created in the face of death. They have the potential to render care more human, meaningful, and enriching for those who receive, as well as for those who provide care services.

In fact, the relationship-centered approach is concerned with the development of large networks of relations among people, professionals, teams, and communities that have the potential to be caring, enriching, and rewarding for all parties involved. Such an approach incites organizations to pay closer attention to the relational aspects of caregiving in order to prevent the marginalization and institutionalization of the dying and the bereaved, and to avoid the stigmatization or idealization of professionals who work in the field of thanatology. Not only should individuals and families benefit from reciprocal and caring relationships, but professionals and teams should also experience satisfaction from collaborating with and supporting each other in the face of death. This renewed focus on relationships aims at rendering dying and bereavement a *social affair* that is shared and experienced as meaningful and humane by those who receive, as well as by those who provide care.

I believe that a shift from a patient- and family-centered approach to a relationship-centered approach requires a thorough and critical review of established ideas and practices, which are often taken as self-evident truth. Whether such a process will lead to new adaptations that will enhance the quality of our services or to a paradigm shift that will involve the reorganization of our knowledge and practices remains to be seen. In any case, a critical review will inevitably involve changes that must occur at multiple levels, three of which, in my opinion, are critical.

At a personal level, it is imperative that we redefine our caregiving role. We are neither practitioners who apply knowledge and skills upon clinical cases nor neutral observers of people's private worlds, which are impacted by death. We are active participants in relationships who affect and are affected by others and by shared experiences. As such, we need to explore our responses to the people we serve, as well as to co-workers with whom we share the caregiving process. An introspective process can be facilitated through appropriate education, supervised clinical practice, and peer review groups, all of which promote self- and team understanding.

At an administrative level, organizations must review their goals and formulate policies that do not thoughtlessly serve their own needs. It is important to create a culture of care that responds both to the needs of individuals and families and to the needs of professionals, who must be held and supported in their work. If the ultimate goal of care is to integrate dying and bereaved people into society rather than isolate and marginalize them, organizations must be responsible for cultivating a web of relationships with other teams, services, and institutions that ensure continuity and quality of care. Relationship-centered care can help organizations become more environmentalized and humane and less impersonal and self-serving.

At an educational level, institutions must offer models of learning that enable students and trainees to develop relationships that are meaningful and rewarding for all participants. An alternative educational approach in palliative care referred to as relational learning (see chapter 11, challenge 2) goes beyond the accumulation of knowledge through didactic lectures in classrooms; it offers a wide repertoire of educational experiences, all of which are situated in direct relationships with patients, families, peers, and colleagues. New challenges emerge when education introduces opportunities for self-understanding, for interdisciplinary collaboration, and for learning from patients and families, whose wisdom is incorporated into clinical practice. Care cannot change without them, nor can it change if professionals do not develop an ability to reflect on and learn from relationships with them.

Changes in the above domains should not be limited to the modification of our views but should involve a progressive reorganization of our values, beliefs, axioms, theories, and models of care. Giving up long-held assumptions and specific ways of thinking and providing care is a threatening process that creates confusion and insecurity. However, this process opens up opportunities for new knowledge and growth that may result from a renewed relation to ourselves, to the people we serve, and to our colleagues. This is a challenge worth undertaking.

A relationship-centered approach, in my view, offers a fresh look at care that is not perceived as a product to be packaged and sold by professionals, and consumed by people in need. It emphasizes the interpersonal and social nature of care that tempers suffering in the face of death, fosters belonging, and allows growth to occur. Such an approach can enhance and enrich relationships that are relevant to health care through both education and practice (Report of the Pew-Fetzer Task Force on Advancing Psychosocial Health Education, 2000).

NOTE

1. SPIKES is a protocol for delivering unfavorable information to patients about their illness through which clinicians fulfill four key objectives: gathering information from the patient, transmitting unfavorable medical information, providing support, and eliciting the patient's collaboration. This protocol involves the following steps: *setting* up the interview, assessing the patient's *perception,* obtaining the patient's *invitation,* giving *knowledge* and information to the patient, addressing *emotions* with empathic responses, and developing a *strategy* of collaboration and a plan for the future—or SPIKES (Baile, Buckman, Lenzi, Glober, Beale, & Kudelka, 2000).

2 A Relationship of Care

Several psychologists have stipulated that we are all born social beings. Through early relationships with significant others, we find our way into life. In a parallel way, through relationships with others, we find our way out of life when we are dying. Our need for safety, love, and belonging at the beginning and at the end of our existence is met through relationships with others. Not only do we seek to satisfy these needs through these relationships, but we also attribute unique meanings to our experiences as a result of our encounters with others. Dying and bereavement are social trajectories that acquire personal meanings within the context of a web of relations.

Based on this assumption, the patient-professional relationship (referred to in this text as the person-professional relationship) is one of many relationships that affect how one's trajectory develops through life and death. It is an ordinary relationship (with distinct characteristics, as described in the following chapter) that sometimes becomes extraordinary as a result of its profound positive or negative effects upon those who seek care and those who provide it. Quality of care is largely affected by what transpires in this relationship.

In palliative and bereavement care, this relationship is often described as a partnership. The traditional asymmetrical patient-professional relationship that emphasizes symptom management and adherence to treatments by people who conform to professionals' orders, guidance, and decisions is replaced by a more "symmetrical" relationship. Despite the fact that the nature of this relationship remains elusive, it is commonly described as one that is characterized by a holistic interest in the uniqueness of each person who is dying or grieving, a concern for the family who is also affected by death, and active involvement, presence, and availability on the part of the professionals who help people make their way through life and death situations.

PARTNERS IN CARE

What does a partnership entail? First, a mutual commitment and active engagement in the pursuit of shared goals. Partners must rely on and trust one another in order to ensure the best possible care. The belief that the provider follows the dying or bereaved person, who leads the way through dying and bereavement, is only partially true. Some people do not know what is in their best interest, others are mistaken in their decisions, and still others mobilize dysfunctional patterns in coping with their suffering. A mother, for example, may avoid informing her children about their father's death in order to spare them from the pain they will experience if they attend the funeral. Or a spouse may believe that the choice to refuse DNR orders is in the best interest of her loved one who suffers needlessly a prolonged death and is deprived of any quality of life.

In a partnership, our role involves helping dying and bereaved people identify what is in their best interest by providing information, offering practical advice, and helping them reflect upon available options before deciding and acting upon a plan. It also involves inviting them to explore their deeper needs and understand their behavior. It comprises the facilitation of communication among family members with conflicting goals and desires in order to reach decisions that benefit the dying or bereaved person, and with which they can live. By assuming an active role, we accompany people in their trajectories and facilitate their transition through one of the most difficult periods in their lives.

Being partners does not make us similar to dying or bereaved people, nor does it render the relationship symmetric, as is often assumed. Our role, experiences, needs, and knowledge about dying and bereavement make us dissimilar from those who need the services that we are in a position to provide. Our partnership is characterized by complementarity, which does not rigidly place care seekers at the receiving end, and professionals at the giving end. As Oliviere (2006) suggests, a partnership must be based on reciprocity, where giving and receiving happen at the same time. Care is not imposed, but co-created by partners.

Viewing care as stemming from partnership has significant advantages: first, it acknowledges commitment between care seekers and care providers, who rely upon each other to shape a shared trajectory through dying and bereavement. Second, it promotes shared responsibility in a situation that is characterized by intense suffering, confusion, uncertainty, ethical dilemmas, and a lack of perfect solutions as to what is appropriate or desired. Third, it reinforces communication and involvement between partners and fosters belonging in a community of concerned fellows. Fourth, it ensures continuity of care in the midst of uncertainty and distress. Fifth, it relieves care providers of the expectation that they must act as authorities and enables them to relate in meaningful and personal ways. Finally, it allows both partners to learn from each other and benefit from a shared process.

While a partnership approach to care appears attractive in theory, it also presents some shortcomings when we mistakenly believe that dying and bereaved people always know what they want in death situations and are autonomous in making decisions about their care. Quite often a person does not have all the necessary information (especially when dying is not discussed openly with the patient), and one's decisions are often determined by family needs rather than personal desires or preferences. Other times, when dysfunctional patterns threaten a person or family with total disorganization, we must assume a directive role and the responsibility of care. To provide our partners with appropriate information and support requires that we hand over some of our control to them, and relinquish some of the security that our intervention plans offer. Partnerships are not easy and require us, the care providers, to be open to surprises and creative in the planning of services that aim to accommodate the needs and preferences of our partners (Farber & Farber, 2006).

When we propose a partnership, there is no guarantee that it will be accepted. There are people who adopt a strictly consumer approach, make use of specific services, and maintain impersonal relationships with us. Others, fearful of involvement, reluctantly cooperate and are ambivalent. Still others avoid forming partnerships because managing the hardships of life alone and suffering with pride and dignity become their trophy. Finally, there are also people who cannot form a partnership because they cling to or develop an enmeshed relationship with us. In summary, people vary in their responses to the idea of forming a partnership in the face of death. However, we also differ in our ability to establish one. Some of us are reluctant to trust our judgment and feel insecure giving up some of the control and security that familiar or planned interventions offer. Others impose services in a coercive or intrusive manner by exerting power and control. Still others expect people to display unconditional faith in professionals, and fail to realize that trust is not a given but is earned in a partnership. In reality, all of us have to prove that we are trustworthy through the competent use of our scientific knowledge and skills, but also through our ability to connect with respect and genuine care for others. Most dying and bereaved people seek to form a relationship with a *professional* who possesses knowledge and skill to assist them with practical needs and concerns, and a *person* who is compassionate, willing to share the reality of death and the suffering it evokes, and trusted with intimate disclosures. While such a relationship can come in the form of a partnership, sometimes it develops into an attachment bond.

THE ATTACHMENT BOND

When does a partnership become an attachment bond? First, when the relationship is experienced by both the person and the professional as special or unique; second, when it gives rise to a set of care-seeking behaviors and caregiving behaviors; and third, when it enhances a sense of belonging to the relationship.

The first two criteria are reflective of what Bowlby (1969/1982, 1988, 2005) described as an attachment bond, while the third criterion reflects the necessity of bond affirmation through belonging advocated by Adler (1923/1971, 1932/1958b, 1933/1964, 1935, 1937, 1958a; Ansbacher & Ansbacher, 1956, Ferguson, 1989), 2000. In other words, a caregiving relationship can function as a secure attachment bond when it enhances the person's and the professional's sense of being unique, significant, loved, and accepted as a result of belonging to a meaningful relationship in which care is offered and received. Not all partnerships end up in attachment bonds. Moreover, whenever they do, these are not invariably secure attachments. Sometimes bonds are reflective of insecure attachments that increase suffering and compromise the quality of care.

To illuminate the bond between a dying and bereaved person and his or her care provider, it is helpful to understand how humans form attachments in loss situations. Bowlby's theory on attachment is enlightening in that respect. It explains how we develop secure or insecure attachments, which give rise to different care-seeking and caregiving patterns in the face of loss, separation, and adversity (Bowlby, 1969/1982, 1973, 1980, 1988, 2005). While Bowlby's work focused on the formation and disruption of the mother-child attachment bond at the beginning of life, his theory is highly relevant to our understanding of the formation, maintenance, and disruption of attachment bonds at the end of life and through bereavement (for readers who are unfamiliar with Bowlby's theory on attachment, a brief description is included in the appendix).

Bowlby's work can help us understand that people have different attachment styles by which they form and maintain bonds with us. Some trust the caring relationship and develop secure bonds (secure attachment), others are mistrusting and dismissive of any help or fearful of intimate encounters (avoidant attachment), and still others become dependent and clingy (dependent/ambivalent attachment). Each of these attachment behaviors triggers different responses that affect our caregiving behaviors. While we respond differently to each person, all our relations are greatly affected by our own attachment style and our ability to develop secure, dependent, or avoidant attachments with the people we serve.

In what follows, I wish to address the following questions:

- What transpires in the person-professional relationship when a person seeks help and assistance in death situations?
- Which are people's attachment needs and behaviors, and how are these reflected in their request for help?
- By which caregiving behaviors can professionals effectively respond to people's attachment needs and form secure bonds?
- How is the relationship between care seekers and care providers affirmed in the face of death, loss, and separation?

My purpose is not to offer absolute answers, but to share some initial thoughts that may enlighten some of the dynamics that characterize the caregiving relationship.

REQUEST FOR SERVICES IN DEATH SITUATIONS

Let's think for a moment what dying and bereaved people usually want when they seek our services. They come to us with a complaint (usually about somatic or psychological symptoms), and an explicit request: "Relieve me of my symptoms." "Help me get rid of my suffering." "Cure this life-threatening disease." "Get rid of my depression." "Treat this physical pain." "Help me have a peaceful death." "Help me get over my grief." "Help me stop drinking." "Give me information." "Help me decide." They direct their requests to professionals, who are perceived as competent to relieve suffering by offering information, guidance, or practical assistance. In other words, they expect us to do something about their condition, which is usually presented in terms of manageable symptoms. While some aspects of their suffering (e.g., physical pain) can be relieved, other aspects can only be accepted, contained, and tempered (e.g., loss of loved person, impending separation), and still others, transformed (e.g., quest for meaning).

Interestingly, dying and bereaved people know that not every aspect of suffering can be relieved. They also know that we cannot spare them from death when they are dying, nor from the pain of loss. So what do they seek from us? Most often a relationship to sustain or hold them through probably one of the most distressing and most unfamiliar periods of their lives. Underlying their request for knowledge and practical guidance is often a "call for a relationship" (Morasz, 1999, p. 115)—not just any relationship, but a secure relationship with someone who can listen, accept, and contain their suffering; take care of them; and genuinely care for them as they strive to cope with issues related to their existence. This unverbalized request for a relationship conveys a message such as "Take care of me," "Stand by me," "Nurture me," "Help me cope," "Help me understand and make sense of this," "Reassure me that I will not be abandoned, be lost in suffering, or disappear," "Assure me that I am important and that I matter to you," and "Reassure me that I belong." Underlying these messages are two basic needs: (1) a need to be accepted as *vulnerable* and in search for safety, nurturance, support, and belonging and (2) a search for be viewed as *resilient* and capable of exploring new and unfamiliar experiences, learning from them, changing, and growing.

In order to develop a secure bond, we need to respond to explicit requests for clinical care, relief, information, guidance, and the like, as well as to the implicit request for a relationship in which individuals seeking care are accepted as both vulnerable and resilient. Let's clarify the concepts of vulnerability and resilience.

Being accepted as vulnerable does not mean that one is viewed as weak, incompetent, or dependent. Rather, it implies that one is recognized as a person who seeks to form attachments with those who can offer safety and comfort and promote belonging in the face of loss and separation. The vulnerable person does not hide or deny reality. Unless his or her vulnerability is not overwhelming, he or she remains open to the challenges of a situation that is perceived as threatening, distressing, or novel and concurrently seeks to establish attachment bonds that provide a secure base, which in turn facilitates explorations into an unfamiliar reality.

Being viewed as resilient and capable of effectively coping with adversities, on the other hand, does not mean that one is perceived as strong or heroic, nor does it mean that one produces success stories about coping with loss. In fact, a person's resilience is compromised when he or she is forced to perform a heroic script or share accounts of bravery over illness, death, and loss in order to spare others from suffering. Resilience is mistakenly associated with stability and equilibrium. However, in my view, resilience is a dynamic process (rather than a personality trait) that takes place through adverse and unfavorable life situations and is enhanced when the person moves forward and uses functional patterns to cope with difficulties and challenges. Therefore, a person who expects to be perceived as resilient wishes to be seen and approached as having the potential to manage the unknown, to tame chaos, to take risks, to learn from successes and failures, to change, and to grow.

In fact, what dying and bereaved people express through their requests for services is a desire to establish a relationship that can function as a safe haven in times of trouble, as well as a secure base from which they can explore distressing and novel experiences and challenges. They do not seek to become dependent upon us but, instead, to become attached to us.

Attachment is distinct from dependency (Bowlby, 1969/1982). A person who is dependent relies on the professional for his or her survival or existence. In some situations (e.g., critical health conditions), this is inevitable. However, in most situations, the person seeks to develop a privileged relationship or special bond with a professional who is physically and emotionally available, in proximity during distressing events, but also encouraging of the person's efforts to cope with novel and unfamiliar situations.

I have always been impressed by patients—even very young children—who, once they come to an awareness of their impending deaths, suddenly stop cooperating with care providers and adamantly insist on returning home. In total disregard of their physical symptoms, pain, and deteriorating condition, they seek a safe and familiar environment where they can contain their suffering and ensure safety and belonging. These patients perceive the hospital as a threatening and unfamiliar setting and often view professionals as limited in their ability to accept, contain, or mitigate suffering in a meaningful way. Their decisions to go home acquire meaning only when understood within the context of a web of caring relationships that address their attachment needs and enhance their sense of belonging in the face of the ultimate separation.

In contrast, others who receive care at home decide during the last day or hours of life to return to the hospital or another facility where they were cared for in the past. These patients are not driven out of a desperate hope for a cure, nor out of a need to deny their dying. This last-minute return reflects an attachment to the professionals who provide them with the safety of a secure base that enables them to explore the unknown of death that lies ahead and offers reassurance that their families will be supported. Occasionally, this last-minute return represents a farewell gift to care providers with whom they shared, and wish to complete, a journey that has been significant to all the parties involved.

In death situations, secure attachments are vital because they ascertain a sense of safety, connectedness, and belonging when death threatens or bestows irreversible separations. Let's explore what transpires in the attachment bond by focusing on people's attachment behaviors and our caregiving responses.

THE PERSON'S ATTACHMENT BEHAVIORS

Attachment behaviors comprise two sets of behaviors that become most apparent when the person experiences a situation (e.g., dying or bereavement) as highly distressing, threatening, or novel:

1. *Proximity-seeking behaviors.* These are referred to in this book as care-seeking behaviors. They comprise a striving for safety, comfort, nurturance, advice, and reassurance that occurs when the individual turns to care providers, who are often perceived as attachment figures. These behaviors are not childish, immature, or regressive, as is often assumed, but healthy and natural responses to a complex, distressing situation that evoke caregiving responses from care providers.
2. *Explorative behaviors.* These are elicited when attachment needs are met, and the person moves on to transform an unknown

situation into a familiar one. Explorative behaviors are reinforced when three conditions are present: (1) the person does not question the security and availability of the care provider, (2) he or she does not experience increased levels of threat or suffering that arouse a persistent striving for safety and security, and (3) the care provider encourages exploratory behaviors in the face of loss and adversity.

Peter, a 42-year-old patient with cancer, had a strong attachment bond with his family doctor. Every time he was confronted with a crisis, he displayed attachment behaviors. He immediately called him up and invited him to participate in consultation meetings with his treating physicians. He used to say: "No matter what the experts say about my condition, the *only* person I trust is my family doctor. I have to get his approval before I consent to any proposed protocol. His presence, support, and advice *are* my medication. They help me walk through hell, fight this terrible disease, and have the confidence that I will beat it."

While most people develop partnerships with several professionals who belong to the same or different teams, often they choose only one (or a few) care provider with whom to form an attachment bond and trust him or her with their innermost concerns and needs. From that professional they welcome support, guidance, and assistance and are receptive when he or she imparts bad news about their condition or impending death. In a similar way, people who experience a major loss in life often return to their ex-therapist or ex-counselor, not necessarily out of a need to engage into a new therapeutic process, but in order to receive the nurturance, support, and encouragement that enable them to confront the losses and challenges that emerge from a new and painful reality.

It is important to note that in death situations, people do not form attachment bonds solely with others but often display attachment behaviors toward specific places (e.g., home, place of birth, native land), a deity or religious faith (e.g., God, church community), or a situation or project (e.g., social contribution), which becomes a source of safety as well as a resource in their explorative approach to novelty and challenge.

Attachment to Others

I have worked in pediatric oncology as a psychologist and had the privilege of accompanying several families through the child's dying process. When death drew closer, these children sought with great determination the presence of a parent, a sibling, a member of our team, or myself. Sometimes they even prolonged their dying until the arrival of a relative or a professional to whom they were attached. Other times, they waited until a parent was willing to accept their death or give them "permission" to die. But it was not only dying children who manifested attachment behaviors. Parents and siblings also did. When death was imminent, parents never left the patient's bedside, and older siblings stayed close by through frequent visits, phone calls, messages, cards, and other tokens of love and affection. Younger siblings, on the other hand, displayed attachment behaviors toward their parents; whenever the latter attended to their needs, these children were actively involved in end-of-life care and engaged in meaningful interactions with the dying child.

Our team's goal was to reinforce the bonds among family members or significant others while remaining fully available to each of them. When death occurred in a safe environment that recognized everyone's needs, pain became more bearable, and the family entered bereavement with comforting memories and increased resources. For them, a good death was determined by the nature of attachments and the content of encounters that had unfolded prior to death.

We must keep in mind that secure attachments are experienced not only with living people, but also with the deceased person, who occupies a central position in the life of the bereaved individual and functions as a guardian angel. His or her presence is felt in times of distress. Dreams of the deceased, searches for signs, and visits to the gravesite are all attachment behaviors that provide the bereaved with reassurance that he or she is cared for by the benevolent and protective presence of an absent person. The deceased is imagined to accompany the bereaved and is invested with caretaking abilities that involve the offering of reassurance, guidance, support, and encouragement to move on into a new reality.

Attachment to a Religion or Deity

Other times, people are strongly attached to a religion.[1] Their attachment behaviors are directed toward some divine element that is cosmic and supernatural. In monotheistic religions this divine element is personified in one God, usually a male attachment figure that is worshiped and perceived as being all powerful, all giving, and all protective, offering endless love, peace, serenity, and comfort. But this God is also perceived as putting His children to the test by encouraging them to cope with challenging situations and inciting them to explore the limits of their faith. The strong bond to a fatherly God or to a maternal Virgin Mary reflects a love relationship similar to a parent-child attachment bond.

Parkes (in press) suggests that falling in love with God is usually a process that develops gradually. However, under extreme stress, some people fall in love with God and convert to a religion within a relatively short period of time, while others suddenly fall out of love with God, who is perceived as distant, unjust, punitive, or insensitive to their attachment needs.

In multi-theistic religions, the bond with a divine element is personified in several gods who serve as alternative attachment figures available to respond to different needs.

Attachments sometimes extend to spiritual leaders, the clergy, or members of one's church or religious community. Collective praying, fasting, and participation in rituals serve several functions: they enhance one's sense of being supported through loss, they offer clear and unambiguous explanations about existential concerns, and they increase one's sense of belonging in the present life, or in a life that exists after death.

Attachment behaviors toward a divine element are evident even among people who declare themselves to be atheists yet remain deeply religious without abiding to any particular faith. Their religiosity stems from a striving to connect with something bigger, a supernatural being to which they feel strongly attached. Being in union with nature or a divine power provides them with the security that helps them transcend loss and cultivates a feeling of cosmic belonging that ensures immortality.

Attachment to Home and Land of Birth

Some dying people manifest attachment behaviors to their home or birthplace, which provides the security and belonging they long for. This safe place functions as a refuge that protects them from intrusions and from obligations to enact an unwanted social role (e.g., as patient, widow, orphan). At home, the person feels free to be him- or herself, express attachment needs, seek cuddles and nurturing, and receive unconditional love and acceptance.

In my country, Greece, it is very common for terminally ill people to express a desire to return home to die and be buried in their land of birth. Attachment to one's home and native land becomes sometimes more important than attachment to people. It reflects a symbolic return to the safety of a womb represented by the place of birth, as well as an affirmation of their belonging to a familiar world associated with their family history. These individuals, who usually live in big cities, keep a special attachment to their homeland throughout life. This is manifested by regular visits, beneficiary acts toward their communities, practical assistance to kin or individuals born in the same village or town, or the maintenance of their voting rights in their birthplace, to which they return to exercise their civil responsibilities. At death, they expect to be buried in their homeland and offered a ceremony that accords them a special status and position in their native community (Papadatou & Iossifides, 2004).

Something similar happens for the bereaved, who come to be attached to the gravesite of their loved ones and organize their lives in such a way so they can pay regular visits to the cemetery. During my recent visit to the areas of the Peloponnese that were burned by devastating fires in the summer of 2007, we met people who, in the midst of the disaster, risked their lives by refusing to leave their villages, where their ancestors were buried. Their homes were less important to them. What was most traumatic was the thought of losing a place that was associated with their family stories. Some of them told heartbreaking stories about olive trees that had been planted by their grandparents, their parents, or themselves the day their children were born in the hope that they will be passed on to future generations. Their family histories and identities were associated with the earth and the trees, to which they were strongly attached.

Attachment to a Significant Goal or Project

Finally, some people manifest attachment behaviors toward a goal or a project, such as a campaign for a benevolent cause, the foundation of a charity, a contribution to the community, the publication of a book, or the writing of one's memoirs. This goal becomes a raison d'être in times of trouble, provides people with a sense of self-worth and orientation, brings order to chaos, and allows them to create some meaning out of an unfamiliar situation. Through this goal or project, they often seek to become integrated into the social fabric of their communities before they die. Their devotion to a goal that ensures a symbolic immortality helps them transcend loss and suffering and attribute meaning to their lives.

THE PROFESSIONAL'S CAREGIVING BEHAVIORS

The dying or bereaved person's attachment behaviors evoke in us caregiving behaviors, which have two basic functions: (1) to provide a *safe haven* to which the person can retreat when feeling vulnerable, threatened, distressed, uncertain, or confused, and (2) to offer a *secure base* from which the individual can move forward and explore the challenges of dying or bereavement, knowing that he or she can always return for comfort, reassurance, or assistance when troubled.

How do we provide a safe haven? First, by acknowledging the person's vulnerability in the face of death, loss, and separation (often manifested through intensified care-seeking behaviors), and second, by responding with sensitivity to the person's attachment needs. According to Feeney and Collins (2004), this process entails the following:

- The regulation of our behavior so that it meshes with that of the bereaved or dying person
- The ability to take cues from the person and plan appropriate interventions, which are paced by him or her
- The correct interpretation of signals and attachment behaviors, and an attuned response to the person's needs
- An awareness of how our behavior affects the other, which enables us to adjust our responses so as to be in synchrony with the person

To create a safe haven, we need adequate time and a relaxed atmosphere (Bowlby, 1988). It is impossible to establish such a haven in an environment where everyone and everything happens in a rush, and constant interruptions and intrusions hinder our ability to listen to stories and preclude any continuity of care. Paradoxically, the more we allow the dying and bereaved to find refuge in the haven of a secure attachment, the less likely they are to become dependent on us. In fact, the opposite occurs: they become more cooperative, trust that they will be helped, gain confidence and become more autonomous in their explorative pursuits.

How do we offer a secure base? First, by recognizing and reinforcing strengths and resources. People move forward in life and change by building upon their strengths, rather than by focusing on their weaknesses, shortcomings, and limitations. Unfortunately, our educations in psychology, nursing, medicine, and other allied professions have overemphasized the dysfunction, the pathology, and the disorder and have made us experts in identifying what is wrong with people that must be fixed or changed. We sadly lack expertise in discovering the immense capacities, creative abilities, and inner resources that people possess. As a result, we cannot reflect back to them the valuable resources they possess that enhance resilience.

Second, we offer a secure base when we provide reassurance and encouragement to engage in explorative behaviors, and when we establish conditions for the achievement of realistic goals. Exploratory behaviors can be outer and inner directed. Those that are outer directed enable the person to meet the practical challenges of dying and bereavement by taking initiative, by developing new skills, by actively participating in decisions, or by exercising autonomy and control over distressing events. Those that are inner directed invite a reflective process that helps the person accept, tolerate, or transform suffering, work through unresolved losses, address existential concerns, or reconstruct a biographical story in the face of loss. We should neither rush a person into being active, assertive, autonomous, or self-reflective nor protect him or her by offering immediate guidance, assistance, advice, or hasty interpretations of his or her behavior. Instead, we must discern when to wait and avoid interfering with the individual's explorative attempts, and when to step in and offer guidance, assistance, or encouragement. Feeney and Collins (2004) eloquently describe our role: "The ability to confidently explore the environment stems from having a caregiver who both encourages and supports such exploration and who has proven to be readily available and responsive when comfort, assistance, and/or protection have been sought" (p. 308).

Where do we learn how to provide care? Obviously from people who served as attachment figures in our early childhood. If we had caretakers who were sensitive to our needs, then we are more likely to use them as role models and inspire trust in people by offering a safe haven and a secure base from which they can confidently explore the challenges of dying and bereavement. In contrast, if our own attachment needs were inadequately met by caretakers whom we experienced as distant or anxious/ambivalent, or whom we had to care for through role reversal, then we are likely to develop relationships in which we find creating a safe haven or secure base more demanding. There is preliminary evidence that our own experiences of early attachment affect our motivation to work in a helping profession, as well as our ability to be available to people's needs and to respond judiciously through caregiving (Fussel & Bonney, 1999; Hazan & Shaver, 1990; Leiper & Casares, 2000).

If we experienced early and current secure attachments, we are more likely to be fully present in our relationships with dying and bereaved people, responsive to their needs, and trusting of their abilities to cope with difficult situations. We do not seek to satisfy unmet personal attachment needs through the care we provide to them. In other words, we do not relate to people for the sake of pleasing them, exerting control, or striving for superiority and significance, nor do we use them as an excuse to avoid developing intimate and social relations in our personal lives. Undistracted by unmet personal needs, we value each relationship and maintain an inquisitive, explorative, and open mind in situations characterized by ambiguity, uncertainty, and no perfect solutions or answers. As secure caretakers, we reap rewards and derive satisfaction from bonds that we perceive as being meaningful and enriching.

In contrast, when we develop insecure attachments, we seek to meet some personal unattended needs through the helping relationship, in which we adopt an anxious/ambivalent or avoidant attachment style. In the case of an anxious/ambivalent attachment, we display patterns of compulsive caregiving and strive to gain the person's or family's approval, admiration, and recognition in order to avoid the rejection or failure that we dread. We attempt to control events, fix problems, find "right" solutions, and avoid situations that evoke feelings of powerlessness, helplessness, and low self-esteem. In the case of avoidant attachments, we focus on practical tasks and neglect or dismiss people's attachment needs. While we actively collaborate with them toward the achievement of commonly agreed-upon goals, we concurrently remain busy, unavailable, and less affectionately supportive in the face of personal disclosures and communications, which are perceived as threatening. Thus, our own explorative activity as care providers is limited to situations that do not cause discomfort and do not have the potential to uncover our increased vulnerability.

A history of early life trauma and deprivation associated with insecure attachments does not necessarily mean that our attachments to dying and bereaved people are always insecure. They remain insecure only if we are unaware of how our personal history affects the caregiving patterns and relations we form with others. To act as secure caretakers, we need to attend to our own loss issues and unmet attachment needs so as to avoid using work relations to satisfy them. This process is facilitated when our job offers a holding environment in which we can process our work experiences and support our exploration into the worlds of the dying and the bereaved, and of ourselves (see principle 7 in chapter 9).

BOND AFFIRMATION THROUGH BELONGING

As has already been suggested, care-seeking and caregiving behaviors are interrelated and complementary. One of their functions is to ensure a sense of belonging to a key relationship that is significant both to the helper and to the person being helped. When both people in the relationship are committed to the shared bond, each occupies a special place in the life of the other. This fosters a sense of belonging that engenders the feeling that one is unique, valued, appreciated, respected, or loved by the other.

The concept of belonging—"to belong, to feel worthwhile as social beings and part of the human community" (Ferguson, 1989, p. 357)—was advanced by Alfred Adler (1923/1971, 1932/1958b, 1933/1964, 1958a), who considered it a fundamental motivation of human beings. Belonging is viewed as necessary for the survival of the human species. If the individual were left to him- or herself, he or she could not survive. Therefore, it is the nature of humans to be social. People are born with a need to belong (referred to as the "urge to community"), but also with a motivation to connect and cooperate with others for the common good. Both of these fundamental human motivations enhance feelings of self-worth and connectedness to others.

In death situations, the need to belong in ways that are meaningful to oneself and to others is experienced with increased intensity. When a person is faced with a world that falls apart and is changed forever because bonds are threatened or irreversibly broken, his or her sense of belonging is seriously compromised, and feelings of insignificance, helplessness, inferiority, and meaninglessness are common. To temper or mitigate some of these feelings, the dying or bereaved person seeks, through a secure attachment, to reconstruct a world, connect with others, and eventually find a special place that fosters belonging. Oftentimes, this process is difficult either because the person has limited energy as a result of his or her condition, or because people around him or her distance themselves and victimize, marginalize, or stigmatize him or her. Dying alone, invisible, and indifferent to others is most tragic. Similarly, grieving alone, unsupported, and alienated from one's community renders bereavement a deeply painful and lonely process.

When we develop secure attachments with the people we serve, we prevent isolation and hopelessness and integrate the dying and the bereaved into a world of meaningful connections that are affirmed. Secure attachments increase trust in ourselves, in others, and in the caregiving process. They foster belonging, which, paradoxically, facilitates separation. When dying people feel affirmed, loved, appreciated, accepted, and reassured that they will continue to live in the memory of others (including our own), they are freer to let go. In a similar way, when bereaved individuals are reassured that they can choose to maintain a cherished bond with the deceased without being excluded from the living, they are able to move on with life and invest in other relationships, goals, and pursuits.

Sometimes a person's striving for belonging extends beyond the caregiving relationship and his or her small world of significant others. It encompasses the larger community, society, or world. Under those circumstances, belonging is ensured through profound achievements, social acts and significant contributions for the common good, or the confirmation that one's wisdom, knowledge, skills, or love has created ripples of influence upon others, who have been enhanced in their growth (see chapter 7). Underlying such behaviors is a striving for a cosmic belonging that tempers one's fear of death and sense of existential isolation.

Cosmic belonging is also reinforced by the person's attachment to a faith or religion, as described above. Most, if not all, religions promise believers a special and unique place in a metaphysical world. In this world, the deceased possesses an immortal soul that interacts with God, with spirits, or with the living. This belief is very comforting to some dying people, who let go with ease into the unknown of death, as well as to some bereaved families, who adjust to loss knowing that their loved one belongs in and occupies a special place in an ideal world.

Bond affirmation through belonging is important not only for people who seek care, but also for those of us who provide it. Not infrequently, we choose to work in death situations because attachment bonds are lived with a distinct intensity and provide an opportunity not only to contribute something significant to the lives of others, but also to occupy a special place in their worlds by which we are enriched.

The following chapter explores some aspects that render the relationship between a care provider and a person who encounters death distinct from other helping relationships.

NOTE

1. Note that the word *religion* comes from the Latin *religio.* In pre-Christian times, the word *religio* had quite a different sense from what it currently means (a creed, belief system, or spiritual affiliation). Connected to the verb *religare,* it meant "to bind." *Religare* had etymological roots in *ligare,* which meant "to tie," "to cement an alliance," "to close a deal," or "to unite in harmony."

3 Distinct Features of the Helping Relationship

"How can you keep doing this job?" "It must be so depressing to care for people who are in mourning." "I could *never* care for dying people." "Isn't your personal life affected?" "How do you cope?" These are common questions and statements that most of us have heard from friends, acquaintances, and colleagues. While these questions express fear, curiosity, admiration, disgust, or concern, they also communicate the fact that something distinct characterizes the person-professional relationship in death situations.

How is this relationship different from other caregiving relationships? In many ways it is an ordinary relationship that addresses "limit experiences," which involve life-and-death issues related to human existence. As a result, this relationship has the potential to become extraordinary for both care seekers and care providers, who are changed by their encounters with death.

There are at least four aspects that render the person-professional relationship distinct from other caregiving relations:

- Exposure to death and mortality awareness
- Inevitability of suffering versus potential for growth
- Experience of an altered sense of time
- Involvement in the caregiving relationship

EXPOSURE TO DEATH AND MORTALITY AWARENESS

While it is impossible to imagine our own non-existence, the death of another person is never abstract in our field of work. It is a real phenomenon. This phenomenon is lived quite differently by those of us who are directly exposed to and witness the death of a person and those who are indirectly exposed and listen to the narratives of bereaved people.

Direct exposure confronts us with human mortality. A person's dying process and death are *lived experiences,* recorded by all our senses. The sight, the sounds, the smells, and the physical touch of the dying person and of the dead body all trigger unique feelings, thoughts, and responses that often leave lasting imprints. Not only does a person die, but our relationship to him or her comes to an irreversible end. We live in the here and now the death of a human being and the finality of our relationship to him or her.

Indirect exposure provides us with a shield. We imagine the death through the account of a bereaved client. While the office setting and the distance from the actual death event protect us from direct exposure, we are still confronted by the raw, acute, or prolonged grief of a bereaved person.

Whether we are directly or indirectly exposed, death remains present in every relationship we develop with a dying or bereaved person. Our relationship is never dyadic. It always involves three participants. More specifically, in terminal care, a relationship is formed among the dying person, the professional, and death with its associated representations. To ignore death or pretend that it has no place leaves us at risk of estrangement and deception and deprives both the dying or bereaved and the care provider of the opportunity to share meaningful encounters in the face of irreversible loss. In bereavement care, the participants in the care relationship involve the bereaved, the professional, and the deceased person, who is brought into counseling or therapy through the mourner's verbalized and unverbalized accounts and occupies a central position. A critical aspect of effective support is to help the bereaved find new ways of maintaining a connection to the deceased.

Death's presence in every caregiving relationship confronts each of us with the realization that we are all mortal and that valued relationships come to an end. While dying and bereaved people have no choice but to cope with this reality, we, on the other hand, have a choice to face our mortality and explore core issues related to our existence. Some of us choose to contemplate our death from a safe distance. Others, too afraid to cope with existential issues, believe that death belongs only to patients or clients and imagine that being helpers or healers offers immunity from death. These professionals do not necessarily deny death. On the contrary, they acknowledge its existence *only* in the world of the seriously sick and the bereaved. This world they visit briefly and often in a detached manner, out of fear of being contaminated by dying or grief.

Is it ever possible to keep death out of awareness when we are repeatedly exposed as a result of our work? When Marcella, a nurse who worked in an intensive care unit, was asked to share her experience with dying patients, she responded, "I encounter death from a very close distance, yet I remain very distant from it." While she acknowledged death, she concurrently recognized her tendency to dissociate from the experience. Asked to elaborate on how she maintained such a distance, she said:

> I participate in a game that is played in our unit and reinforced by society. The game is called Life Preservation. The goal is to preserve life, at any cost.... This game has only one rule: to keep the patient alive, even if he left this world a long time ago. We fool ourselves, believing that with our sophisticated interventions, we can stop time, prevent death, and spare ourselves from the fear that someday—sooner or later—we are going to die too.

Through her insightful account, this nurse recognized her anxiety over both her patients' deaths and her own mortality. She actively participated in a collective effort to keep death at a distance from both her patients and herself.

Marcella's account raises a question: Can we be truly effective in helping people accept and cope with their dying and bereavement if we avoid facing our mortality and their death experiences?

Some years ago, I was invited to give a presentation to the staff of an adult oncology unit. Following my presentation, I was asked to attend the staff meeting before joining a Christmas celebration on the ward. I gladly accepted and sat silently in a corner, observing care providers discuss their patients. A physician reviewed the illness trajectory of a 52-year-old patient who had just died, and care providers discussed the effectiveness of the medical and nursing care that was provided to him at the end of his life. Satisfied by their interventions, the case was closed. Then the head nurse addressed some concerns with regard to the alleviation of symptoms in a critically ill patient, and a detailed plan was developed for the management of his pain. Someone mentioned his spouse, who had become hostile toward the staff member who told her that "there was not much left to offer" her husband. The discussion proceeded immediately to another patient who had repeatedly asked a nurse if the relapse of her disease was an indication that she was dying. The nurse shared how awkward she felt, and how skillfully she avoided answering by turning her attention to symptom management and spending Christmas at home. Team members appeared confident of their interventions, which rendered their patients' critical conditions manageable and efficiently controlled.

Throughout the staff meeting, no one alluded to the psychological or spiritual pain of patients, nor to the suffering of family members. Moreover, none spoke about the impact that the dying process and death of these patients had upon them. It felt as if death, to which they were all exposed, was absent from their relationships with the people they served.

The most intriguing part of this staff meeting occurred once discussions about patients ended and team members began to chat informally. One care provider said with annoyance that she had lost, for a third time, her glasses, which she despised wearing because they reminded her that she was growing old. This triggered jokes about old age, and staff members shared numerous examples of physical symptoms indicative of their loss of youth. The discussion was interrupted by the unit's director, who expressed concern about the prolonged absence of a colleague who was scheduled to undergo some medical tests. Hopes and worries about the possibility of a "CA diagnosis" (the word *cancer* was avoided) were shared. One care provider responded by knocking on wood, another crossed himself, and a third accused the physician of being a pessimist and of creating negative vibes. Someone volunteered to call their colleague later in the day. Soon the discussion became animated, and people made general statements about the uncertainties of life. This led a team member to describe how she panicked earlier that morning when the unit's secretary told her that she had received a phone call from her adolescent son's school. Catastrophic thoughts had crossed her mind until she called the school back to find out that her son had had a minor accident during sports activities. Senior members shared how work had made them more anxious over the safety and health of their loved ones and aware of the fragility of life.

I was observing and listening attentively. Death was fully present in that room. While during the staff meeting the event of death was objectified and became part of a scientific discourse, it is only through informal discussions that death acquired personal meanings. Fear of death was the common theme of intimate sharing. It was expressed in accounts that addressed the fear of growing old, the fear of becoming seriously sick, and the fear of unexpected harm and was reinforced by the realization of the fragility and preciousness of life. Death, which was efficiently managed in the care of dying patients, was dreaded by the professionals, who were, nevertheless, challenged to address some existential concerns.

Exposure to death has a profound impact, whether we recognize it or not. What we often dismiss is that our confrontation with death can be potentially enriching. Dying and bereaved people offer us a gift: the opportunity to reflect upon the fact that what is reversible in life becomes irreversible in death. They invite us to face our mortality and review our lives. Despite the anxiety that such a process often entails, it has also an empowering and life-affirming effect. It makes us aware of the freedom we have to determine how to live a life that is worth living.

But can we really contemplate our own death? Freud argued that it is impossible to imagine our own death. What he really meant was that it is impossible to grasp the concept of our non-existence. Death exists somewhere, where we do not have consciousness, and as a result, it becomes impossible to experience the self as non-self. We do not possess similar experience with which to compare or contrast it. Instead, we create representations that help us transform the unknown of death into something familiar.

On the first day of the graduate courses I teach on dying, death, and bereavement, I invite students to draw death as they see it. For some, death looks like a totally black piece of paper or is represented by the figure of the black reaper or a threatening monster. For others, death is personified as a conniving stranger that plays tricks upon people or as an abstract violent force that takes life away. Some draw a door or a window leading to a new reality that is clear, ambiguous, or unknown. Many represent death and life as opposing realities: life as colorful versus death as black, or life as filled with struggles and hardships versus death as idyllic. Other students focus on the passage or journey from life to death, which is perceived as peaceful or as filled with turmoil. The finality of death is sometimes represented by a dead body or a graveyard or the suffering of bereaved people, who are left empty, lonely, and in deep pain. Still others draw representations of an afterlife or a connection with the deceased. These representations take endless forms.

Each student is then invited to give his or her drawing a title and present it to the class. All drawings are placed on the wall, and key themes are identified and discussed in terms of how they are brought into relationships with dying and bereaved individuals. Then I invite students to take a step back from their drawing and imagine that the mural they created together was made by terminally ill or bereaved people. I ask them to choose one drawing that reflects the death representation of the person whom they would feel most comfortable accompanying through dying or bereavement, and the drawing of the person to whom they would feel least comfortable relating, because of his or her death representation.

For example, a nursing student who drew a big question mark as her own representation of death said she would have some difficulty supporting a patient whose representation of death comprised a black and hopeless trajectory from life to the unknown of death; it reminded her of the darkness that she experienced over an agonizing quest for meaning following the death of her cousin several years ago. In contrast, she was attracted by the drawing that represented death as a butterfly that flew freely out of a cage toward a destination that was bright and joyful. She felt that she could learn how to answer some of her own existential concerns from a person with beliefs in an afterlife and admitted to a need to make sense of her own loss though the care of such a patient.

Death representations that are attractive to some participants for personal reasons are repulsive to others. Not only are students affected by each other's representations, but they also realize that in the intersubjective space of their peer group, they experience new representations that affect their approach to care. At the end of the course, they revisit their drawings to discover if the way they think about death has changed, has been reinforced, or has been enriched and how their perceptions of providing services to dying and bereaved people have been affected.

In the first drawing, Thanassis, a male nurse, depicted dying and bereavement as the lonely voyage of a bird (see Illustration 3.1). At the end of the training, he added a second bird to his picture (see Illustration 3.2) to illustrate that dying and bereavement do not need to be a lonely process but instead a rich journey that is shared with another person who really cares. Thanassis acknowledged that such sharing between the dying or bereaved person and the professional is of critical importance. However, he also noted, that equally significant is the sharing among care providers who support each other through the process of caregiving in death situations.

In her first drawing of death, Eleni, a nurse in cardiology, depicted her sadness over the death of her patients (see Illustration 3.3). At the end of the training, added some grass to her initial drawing (see Illustration 3.4) and described the personal changes she had experienced when

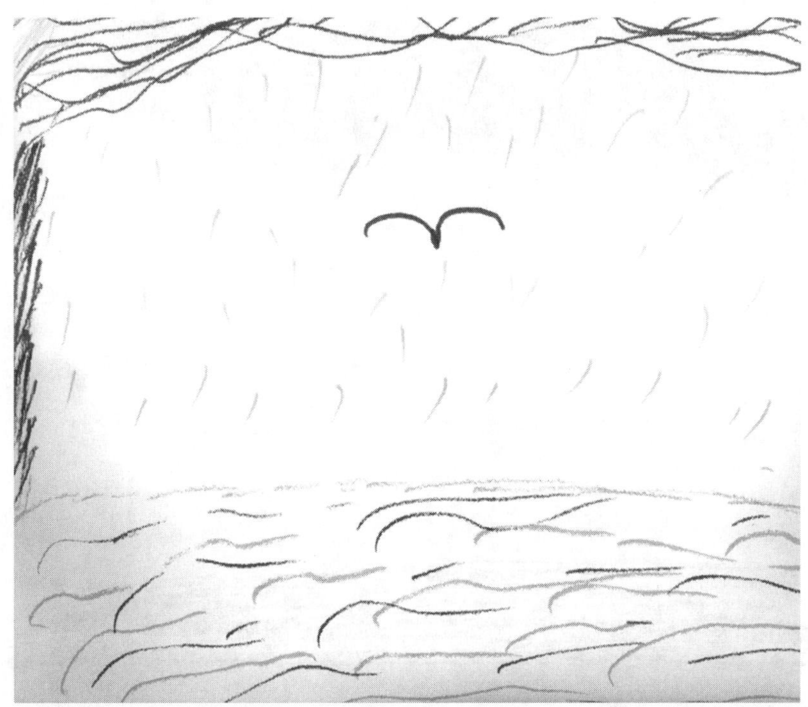

Illustration 3.1. Thanassis' representation of dying and grieving before the training.

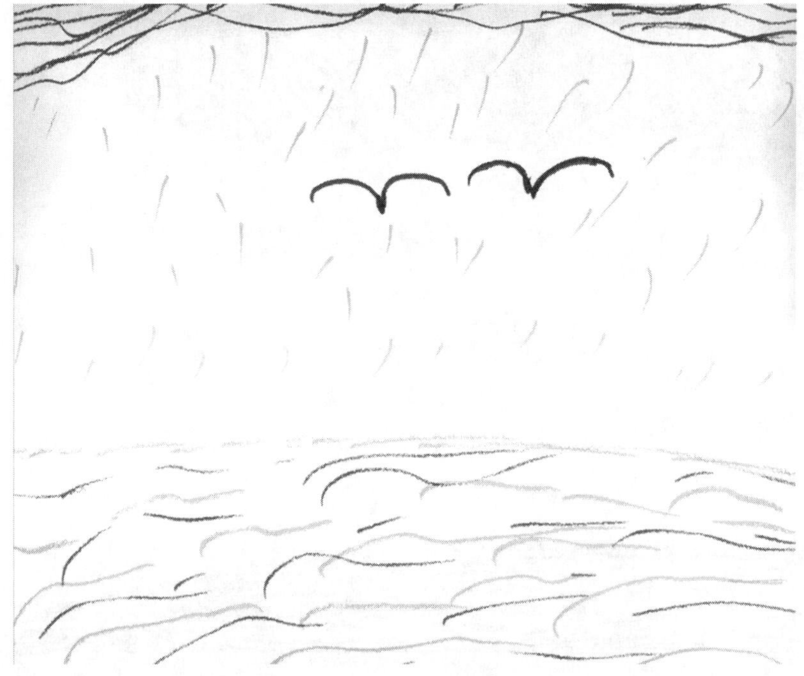

Illustration 3.2. Thanassis' representation of dying and grieving at the end of the training.

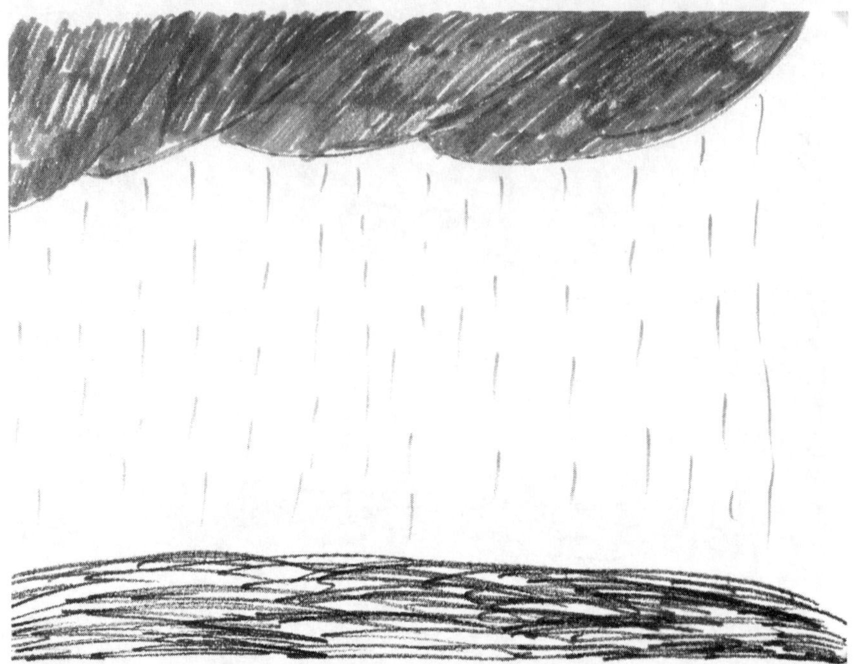

Illustration 3.3. Eleni's representation of the impact of death before the training.

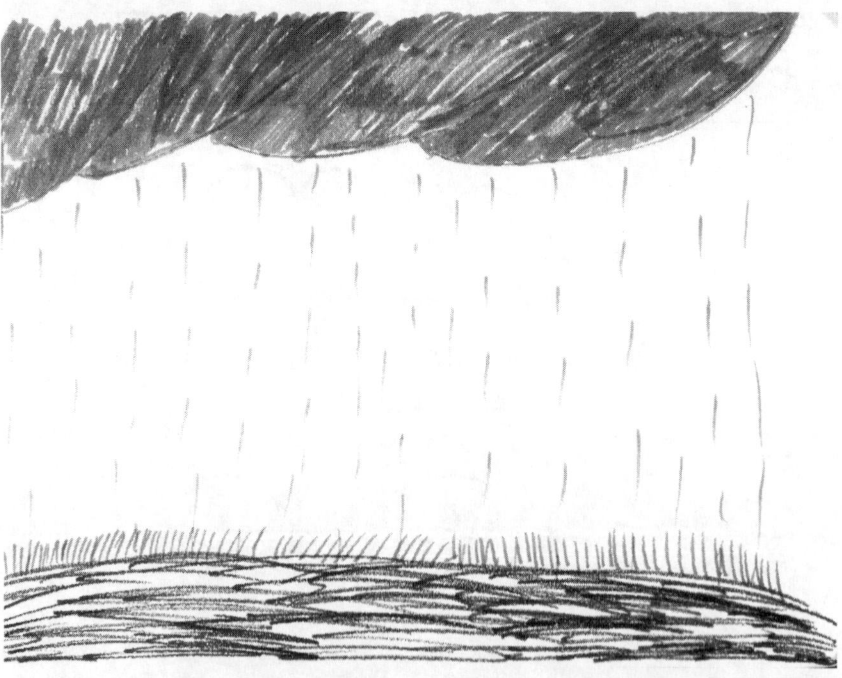

Illustration 3.4. Eleni's representation of the impact of death at the end of the training.

she began to confront, accept, and address her grief over a personal loss that had remained disenfranchised. One of her most profound realizations was that suffering provides the potential for growth.

INEVITABILITY OF SUFFERING VERSUS POTENTIAL FOR GROWTH

The experience of the suffering that is inevitable and integral to death situations also makes our relationship with dying and bereaved people different from other helping relationships. This suffering, however, is associated with profound possibilities for change and personal growth. Unlike our colleagues in other fields of care, who are expected to relieve people of suffering, we assist people in bearing suffering of a different nature.

Defining suffering is not an easy task. Different concepts are used in bereavement and palliative care to describe the same phenomenon. In bereavement, for example, suffering is traditionally associated with the concept of grief, while in end-of-life care, it is associated with the concept of "total pain," which has physical, psychological, social, and spiritual dimensions. The problem with most definitions is that that they view suffering as the outcome of one's exposure to impending or actual death; as a result, models of care propose how to manage specific aspects of suffering that are usually perceived as located within the individual. Suffering, in my view, is a process that stems from and is transcended through relationships. Therefore, suffering in dying and bereaved people occurs at different levels:

- *Through one's relationship with one's body.* Suffering is of a physical nature, manifested through bodily disintegration in the dying and an increased health vulnerability in the bereaved.
- *Through one's relationships with others.* Suffering is of an interpersonal nature and occurs when bonds are threatened or severed. It is the price all humans pay for loving, being loved, and belonging to a community that cares for the welfare of its members.
- *Through one's relationships with self and one's human existence.* Suffering is of a personal and existential nature and occurs when core assumptions about oneself and the world are challenged or disrupted. It is usually manifested in a quest for meaning over life-and-death issues and one's existence in the present world and/

> or in a spiritual or cosmic world. Questions such as "Why me?" "Am I going to die?" "What is death?" "Is there any purpose in suffering?" "Is there any meaning in a life that is torn apart as a result of my impending death or the loss of my beloved one?" "Does life have a purpose?" and "Is death better than life without meaning?" are indicative of a suffering that is of an existential nature.

The suffering of dying and bereaved people cannot always and should not be invariably eradicated. While its mitigation at a physical level must always remain a priority, the total alleviation of suffering at a relational and existential level is unrealistic and sometimes even detrimental because it prevents the dying from preparing for death, and the bereaved from adjusting to loss. Both processes involve an active grieving process that is healthy and necessary. This process can lead to major intrapersonal, interpersonal, and spiritual reorganizations that contribute to personal growth and fulfillment. Growth in the midst of suffering is more likely to occur when we acknowledge, accept, and contain the person's suffering and facilitate its tempering and/or transformation.

This is expressed eloquently by Rehnsfeldt and Eriksson (2004), who suggest that the transformation of suffering develops in three "acts": the first act involves the confirmation of a person's suffering by care providers; the second act involves the person's experience of being in suffering while being heard and accompanied; and during the third act the individual is described as becoming in suffering through a renewed sense of self that leads to personal growth. Each act requires the presence of a compassionate other who allows suffering to exist but also contributes to its transcendence by facilitating the construction of meaning in communion (Fredriksson & Eriksson, 2001; Lindholm & Eriksson, 1993).

Being in suffering with another demands that we, the care providers, acknowledge both the violent impact of death upon relationships, which are threatened, broken, and severed forever, and the vitalizing force it engenders, which can lead to profound changes, transformations, and enriched experiences. Thus, the caregiving relationship becomes the recipient of such violence, as well as the source of significant growth.

We usually become aware of the violence when we bear witness to deaths that are dramatic, sudden, unpredictable, or perceived as unnatural and untimely; we observe families being torn apart; or we listen to traumatic and chaotic accounts that communicate—beyond words—an excruciating pain that we can barely withstand. Tedeschi, Park, and

Calhoun (1998) use the metaphor of an "emotional earthquake" to describe the trauma experienced by people in highly distressing situations. Death is like a seismic event that shakes, threatens, and damages existing psychic structures that involve fundamental components of their view of themselves and of the world.

Some of us cannot bear such violence and destruction and, as a result, deny, displace, dismiss, or desperately strive to control it. We keep busy and unavailable to people, we become impersonal or indifferent, we seek to control dying conditions through futile interventions, or we force the bereaved to move on with life and quickly "resolve" their grief. In so doing, we introduce an additional form of violence that increases their suffering, which becomes more devastating than death itself. The person ends up dying alone, resentful, or in despair; the bereaved are isolated and exiled from a world of meaningful relationships; and we remain dissatisfied with the services we provide.

Care providers who are able to contain the violence and destructive effects of death can also experience its vitalizing and transformative power. This becomes evident when, for example, a person confides to us that the time since his or her diagnosis has been the best of his life. Despite the rapid deterioration of one's body, his or her psychic, social, and spiritual worlds regain a vitality that unleashes explorative and transformative processes. In a similar way, the bereaved, whose worlds have fallen apart, become conscious of the transience of life and are awakened to an enriched life. Dying and bereaved people plunge into life and bring some of this vitality into their relationships with others.

To return back to Tedeschi, Park, and Calhoun's (1998) metaphor of an earthquake, we see the dying and bereaved remove the remains of old structures, consider new plans, and build new foundations that can withstand the aftershocks of subsequent earthquakes. Through this transformative process, they reconstruct a life narrative and develop a new sense of self, relate differently to others, and relearn the world, which comes to acquire new meaning. This process can develop within a very short period of time, can be profound, and can lead to personal growth beyond one's previous levels of psychological functioning (Attig, 1996; Hogan & Schmidt, 2002; Janoff-Bulman, 1992; Neimeyer, 1998; Nolen-Hoeskema & Larson, 1999; Parkes, 1971; Tedeschi & Calhoun, 1995, 2004; Tedeschi et al., 1998).

If we perceive our relationships with dying and bereaved people as being solely submerged in suffering, then we neglect the immense potential for self-actualization and growth and deprive those we serve of hope and the possibility of change. In addition, we deny ourselves the opportunity to learn from them how to live, appreciate and value life, as well as our existence in the world. Affected by their experiences, we are often challenged to review our role, our relationships with others, and our values and priorities in life. The positives of such a review are evident in a changed sense of self (e.g., greater strength or vulnerability but also increased compassion for others), changed relationships with others (e.g., greater closeness and appreciation), and a changed philosophy of life, which is valued, cherished, and lived more fully (Tedeschi & Calhoun, 1995). We develop what Adler described as a "social interest" by being more humble and by striving to contribute to the welfare of others (Ferguson, 1989).

EXPERIENCE OF AN ALTERED SENSE OF TIME

The third aspect that makes our relationship distinct from other caregiving relationships is related to the experience of time, which is affected by the reality of death. According to Hartocollis (1983), "Time objectifies human experience, keeps score of a person's life, delineating its limits, its progress, its existence" (p. 205). To illustrate this point, he offers the example of patients who awaken from anesthesia, sedation, or comma. The first thing they usually ask is: "What time is it?" "What day is it?" "When did the accident happen?" In this way, they try to reestablish contact with the world of the living and reintegrate themselves into a life with a time trajectory: a past, present, and future.

In a similar way, people who are diagnosed with a life-threatening illness or informed of their deteriorating health condition usually ask: "How much time have I left?" or "For how long will my life be prolonged with this treatment?" or declare, "I want to make the most of each day that is left." In the face of an imminent death, they experience time and their existence in the world differently. For some, the time they have left is perceived as too long, especially if they experience unrelenting suffering; for others, it is just enough if they have lived a full life and are prepared to move into the unknown that lies ahead; still others perceive the time left as too short to achieve important goals or attend to personal issues.

Bereaved people also situate their experiences in an altered time perspective. Their entire lives are divided into a time before and a time after the death of their loved person. Experiences acquire meaning in relation to a perceived time that heals or prevents a meaningful existence in the world.

Time becomes the organizing pivot of the experiences of the ill, the dying, and the bereaved (Sourkes, 1982). It often becomes the organizing pivot of the experiences of care providers as well. We set goals and plan interventions in relation to time. Time is experienced as moving too quickly when death threatens our plans to prolong life or help families have meaningful experiences; it is perceived as moving too slowly when our resources have been exhausted and we feel helpless to relieve a person's suffering; it is perceived as sufficient when we are able to determine the duration of our services to the bereaved (e.g., 6, 10, or 12 sessions of group counseling). Encounters with death affect our subjective experience of time.

Peter was a social worker in an adult hospice. His professional and personal life were profoundly affected by his work with dying patients and bereaved families, which led to an altered sense of time. This was expressed in the following account:

> My work in the hospice has helped me to develop an acute awareness of time. It's the present moment that matters, and how this moment is used to relate, to communicate, or to be with another person. Life for these patients and families is *lived,* because time is made to count, not in terms of hours, but in terms of meaningful interactions and experiences that help them transcend suffering and pain.

Peter perceived his role as one of "helping people invest time with meaning." He believed it was unrealistic to expect them to invest their entire lives with meaning when they were close to death.

> You see, contrary to my colleagues, I do not expect them to address and solve all their problems and cope with unresolved issues, especially since most of them are ravaged by grief and depleted of energy. So I try to make time, for a family, count. Sometimes something special and unique occurs that remains unforgettable in their lives and in mine.

Peter went on to describe how, in his personal life, time with his children, his spouse, and his elderly parents was made to count. Without taking relationships for granted, he learned to live in the present moment with an acute awareness and aliveness.

Life, death, and time are interrelated (Dossey, 1984). It is impossible to separate them. Confronted with death, we realize the inevitability of life's limits, and our sense of time is often altered. We strive to prolong time, to slow it down, to stop, to accelerate it, or to make the most out of it, like Peter. Death evokes in each of us a desire to eliminate time, to escape from time, or to generate time. Let's consider some of the ways in which we alter our sense of lived time.

How Do We Subjectively Eliminate Time?

We subjectively eliminate time by altering our sense of its flow. If there is no flowing of time, then there is no loss, and consequently no death (Dossey, 1984). As pointed out by Mann (1973), "If one can eliminate time sense, one can also avoid the ultimate separation that time brings: death" (p. 6). We can make death disappear from our consciousness in two distinct ways: by accelerating the flow of time or by stopping it altogether (see also principle 4 in chapter 9).

We accelerate time's flow by moving frantically from one activity to another, from one event or task to another, from one patient to the next. Time is filled with an avalanche of experiences, events, tasks, or crises episodes that are managed with a sense of urgency, with no opportunities to reflect upon experiences, especially since they involve suffering, loss, and death. We have a sense not of a unified linear time, but of several "parallel times" that are experienced as fragmented. Experiences are hardly situated in time. "Time flies," we admit. "Where did it go?" we ask ourselves. In reality, we subjectively make it disappear by fragmenting it, along with the awareness that it leads to the end of human existence.

Our relationships with dying and bereaved people remain superficial, while the time that is spent with them focuses on the management of practical challenges imposed by an "outer" reality. We avoid becoming acquainted with the dying person's body and psyche, which know when life is coming to an end. In a similar way, we rush the bereaved through bereavement and deprive them of the arduous process of grieving and of confronting mortality.

But we also strive to eradicate time by experiencing it as frozen, stopped, arrested. We achieve that by avoiding situations that involve loss, separation, or any other form of change and by staying away from relationships with individuals who may die or grieve. We find refuge in a rigid routine, suspend decisions, inhibit changes, and avoid dreaming, projecting ourselves into the future, and hoping for the people we serve.

How Do We Subjectively Escape From Time?

We subjectively escape from time by becoming involved in activities such as arts, poetry, meditation, reading, gardening, and other hobbies or recreations in which we lose any sense of temporality. The subjective sense of escaping the boundaries of time allows us to cultivate—even momentarily—the illusion that we can escape death. A similar state is attained through the use of drugs, alcohol, or other addictive substances, as well as through the development of symbiotic relationships with others. With regard to the latter, we experience a sense of oneness with the people we serve and develop enmeshed relationships with our children, partners, or lovers. In that way, we transcend the threat of loss and separation by cultivating the illusion of an eternal bond that does not obey time limitations. According to Hartocollis (1983), most religions achieve this by promising an eternal afterlife and a union with a divine force that transcends death, loss, and separation and preserves the illusion of an immortal self, whose existence is not limited by the barriers of time.

How Do We Subjectively Generate Time?

We subjectively generate time in two distinct ways: first, by situating our experiences in a temporal perspective that expands our sense of living (past-present-future), without excluding the possibility of loss, separation, and death, and second, by living in the present moment with an acute awareness. In both situations, we make time count, as eloquently described by Peter.

In other words, we acknowledge that objectively measured life time has an end, and strive to expand the here and now (subjective time) by rendering it conscious and worth living. When we generate time, we create history—with a past, present, and future—that provides opportunities for meaningful encounters and the realization of goals and activities that are significant to us and to others. Each here-and-now moment becomes a lived moment that is distinct and unique. Paradoxically, it is never isolated in the present, since the clarity and consciousness by which it is lived engrave it in memory (past) and multiply opportunities for growth (future). In other words, a lived moment (or a moment that counts) transcends the chronological barriers of time.

We are more likely to generate time when we develop relationships with dying and bereaved people in which *doing* becomes less important than *being with*. *Being with* allows us to honor the present moment as well as the relationship that can contain it. When we allow ourselves to be with another person in death and bereavement, then the patient-professional relationship fades away and emerges as a person-to-person relationship. In such a relationship, time is worth living because it holds the potential for changes and transformations that can be profound. Paradoxically, such changes occur within a second, an hour, or a day and are profound for the other and for us.

INVOLVEMENT IN THE CAREGIVING RELATIONSHIP

The fourth aspect that is unique to our relationship is the nature of our involvement with people who, through their dying and grief, experience processes that are integral to being human. While we are challenged to relate as professionals who possess expert knowledge and skills, we also connect to them as equal human beings who are mortal and bereft when we lose valued relations. This realization has led clinicians in palliative and bereavement care to describe the nature of our involvement with the dying and the bereaved. Some have emphasized the importance of a personal or emotional involvement; others have described the need for active engagement through the use of counseling skills and behaviors; still others have proposed the display of professional friendly interest, while several support the adoption of an attitude of detached concern that ensures a "perfect" distance—not too close or too distant—from dying and bereaved people. Although consensus has not been achieved, it is worth exploring how each of these views illuminates our involvement in the caregiving relationship.

Emotional Involvement

In her description of her psychotherapy practice with a patient who was dying from metastatic breast cancer, Janice Norton (1963), a psychoanalyst, identified distinct moments when the issue of involvement and separation between her and the patient came into sharp focus. Norton had made herself widely available to her patient when her condition became critical; in response, the patient experienced her therapist as being with her 24 hours a day and carried on imaginary conversations with her, even in the analyst's absence. When death became imminent, the woman expressed distress at the thought that her analyst would not be dying with her, and that death was something they could not share. She disclosed her fantasy of carrying the therapeutic relationship into death, as well as her desire to extend her existence through her therapist, to whom she offered, as a parting gift, a red dress that she had bought before becoming too ill to wear it, with the hope that "the dress [would] have some fun."

This brief example illustrates how involvement in death situations can become personal and intimate. Such involvement evokes intense feelings of love and anger, of hope and despair, as well as fantasies of moving between the world of the living and the world of the deceased. It fosters intimacy and rich encounters that are valued by the dying, the bereaved, and us. In fact, the opportunity for intimate encounters attracts some care providers in this field of work, while it causes others to turn away or resist any form of involvement.

Palliative and bereavement care consider personal involvement as necessary, since it humanizes care by introducing emotions into the helping relationship that have been denied a place by traditional medical practice. Such an involvement implies a certain degree of intimacy that is assumed to be appropriate, as well as desirable.

But is such an assumption true? Not all care providers wish to become personally involved or are appropriately trained to support people through intimate encounters. Moreover, not all people desire emotional involvement with professionals, especially during a transitional period when they strive to cope with loss and separation. Randall and Downie (2006) challenge some of the prevailing practices that impose involvement and intimacy upon the dying patient and the grieving family and question whether a professional "has any *right* to thrust a close relationship on a reluctant patient" (p. 153). They criticize the imposition of intimate and personal relationships through the use of assessment tools, structured questionnaires, and interviews that assess people's physical, psychosocial, and spiritual needs and force them to make personal disclosures that they may be unwilling to offer or have not consented to.

Engagement Through the Use of Counseling Skills and Behaviors

Other clinicians foster personal involvement through the use of counseling skills and behaviors. Parkes, Relf, and Couldrick (1996), for example, view the relationship between a dying or bereaved person and the care provider as similar to the counselor-client relationship described by Carl Rogers. They believe that even people who do not seek formal counseling when they are dying or grieving can benefit from a personal relationship with care providers who display empathic understanding, unconditional acceptance, and genuineness. They describe engagement in the following terms:

> It is not a passive process but an active engagement. It requires the use of all our senses. It means listening with our ears to what is being said and to the tone of voice, listening with our minds to understand the message contained in the words, listening with our eyes to what is being conveyed through the client's posture, bearing and gestures, and listening with our hearts to the human being we are trying to understand. Listening in this way enables clients to feel that we are really there with them and value who they are. (p. 60)

Counseling skills—referred to as "helping strategies"—enable the individual to identify goals that are significant to him or her at a given time and receive support from a care provider who avoids giving advice, information, or reassurance, as is commonly done in the traditional asymmetrical patient-professional relationship. The ultimate aim is to decrease the person's perception of isolation or hopelessness and increase autonomy and control over his or her terminal or bereavement condition.

Maguire and Pitceathly (2005) propose a more rigidly structured counseling approach that is determined by specific goals, is of limited duration (from one to six sessions), and makes use of prearranged meetings during which care providers are expected to refrain from becoming emotionally involved in order to reduce the risk of professional burnout. To minimize involvement, they offer a list of strategies of what to do in death situations when people experience fears; are in denial, in despair, angry, or withdrawn; and display various responses that result in what are described as "difficult situations." Their approach emphasizes appropriate assessment and problem solving through a relationship that protects the professional from the chaos, uncertainty, and suffering that death engenders.

Friendly Professional Interest

Randall and Downie (2006) borrow the concept of friendly professional interest from Brewin, who suggests that care providers must combine professional competence and a friendly attitude that is characterized by genuine concern and understanding. They argue that we should not be trained to *look* concerned and understanding through the use of specific communication or counseling skills but should experience genuine interest in the person who suffers. Such an interest does not require assessment, intervention, or treatment, but ordinary human interactions, sensitive explanations, and advice based on professional knowledge and experience:

> In our view competence in professional skills and knowledge should be regarded as essential—neither an attitude of caring and compassion, nor the establishment of a particular relationship with the patient will achieve the goals of health care, even in the context of incurable and fatal illness. (pp. 152–153)

They give priority to professional knowledge and skills yet urge us not to hide behind tools, questionnaires, protocols, and evidence-based research, all of which aim to create an objective science of emotional, social, and spiritual care. Instead, they propose a caring relationship in which the provider is both technical and human—that is, able to observe and explore a person's condition and private world from a scientific perspective, while relating to him or her as a human being. What Randall and Downie do not address is how "humanness" is cultivated, displayed, and maintained in death situations, and how it affects providers, who are invited to give up some of their "technical professionalism" in order to relate authentically to the people they serve. Their ideas echo Hippocratic writings, according to which the healer is expected to develop *philia* (friendship) with the people who seek his or her services. According to Randall and Downie, friendship, which is characterized by pure feelings for another person, and an impartial concern for all human beings allow care providers to relate with concern and to view themselves as more similar to than different from people who, like them, are affected by death.

Involvement Through Detached Concern

Detached concern is a controversial concept that was promoted in medicine in the late 1950s and early 1960s (see Halpern, 2001, for a comprehensive review) and continues to be prevalent in the education of physicians, nurses, psychologists, and social workers. It suggests that both emotional engagement and emotional detachment are detrimental to the helping relationship and should be avoided. A middle ground is therefore found in a detached concern that promotes emotional detachment and rational understanding.

An approach of detached concern expects that care providers remain emotionally detached yet display concern and empathic understanding toward people who seek their services. Empathy is misperceived as a purely intellectual form of understanding of the person's experiences and private world. Emotions are avoided and viewed as subjective and therefore dangerous, harmful, and unscientific since they cloud clinical judgment, which should always be impartial and objective.

It is assumed that detached concern protects professionals from burnout, from biased judgments, and from being accused of being impersonal. Clinical experience as well as observational and qualitative studies all indicate that none of the above is achieved (Halpern, 2001). First, burnout is not prevented. In reality, emotional detachment is associated with lower degrees of job satisfaction, which contribute to and aggravate burnout. Second, emotional detachment does not render us more objective or rational in our reasoning. Our reasoning is never solely cognitive; it relies heavily on how we experience reality through our emotions, physical senses, and bodily reactions. When we selectively focus on some aspects of another person's experience while casting other aspects into the shadows, we end up more vulnerable to biases, prejudices, and errors of judgment.

In our effort to develop an attitude of detached concern we are faced with a bind: to be both involved with and detached from the people we serve. In other words, we strive to be close to dying or bereaved people by displaying understanding, concern, and compassion and simultaneously distant in order to be objective and protect ourselves from being affected by their experiences. It is mistakenly assumed that there is a perfect distance to be found that ensures objective professionalism, along with compassion, and offers immunity to suffering. Unfortunately, when we spend all our energy trying to find this perfect (illusory) distance, we become blind to the rich exchanges that unfold in the face of death.

Clinical experience shows that the "correct" amount of involvement varies. A distance that feels right to one person may feel uncomfortable to a different individual, or to the same person at another time. We must realize that there is no perfect closeness or distance, no perfect involvement to be achieved. The only thing we can fully determine is how distant we wish to remain from our own inner selves and from an awareness of how we affect and are being affected by the relationships we develop with dying and bereaved people in death situations.

It becomes evident from this conceptualization of our involvement with the dying and the bereaved that the issue is far from being resolved.

Involvement with dying and bereaved people is not a matter of emotional versus rational engagement. Assuming that reason is distinct from, independent of, and opposed to emotion fosters the illusion that we can relate to people by switching off our emotions and turning on rational thinking, or by switching off rational thinking and turning on emotions, at will. This reason-versus-emotion dualism is not new. It has always permeated the education and training of physicians, nurses, psychologists, and social workers and contributed to the development of unrealistic expectations with regard to their involvement with people in need.

We are challenged to recognize that we relate to others through all our senses, with our bodies, feelings, thoughts, and actions, which are all interrelated. It is through an embodied experience that we understand reality and establish relationships that sometimes are personal and intimate and other times are more distant and disengaged but, nevertheless, effective. Involvement is a holistic experience and the outcome of an interactive process that unfolds between us and the people we help as we both face death and remain committed to each other through dying or bereavement.

The following chapter explores how this embodiment is achieved when we assume the role of companion to people experiencing a painful yet normal and unavoidable period of life. Special emphasis is placed upon the conditions that facilitate companioning and enrich our encounters with them.

4 The Accompanying Process

THE MYTH

Sometime between 3000 and 1400 B.C., Minoan civilization flourished in Greece under the rule of King Minos, who lived on the island of Crete, where the port of Knossos was a popular stop for the seamen who traveled from Greece to North Africa and brought aspects of Minoan culture, commerce, art, and architecture to surrounding Mediterranean and Eastern countries. The port of Knossos was renowned for the palace of Knossos, an exceptional architectural structure inhabited by King Minos and Queen Pasiphae. The beauty, grace, and splendor of the palace made it the foundation for the myth of the labyrinth. To this day, there is no evidence that a labyrinth ever existed, but inhabitants of Crete used its image on their coins, floor mosaics, and wall paintings in the palace of Knossos and built a myth around it.

According to the myth, when Queen Pasiphae mated with the beautiful white bull that Zeus sent Minos as a token of support for his ruling over Crete, the Minotaur was conceived. The Minotaur was a ferocious creature with the head of a bull and the body of a human. Afraid of offending the gods, King Minos did not kill the Minotaur but instead ordered Deadalus, a genius master builder from Athens, to build a labyrinth, in which the Minotaur was imprisoned, waiting to devour people when they fell in (Kakridis, 1986).

When the son of King Minos, Androgeos, was killed by Athenians during some athletic festivities, his father besieged the city of Athens with his fleet. In exchange for releasing Athens from its siege, he demanded that every nine years the inhabitants of Athens send seven young men and seven maidens to Crete to be thrown into the labyrinth. Lost in this chaotic edifice with interwoven walls and paths, crossroads, and dead ends, these young men and women were devoured by the Minotaur. Not only did they fear the dreadful monster, but they were also terrified by the journey through the labyrinth, in which threats loomed at every corner.

One year, the sacrificial party included Theseus, the son of the Athenian king Aigeas. Ariadne, the daughter of King Minos, fell in love with Theseus and, transgressing her father's orders, decided to help him confront and kill the Minotaur and free Athenians from their heavy debt to her father.

According to the legend, Ariadne handed Theseus a yarn of thread (known as the *mitos*) to help him find his way in and out of the labyrinth and retreat in case of danger. Equipped with a lifeline of safe exploration and safe retreat, Theseus entered the labyrinth, confronted and killed the Minotaur, and freed Athenians from their debt.

His triumph over the beast not only was perceived as an act of bravery but also required him to engage in profound assessment and consideration of the challenges that he encountered during his journey. Supported by a woman who loved him and cared for his well-being, he was able to confront a seemingly invincible threat.

Ariadne was not only clever and knowledgeable of the challenges that needed to be mastered, but she was also a woman filled with passionate love. She did not walk through the labyrinth with Theseus but served as his companion through the trajectory and remained attached to him by means of a thread. She gave Theseus both the security of a world he could return to if he came to be lost, and the confidence to move forward, explore the unknown, and confront the Minotaur.

Maze or Labyrinth?

One of the interesting aspects of the myth is that while we are told that Theseus must journey through a labyrinth, the myth describes a maze rather than a labyrinth. What is the difference between a maze and a labyrinth?

A maze comprises several paths and crossroads, false turnings, blind lanes, and dead ends that make the journey dangerous, unpredictable, and filled with challenges and surprises. One is constantly faced with choices. A chosen path may turn out to reach a dead end or lead one astray. A maze is believed to symbolize the multiple pathways of thought and action from which humans must choose in the journey through life.

In the myth, Theseus needed Ariadne's thread to avoid losing his orientation and find his way out. This thread would not have been vital to his survival if he had had to walk through a labyrinth rather than a maze in order to face the Minotaur. Why? Because the labyrinth is unicursal, having only one unbranched pathway, which—after many curves and detours—leads to the center, and from there back to the point of departure. The sharp twists and turns of a labyrinth force the traveler to change direction, face new challenges, and seek new hope. Each turn presents a new perspective of the surrounding space and of reality. The center of the labyrinth remains always in view, and one's destination is eventually reached.

The journey through the labyrinth is characterized by rhythm and swing from one detour to another, since the voyageur does not have to choose between right and wrong directions. As the traveler meanders through the paths he or she has the opportunity to view reality from different points of view. It is not by chance that Hermann Kern (2000) postulates that the origin of the labyrinth is dance. This spiral dance that moves toward a center and away from it through a number of meandering paths is a symbol of a cyclical time, of rhythmic movement in space, often related to life and death rituals. It represents a journey that starts in the outer world and moves into the inner world before returning to the outer world. In contrast, movement in the maze is characterized by discontinuity, because the flow is interrupted by choices and doubt about whether one has moved in the right or wrong direction. The symbol of the labyrinth is not uniquely Greek. It has been found in other cultures, in central India, Africa, America—among the Hopi and Navaho—and Europe during the Roman period. While most historians believe that the labyrinth symbolizes the journey through life, others suggest that it represents a journey into the psychic world. It is a symbol of self-discovery and of the search for the center of intellectual, emotional, and spiritual life. With the rise of Christianity, the labyrinth became a symbol of man's journey toward divine salvation and was often depicted on the floors and ceilings of churches.

The Myth's Lessons

This myth, like so many others, can be interpreted in many different ways. Viewed in light of the care we provide at the end of life and during bereavement, it communicates three messages that illuminate aspects of the context in which a caring relationship is formed, and the process in which accompaniment unfolds.

The first message relates to how each dying or bereaved person travels through this challenging period of life. One's confrontation with death forces him or her to enter unknown territories, where he or she encounters unfamiliar challenges and symbolic Minotaurs. These may include the threat of impending death, the irreversible loss of life, the overwhelming suffering, the emergence of an old trauma, or the triggering of an existential crisis.

Some people experience their journey as a maze that presents them with difficult choices, disasters, and dead ends. They seek professionals' help in determining the "right" solutions to problems in their attempts to gain control of a reality that appears uncertain, confusing, and terrifying. Their narratives are often chaotic, broken, and filled with threats and inescapable disasters.

Other people experience their trajectory as a labyrinth with turning points, changes of direction, and opportunities to revisit the past, ponder the present, contemplate the future, and change their view of themselves, others, and life. Their stories are usually characterized by a back-and-forth movement in a quest for meaning. This movement enables them to transform the pain, confusion, or uncertainty they are experiencing into ordered thinking that allows for new realizations and insights, as well as novel orientations. Like Theseus, they are able to stand in the darkness, the chaos, and the suffering that is associated with dying and bereavement and learn to temper the anxiety that is elicited by death through intimate relationships with those who accompany them on their journey. Traveling through their labyrinth, both literally and symbolically, enables them to go into their inner worlds to confront their Minotaurs and return to the outside world changed by the voyage.

Finally, there are some people—if not the majority—who move back and forth between a maze and a labyrinth and back to a maze before they find their way into the world, changed and transformed.

The second message of this myth relates to our caregiving role. We are helpful to dying and bereaved people when we assume a role similar to that of Ariadne. We do not fix or solve the problem or kill or eliminate the Minotaur on their behalf. Instead, we offer a relationship that facilitates their coping with the inevitability of death, the awareness of mortality, and the pain of loss.

In the myth, Ariadne did not walk Theseus' path; she symbolically walked alongside him and remained attached to him by means of a thread. In a similar way, we do not walk others' paths; we do not live their impasses, nor do we become lost into the dark corners of their maze. Instead, we find a way of being with them, as long as they wish to have a companion on their trajectory. We use our knowledge, skills, and clinical experience to help them discover their own paths and experience a trajectory that is meaningful to them. By listening to their concerns, by offering information, by discussing options and decisions, by sharing our observations and guidance but also by remaining silent and allowing them to confidently stand alone, without feeling deserted or overprotected, we facilitate their journey through the pathways of life.

Like Ariadne, we are faithfully present and committed. It is our availability, presence, and commitment that cultivate a sense of security, of continuity, of belonging, and of hope. More specifically, we enhance *security* by developing a secure bond that is able to contain painful experiences in critical times and allows for exploration of existential concerns as well as new avenues of thought and unfamiliar experiences. We ensure *continuity* by remaining physically and psychologically present during a time when relationships are threatened by death, loss, and separation. We foster *belonging* by facilitating the integration of the dying and bereaved person into a world of meaningful and rewarding relationships. And last but not least, we instill *hope* by minimizing or tempering suffering, or by transforming it into opportunities for change and growth.

The third message of this myth relates to the potential for growth and development in the face of death. Not only was the thread used by Theseus to find the exit—it also enabled him to transform his journey from one through a maze with branched paths, crossroads, and impasses into one through a labyrinth with a single path.

In a similar way, we provide people with opportunities to transform a journey that is often experienced as a maze (described in their narratives as a "prison," "impasse," "nightmare," etc.) into a journey that is experienced as a labyrinth (described as an "awakening," or a "healing" or "enriching" experience). This transformation is facilitated by means of a strong and sturdy thread that is symbolic of two basic functions:

1. The development of a secure bond between the person and the care provider. As already discussed, such a bond does not cultivate dependence but offers a haven in times of trouble, and a secure base for the undertaking of explorations into new territories and experiences (see chapter 2)
2. The development of thinking and reflection in one's quest for solutions to problems and desire to illuminate the darkness of the unknown by attributing meaning to experiences and existential concerns (Potamianou, 2003)

Does thinking involve solely a cognitive process? It does not. In ancient Greek, the word for thinking (*skepsis*) refers to "a perception by the senses" (Liddell & Scott, 1994), thus reflecting an experience that is not solely cognitive but holistic. It involves shifting one's gaze from the challenges of an external reality that imposes choices and solutions to practical problems (often similar to the multiple paths of a maze) to the challenges of an internal reality that is illuminated through a reflective process (similar to the single path of a labyrinth), and vice versa. To facilitate this shift between the external and internal reality, it is important that we, as care providers, maintain a broad view and move swiftly between the individual's perspective (Theseus's perspective) and our own perspective (Ariadne's perspective). In other words, we must have the capacity to enter the person's private world but also stand outside and view his or her journey from a distance. By mirroring back both perspectives (his or hers and our own), we offer a *miton* that enables dying and bereaved people to acknowledge their experiences; to reflect on these experiences and make connections between past and present events and future aspirations; to cope with current challenges, mend old wounds, and contemplate the future by assigning new meanings to their experiences; and to relate to others in ways that enhance belonging and integration into the fabric of humanity.

Kata miton means "thread by thread" in Greek. People validate or reconstruct, thread by thread, a world with meaning that sustains them through loss and grief. Our role is to facilitate the threading process that leads to changes and transformations. This process is almost always enriched when it is shared.

Clinicians in palliative care (e.g., De Hannezel, 1995; Yoder, 2005) and in bereavement care (e.g., Heustis & Jenkins, 2005; Wolfelt, 2006) suggest that the key function of our role is to accompany people who are faced with impending death or who strive to adjust to the loss of someone they loved. Wolfelt (2006) proposes the term *companioning* to describe both the process of caring as well as the role of professionals who serve as companions to dying and grieving individuals. The word *companion* stems from the Latin roots *com,* which means "with," and *pan,* which means "bread." A person "breaks bread" with his or her companion by sharing personal stories. Wolfelt describes the art of companioning as one "of bringing comfort to another by becoming familiar with her story" (p. 19).

In this book the terms *accompaniment* and *companionship* are used interchangeably. There is limited knowledge about what companioning entails, which conditions facilitate its unfolding, and what the effects are upon those who accompany and those who are being accompanied. The purpose of this chapter is to explore these issues in the hope of contributing to the discussion that is currently unfolding in the field.

FROM MYTH TO REALITY: ASSUMING A COMPANIONING ROLE

There are two critical periods in an individual's life during which we, as care providers, assume a role of facilitating a natural process to unfold: at the birth of a human life and at the end of an individual's living existence. During these periods, bonds are formed, severed, reviewed, or redefined and both the person's and family's life stories are being reconstructed. Through these transitional periods, we accompany people and help them pave their way into life (in birth), pave their way out of life (through dying), or pave their way into an altered mode of living (through bereavement).

We can learn a great deal about companioning if we focus upon the birth of humans. Since ancient times, the midwife has assumed the role of companion to the woman who is giving birth. Her role is to facilitate the unfolding of a natural yet painful process. Assuming that the birth of a child is solely a happy and joyful event is naive. In most situations it is experienced and remembered as such. But this transitional period is characterized by radical changes and a profound vulnerability that is experienced by both the infant and the mother.

For the infant, the passage from the safety of its mother's womb to an unknown and unfriendly world always contains risks and is lived with increasing anxiety. When we, the professionals, create delivery conditions that are amenable to the newborn (e.g., Frederick's Leboyer method of childbirth) and help the mother respond with love, care, and affection to her infant's anxiety, then the baby enters life with less distress and more confidence.

Like the newborn, a woman also experiences increased vulnerability throughout pregnancy, labor, and the postpartum period that stems from hormonal and bodily changes as well as from major psychic reorganizations. The latter are triggered by concerns such as "Will my baby be okay?" "Will it be as I fantasized?" "What is the place of this child in my life?" "What will the life of my child be like?" "Can I be a good parent?" "What did I learn from my parents about parenting?" and "How will my life be changed?" Introduced to the world of motherhood (especially if the woman is giving birth to her first child), she assumes a parenting role that demands that she construct a new sense of self. Her ability to parent the baby and be responsive to his or her attachment needs is largely determined by her own early attachments to her own parents, which are revisited and reviewed around the time of birth.

A midwife, who accompanies the woman through pregnancy, labor, and the postpartum period, helps her review these early attachments and facilitates the establishment of a bond with her "real" child, who progressively replaces the child held in her fantasy to which she came to be attached during her pregnancy. In addition, the midwife helps her construct a positive view of herself as a mother who is able to respond with sensitivity to the needs of her newborn, while containing both the infant's and her own anxiety during a transitional period that changes her life forever.

Something similar happens at the end of life and through bereavement. Like a midwife, we facilitate the unfolding of a natural yet painful process that is analogous to a second birth. Dying and bereaved people experience transitions from living together to living apart, and from belonging to a physical world to belonging to the memory of others. During these transitions they are highly vulnerable and often experience inner reorganizations that shake their assumptive worlds and force them to redefine themselves, review relationships, and revisit goals, values, and priorities in life, and their belonging to the world. Suffering and change during these transitional periods are inevitable. They invariably evoke existential concerns and occasionally an existential crisis. While some people face this crisis with anxiety, guilt, or remorse, others construct a new sense of self that helps them live more fully and meaningfully.

Similar to a midwife, our professional role is to facilitate these transitions by providing a safe environment and by exercising the art of maieutic, known as the art of midwifery. The maieutic is an aspect of the Socratic method according to which, instead of giving information about a new experience, we pose a series of questions and invite reflection, which allows us to formulate personal beliefs, views, and concepts that lead to the discovery of new knowledge. What knowledge?—Knowledge about ourselves, others, and life, as well as about the limits of knowledge in death situations. Therefore, a key aspect of our role is accompanying people through the discovery of personal knowledge that enables them to lead a life that, to them, is worth living.

What is a life worth living? We mistakenly assume that it is life that involves doing something profound or socially meaningful. While in some situations this is the case, in others it involves participation in *ordinary activities* (e.g., returning home, participating in decision-making, praying, creating a ritual or a work of art, writing, visiting a special place) and/or the maintenance of *ordinary relationships* (e.g., sharing, confiding, or expressing love or regrets). What is, however, different about these ordinary activities and relationships is the fact that they are experienced as extraordinary and relived with a sense of consciousness, acuity, and vitality. This enables the dying and the bereaved to temper the pain of physical deterioration and of separation, and offers new opportunities for an altered experience of one's existence in the world.

Seeking a life worth living is at the core of companioning people through dying and bereavement. It does not entail striving for a perfect death or a quick recovery from bereavement; instead, it involves the facilitation of one's transition through critical experiences that can be both painful and growth enhancing. How do we facilitate these transitions through a companioning role?

- By containing a suffering that is unavoidable, and by promoting conditions that enhance personal growth
- By acknowledging and responding to the person's attachment needs, which are intensified in the face of loss
- By reinforcing explorative behaviors in unfamiliar situations
- By assisting with practical issues, decisions, and challenges in ways that promote control, self-esteem, and dignity, as defined by the person and his or her family
- By freeing an individual from physical pain, so as to generate time for relating meaningfully to him- or herself and to others

- By facilitating a reflective process that provides opportunities for insights and new understandings about oneself, others, and a life that is vested with positive meaning and experienced as being worth living
- By affirming bonds that ensure belonging, thus rendering dying and bereavement a social and humane process.

In summary, we assume different functions in our role as companions. Sometimes we become the *container* of a person's suffering by creating a space in which he or she can feel safe enough to express whatever feels unsafe or threatening. Other times, we function as the *facilitator* of a reflective or explorative process over daily challenges, changes, and adaptations. And, almost invariably, we act as an *enabler* of transformations that enhance self-esteem and connectedness with others. These functions derive from an approach that avoids victimizing dying and bereaved people and empowers them to discover and use resources that are conducive to growth.

In order for us to be effective companions, three things are critically important. First, we must be willing to share the dying and bereavement journey, and the people we serve must want to invite us into their world. Such mutual agreement is necessary for the establishment of a partnership and possible bond. Second, we must possess knowledge and skills that help dying and bereaved people confront, temper, and/or transform suffering and promote meaningful living. Third, we must give up our striving to treat the person or to fix problems and remain open to change and growth that are evoked by existential concerns and mortality in the people we serve as well as in ourselves. Only then, can the process of dying and bereavement be transformed from a frightening, lonely, isolated, or marginalized experience to a shared, social, and humane endeavor. In this section I analyze four conditions that are critical in fostering an accompaniment.

CONDITION 1

Establishing an Appropriate Frame

Let's return to the myth of Theseus, the Minotaur, and Ariadne. The plot unfolds in a well-defined frame represented by a given structure. In this frame, the action takes place and two significant processes become apparent: a collaborative alliance is established between Theseus and Ariadne in order to face and kill the Minotaur, and a process of accompaniment unfolds by means of a thread. The journey is challenging and risky but ends in triumph for Theseus, who kills the Minotaur, and Ariadne, who gains her hero's love and respect and embarks on a journey away from Crete with him.

A similar frame is necessary when we strive to develop a collaborative alliance or partnership with the people we accompany through their trajectories. But what is a frame? A frame is both the real and symbolic space in which relationships are developed and care is offered and received. Frames have a structure, boundaries, and rules that distinguish the inside reality that is shared by care seekers and care providers from the outside reality. Why is a frame necessary? Because it enables the development of a "holding environment" (Winnicott, 1960/1990) or a "secure base" (Bowlby, 1988, 2005) in which the dying and bereaved can begin to share experiences that are too painful, taboo, or embarrassing to reveal in other contexts. In a death situation, which disrupts relationships and creates irreversible loss, a frame can contain chaos and suffering. It does not bring order to chaos but enables people to tolerate it; work through powerful feelings, thoughts, and existential concerns; cope with current or impending losses; and progressively reconstruct narratives that are meaningful to them. Without a frame, individuals are likely to become overwhelmed by the bottomless pit of suffering and experience increased anxiety as a result of the frameless context in which dying and grief occur.

The frame is not only helpful to the people we accompany but also valuable to us, the care providers. It provides us with a sense of safety and a context determined by a clear structure, boundaries, and rules that orient our actions and allow us to become creative, take risks, and explore unknown territories. Without a clear frame, we may experience increased anxiety in the face of death and avoid accompanying people on their journeys.

The significance of the frame has been extensively described by psychotherapists in relation to specific ground rules that determine the context within which therapy occurs. Rules relate to confidentiality, privacy, and consistency manifested in a set location and at a set time for an agreed-on fee. Psychoanalysis imposes additional rules by expecting therapists to be neutral, while existentialists and phenomenologists encourage creativity, authenticity, and personal involvement with people and an approach that incorporates thoughtful self-disclosure (Yalom, 2001, 2008).

In grief counseling and therapy the above rules are common, and readily applied. In contrast, at the end of life, rules of confidentiality, privacy, and consistency are often challenged. The hospital, hospice, or home environment, although sustained by a stable routine, is an unpredictable setting in which anything can happen to overthrow the frame's stability. People are mobile one day, and confined in their beds in a confused or semiconscious condition, with energy that varies, the next. They live in a space that is public, with staff members intruding for various reasons (e.g., to offer treatment, to provide bedside care, to empty the trash, or to announce a scheduled procedure), while discussions about medical, psychological, or spiritual issues take place in the presence of other people, often transgressing rules of privacy and confidentiality. Moreover, the person's fears, concerns, or preferences are often revealed to relatives, whose decisions and needs are given equal, if not greater, importance. Usually it is relatives who determine whether their loved one will be cared for at home, in a hospice, or in a nursing home. It becomes evident that maintaining a frame with clear boundaries and realistic ground rules at the end of life may prove to be a challenging, if not an impossible, task. However, striving to develop one is critically important when we seek to accompany people through their journey. There is no ideal or universal frame in death situations. However, there are certain characteristics that can render a frame effective in facilitating the occurrence of an accompaniment process. Such a frame is co-created rather than imposed; is secure and stable, yet also flexible; has clearly defined boundaries, which are, nevertheless, subject to modifications and negotiations; is continuous when needs and circumstances change in the face of death.

Co-Creating a Frame

It is important not to impose a frame but rather to discover and create it along the way. Saying that we create a frame suggests that this takes time and that we must negotiate with individuals and families the context, boundaries, and rules within which we develop a partnership with them. When we are inexperienced or highly anxious, we hastily impose a theoretical or clinical model of intervention that we use as a symbolic frame to manage anxiety, as well as the disorder and unfamiliarity that loss and separation trigger in us. Moreover, we rigidly determine rules of interaction and prescribe specific conditions under which care is to be offered. We avoid modifications that accommodate the changing needs of dying or bereaved people, and as a result, they often feel misunderstood and alienated in relation to us.

Imposed frames serve mostly our needs, rather than those of others. However, if used only temporarily, they can be useful, particularly in crisis situations, since they help us cope with the chaos and pain that death elicits. Let me share an example. Following a traffic accident that killed seven 15-year-old adolescents during a school excursion, our nonprofit organization for the care of children and families facing illness and death, called Merimna (www.merimna.org.gr), was invited by the Ministry of Education to organize a psychosocial intervention in the nine elementary and secondary schools of a small community in central Greece. Even though these schools had not extended a formal request for support, they welcomed our arrival a day after the accident, before the school reopened. We relied on a community crisis intervention model that was more or less imposed. However, we made sure to adjust it to meet the immediate needs of the educators who were empowered to deal with the crisis, prepare for and facilitate the students' support, and cope with some urgent issues that arose as a result of the media coverage. We used our expertise not to "run the show" but to provide useful information and form a partnership with members of each school community in order to attend to their individualized needs during the crisis. We helped educators through this tragedy to discover new ways of relating to and communicating with their traumatized students and remained available, in the background, to all members of the community during these first few days following the event.

Following the crisis, educators began to investigate the possibility for an ongoing collaboration with our team. This time, a new frame was co-created, and new boundaries were delineated while commonly agreed-on goals and rules were established. Psychosocial support was offered to all members of the community and became integrated into the schools' programs and life. At times, the frame was challenged, reviewed, renegotiated, and modified to accommodate the changing needs of educators, students, and the transfer of psychologists. Eventually, it was enlarged to include the needs of parents and other members of the larger community, who benefited from the services we offered over a 3-year period.

To illustrate the value of co-creating rather than imposing a frame, I wish to describe the initial steps we undertook in our encounters with reluctant students who had never been exposed to mental health professionals before or were biased against and mistrustful of us. Psychologists took plenty of the time to explain their role, to correct prejudices and misperceptions, and to offer students the opportunity to get to know them before establishing a frame within which support could be offered and received. The professionals' regular presence on the school grounds twice a week led groups of students to approach them during the break and informally chat with them. Eventually they began to schedule appointments in twosomes and threesomes, during which they began to talk about their traumatic experiences in the presence of their peers. These mini-group sessions lasted for a month before students began to seek individual counseling. As students moved from the courtyard to a private school office, and from group meetings to individual sessions, they progressively negotiated a new frame that felt safe enough to allow them to begin addressing their trauma and grief. Their needs varied. Those whose lives had been threatened and who had lost their peers in the accident chose to meet as a class. Each class created its own frame in which sharing was allowed and support became available. In one, students processed their suffering through discussions and creative activities that reinforced mutual understanding and support. In the other class, sharing proved to be highly distressing, and students chose to address their experience through symbolic rituals and action-oriented activities. By the end of the year, both classes created a DVD dedicated to their deceased classmates in which they narrated their own version of the tragic event, read poems, shared memories of their friends, and sang songs. The DVD also depicted a community protest that they organized against law transgressions and inadequate political action regarding road and traffic regulations.

During the two following years, the frame was renegotiated to expand services to other members of the local community. Its stability allowed students who were previously reluctant to seek support to attend groups, participate in collective activities (e.g., the construction of a labyrinth), and seek individual counseling. Not only did they benefit, but they also displayed impressive signs of personal growth. Shortly before high school graduation, students who had survived the accident expressed a desire to participate in a documentary that would teach other youngsters and educators about coping with traumatic events and disasters that affect school communities.

Frame Stability and Flexibility

Another characteristic of a frame that facilitates companionship is the stability and security it inspires in dying and bereaved people. A stable frame is clear, reliable, and predictable. It exists despite challenges, threats, or disruptions and facilitates the establishment of relationships in which experiences can be voiced, shared, and contained.

When I started working with seriously ill children, I realized how important time was for them—not only in a literal sense, but also in a symbolic sense. They did not have watches or look at a clock but knew when I was supposed to appear on the ward and at the outpatient clinic. Any circumstantial delay or absence due to other professional responsibilities was met with anger, sadness, or resentment by some children. Their lives were already filled with uncertainty, and time was precious to them. They were reluctant to invest in relationships or activities that did not offer a secure space in which they were not threatened by intrusions, abandonment, or loss. As soon as I began to inform them of any anticipated delays or absences, the depth of our bond increased. With the establishment of a stable frame, time was experienced as continuous rather than discontinuous, and companioning was facilitated.

While frame stability is important, it must be accompanied by flexibility, which facilitates adjustment to the challenges, changing needs, and unexpected developments that are inherent to dying and bereavement. Sometimes the frame is enlarged to encompass new people (e.g., relatives occupying a key position or specialists in palliative care), while other times, it is restricted to a few individuals who can share the suffering. Occasionally, inevitable changes occur—some of which are planned, and others unexpected—that alter the frame and affect the experience of dying or bereavement.

A rigid frame dictates the exact location, duration, and timing of care services. While such a frame is welcomed by bereaved people, who negotiate with a counselor or therapist the duration and frequency of the sessions, it is often unrealistic and sometimes inappropriate in the care of terminally ill patients. Companioning under those circumstances cannot be limited to a particular office or room, and its timing and duration cannot be predetermined.

Markos, a reserved 5-year-old boy, was hospitalized because of a serious relapse of his cancer. His condition was terminal, and his parents decided to keep him in the hospital until the end of his life. I saw him daily, and even though he spoke very seldom, he willingly participated in play activities, through which he symbolically communicated his awareness of and feelings about dying. One day, he expressed the desire to go to the zoo and insisted that I go along. His parents were very reluctant to leave the hospital and tried to convince him that I could not go along, because many other sick children were expecting me. Pondering Marko's insistent request, I hesitated. Should I transgress the boundaries that defined the space of my work and interactions with the family? Should I respond to the personal invitations of terminally ill children? How would the transfer of our relationship from the hospital setting to another context affect my patients and myself? Would the boundaries of a therapeutic frame be lost or changed, and with what consequences?

I decided to accept Marko's invitation, mostly because I wanted to encourage the parents to take the trip to the zoo and have a memory of their son enjoying the small pleasures of life beyond the confines of a hospital room. Markos was delighted to see me without my colorful hospital blouse, and proud that I accompanied him. As we visited the animals, he became unusually verbal and directed all sorts of questions to me. Did I have children of my own? Had I ever gone to the zoo with any sick child? Would I come back to feed that zebra for him, in case he was very ill? Would I continue to love him if someday he left the hospital?

It was precisely this excursion to the zoo that allowed this 5-year-old boy to ask personal questions, to express his love, and to confirm that our relationship was also very special to me. By flexibly enlarging the frame of care our relationship grew deeper in the face of impending separation.

When we accompany people through dying and bereavement, we must acknowledge that the wider context has a significant impact on what transpires in the narrow context of caring relationships. As a result, the frame we develop must be both stable and flexible so that it can encompass both.

Clarity of Boundaries and Frame Modification

An effective frame is characterized by clear and well-defined boundaries that are neither too rigid nor diffused. These boundaries may be subject to change when new needs or priorities come to the forefront as a result of the imminence or reality of death. Boundary crossing and frame modification may be justified under those circumstances.

Consider the example of a patient who asks his favorite nurse to sit by his bedside after the end of her shift and wait until he falls asleep. By transgressing established boundaries, she responds to his explicit and implicit request and accompanies him in his sleep. Aware that this may be one of few nights left—if not the last night—of his life, the nurse acknowledges her desire to reciprocate her affection and spends a few hours at his bedside. The safety of the frame allowed this patient to cross the boundaries and voice an out-of-the ordinary request that, in turn, incited the nurse to respond with an uncommon acceptance that transgressed her own and the team's familiar mode of operation.

Crossing boundaries may be salutary at times, neutral at others, and occasionally harmful. Luca (2004) suggests that "involving patients in frame modifications makes it less of an imposition and demonstrates respect for the patient's own life and other commitments" (p. 18). Rescheduling lab exams in order to allow a seriously ill patient to enjoy a family celebration, holding a counseling session in the hospital or at home when the patient's condition is deteriorating, and accompanying a bereaved adolescent to the grave of his sibling are a few examples of frame modification through boundary crossing. When boundary crossing is negotiated and clearly defined for all parties involved, then it increases the likelihood of an enriched relationship between the person and the care provider.

Strict and rigid adherence to boundaries should always incite us to question whose needs we serve: Our own? Others'? Our team's? The organization's, with its need to control dying and bereavement and protect its employees from suffering? Rigid adherence imposes conformity, limits creativity, and constricts care providers' abilities to maintain relationships that are sensitive to the changing and complex needs of dying and bereaved people. It prevents the development of partnerships and secure bonds.

One of the greatest challenges through the accompanying process is knowing why and when to cross or modify boundaries and how to undertake such a process, in consideration of its impact upon the person-professional relationship. Such knowledge comes with experience, maturity, and the ability to tolerate uncertainty, confusion, and the unknown evoked by death. It is my belief that before we transgress or modify boundaries, we must first learn how to establish and maintain them without putting the accompanying process at risk.

Portability of Frame

Continuity of care is ensured when the frame is carried within by both care seekers and care providers, and adapted to the circumstances of a changing reality that is affected by death and separation. Smith-Pickard (2004) refers to a "portable frame" that we, the professionals, should carry into our encounters with the people we serve when boundaries are broken, transgressed, or expanded. Such a frame helps to maintain an internal concept of what is helpful and what is not and ensures continuity of care in the face of loss or disruption.

A portable frame becomes particularly imperative in end-of-life care when the dying person moves from the hospital to a hospice or his or her home. In an ideal world, continuity of care could be ensured by professionals who provide both cure and end-of-life care to their patients, and ongoing support to the family both prior to and after a person's death. In the real world, however, this is rarely feasible, because care is fragmented among experts with distinct specializations and because of the rigid administrative regulations that characterize most health institutions and services. Nevertheless, continuous care can be facilitated when providers who belong to one organization facilitate the smooth transition of a person or family to another organization or service. This requires open communication among colleagues who work in different work settings and the coordination of their services through open teamwork (see principle 7 in chapter 9). Following up on referrals ensures that needs are appropriately met, while key relationships among patients, families, and care providers, although altered, continue to be maintained. As a result, companioning unfolds through an enlarged or modified frame that does not fragment care or relationships by creating discontinuities but ensures continuity in the face of death.

Stephen, a 42-year-old widower dying of cancer, was grateful to members of the palliative care team for providing him with "outstanding" care at the end of his life. His major concern was that his children and parents refused to accept his dying and continued to believe that he was facing one more of the "big nasty crises" that he had successfully overcome in the past. Stephen felt guilty for "dying on them." During a staff meeting, care providers discussed his concern and invited Stephen to assist them in supporting his family beyond the confines of the hospice. The psychologist offered to visit the children's elementary school and assist teachers in supporting them through this difficult period of their lives. The team's pastor volunteered to visit Stephen's church and, in collaboration with the local priest, invite members to stand by his parents, who were reluctant to accept his impending condition. The unit's physician and head nurse offered to plan a Circle of Family and Friends' meeting that would include people who were important to Stephen and his family in order to provide accurate information about his terminal condition and build a supportive network that would be available to his loved ones before and after his death. This meeting was attended by Stephen, a few relatives, some friends and colleagues, a neighbor, and the children's baby-sitter. Questions were raised and answered, feelings expressed, resources identified, and suggestions about how to assist Stephen's children and parents in both their practical and emotional short-term and long-term needs considered. The frame was enlarged to include members of the wider community, who assumed an active role throughout the terminal period and subsequent bereavement. Bonds were affirmed, and Stephen died relieved and surrounded by his family, who was supported by a caring community.

No single frame is perfect. In our work with the dying and the bereaved we establish alternative frames that may prove to be more or less effective in facilitating the unfolding of an accompanying process. Frames that are secure, flexible, continuous, and adaptable to changing needs and circumstances are more likely to benefit dying and bereaved people and to function as a source for rewarding experiences for care providers.

CONDITION 2

Being Fully Present

Establishing a frame that is secure, flexible, and adaptable to changing circumstances is important, yet it is not enough. Another critical condition of companioning relates to our ability to be fully present in our relationships with dying and bereaved people. Ariadne was fully present for Theseus in the Greek myth and kept an ongoing connection to him by means of the thread she gave him. Her presence was interiorized by the hero, who used the *miton* to create a path that led to the confrontation with his terror and his safe return to the outer reality.

Being present for another person calls for involvement with all aspects of ourselves (physical, cognitive, emotional, and spiritual), thus preventing any fragmentation and the leaving out of various aspects of our experience (e.g., emotions over rational logic). It also requires an availability, openness, and commitment that are explicitly or implicitly communicated through a promise that "No matter how much suffering you may experience in your encounter with loss and death, I will not abandon you." The power of presence is critical and central to the formation of a meaningful connection with others. While physical and psychological presence are inseparable, they are discussed separately here so that readers may better understand them.

Physical Presence

When we are physically present, we exchange verbal and nonverbal messages with others that affect our transactions and relationships with them. Sometimes it is our physical absence that is loaded with powerful messages. Early studies in the field showed that care providers avoided entering the rooms of people who were dying or responded with considerable delay to their calls. Their physical absence, which was interpreted as rejection and abandonment by patients and families, served as a shield against discomfort, powerlessness, and helplessness and communicated the message "I do not want to be hurt."

Even though, nowadays, the significance of being physically present at the bedside of a dying patient or grieving relative is overstressed in the literature, such presence is rarely practiced, not because care providers do not wish to be present, but mostly because they feel uncomfortable. They fear that by being physically present, they risk being affected by the suffering of others and exposing their vulnerabilities. It is not uncommon for students and young practitioners to raise questions about how to manage physical responses that are indicative of their emotional state: What if my eyes fill up with tears and the other person sees me crying? How can I hide my physical discomfort when people begin to grieve? Should I go away? Unfortunately, young practitioners are trained to enter relationships without a body. They are taught to focus on knowledge and skills and ignore the richness of communication that is received and conveyed through their physical responses, facial expressions, gestures, touch, and somatic reactions. They dissociate from their bodies and become unaware of how their bodies react to other people's experiences. Thus, they develop disembodied encounters in which they perform professional tasks while remaining physically absent from the relationship.

In embodied encounters, in contrast, the physical body is not separate from the caregiving relationship. We identify and understand our physical responses and avoid projecting our feelings and thoughts on others. We use these responses (e.g., blushing, tears, palpitations, sweating, muscular tension, physical revulsion) to understand the other person, ourselves, and our encounter in a given situation. According to Shaw (2003), bodily experiences reflect an empathic process. He describes "body empathy" as a form of heightened body awareness through which we become attuned to and pick up information that helps us understand the other person's experience, as well as our own.

Imagine, for example, that you listen to a seriously ill patient complain about physical pain as he registers in a home care program that offers palliative care services. When you ask him about his choice, he reassures you that 'this is the best solution for everyone'. Aware of your physical tension resulting from the patient's unusually rigid demeanor, you ask more questions that allow him to express his resentment over being "pushed" into deciding to return home, as well as his anger at being "deserted" by care providers and family members who "gave up" on him. This brief example illustrates how the body can function as both a receiver and a provider of nonverbal information that can deepen and enrich encounters. When we are receivers of nonverbal information, bodily responses confirm or disconfirm our assessment of a person's experiences. For example, our physical discomfort when we listen to a story of how bravely a bereaved spouse coped with his loss helps us identify the person's latent and hidden anxiety. When we are providers of nonverbal information, the body transmits messages of our intentions and feelings. When we mirror, for example, an individual's gestures or when we smile, grimace, turn our back, or gently touch the other person, we convey a wealth of information that affects our relationship. Occasionally, our nonverbal responses provide us with information that enables us to learn something new about ourselves, as in Laura's case.

Laura was a young social worker who experienced butterflies in her stomach to the point of becoming nauseous every time she visited a terminally ill 2-year-old whose pain and discomfort were managed with great difficulty. She was startled by the intensity of her physical responses, which she did not experience with other young patients, and felt guilty that she avoided being around this little boy and his distraught parents. In supervision, she described her responses as feeling "sick to death" and "helplessly petrified." When her supervisor asked Laura to mentally rehearse the circumstances that evoked such strong physical reactions, she referred to her experience that morning. She was standing in front of the child's room when she began to experience butterflies in her stomach and started to perspire; when she entered the room, she kept the door open so that she could escape from a situation that a few minutes later became too overwhelming for her because of nausea.

Where did these sensations originate for Laura? From empathizing with her patient's discomfort, the parents' grief, or her own personal story? She did not experience similar reactions when she attended to the care of other young patients. Stuck in an impasse, Laura fled her supervisor's office. When she returned from the restroom, his door was half open. She stood hesitantly at the doorway, when suddenly she experienced butterflies in her stomach, which she later associated with an early life recollection. In that recollection, at age seven, she stood behind a half-open door, looking at her mother, who was silently crying as she tended to her baby brother, who was very sick. Overwhelmed by her own grief over her brother's serious illness, she hid her feelings to protect her distraught mother. Petrified and powerless to undo the suffering of her mother and the distress of her sick brother, she stood at a safe distance. Later in life, she chose a career in nursing in the hope that she would overcome her powerlessness and the threat of death. Her high motivation and striving made her a dynamic, energetic, and dedicated nurse who is much loved by children and parents. However, it was only when she was confronted with this little boy and explored her physical responses that she realized the depth of her neglected suffering, which acquired personal meaning in supervision.

Situations such as Laura's are unique experiences that happen only once in awhile; however, there are several daily situations in which awareness of nonverbal communication can increase our awareness of what we bring to our relationships with the dying and the bereaved. How do we use the space around a patient's bed or room? How do we maintain or avoid eye contact? When and how do we use physical touch? How do we respond nonverbally to a long silence, or to a person's anger, crying, or despair? When do we get sick, or what do migraines tell us about the source of our distress? What purpose does their repeated occurrence serve in our work with dying and bereaved people?

Physical responses are reflective of a personal body narrative and, along with the patient's body narrative, contribute to the creation of a story that is neither ours nor the patient's. This story stems from our relationship and is affected by whatever transpires in the intersubjective field that we share (see chapter 1).

How do we incorporate a body narrative in our encounters with those we accompany? One way is through the disclosure of personal information about aspects of our physical responses that we tend to interpret in emotional terms. We do not pretend that our bodies are neutral or inexistent but acknowledge our experiences. If deemed appropriate, we openly reveal to the other person that our blushing, for example, reflects our excitement over his incredible growth through trauma, or that our teary eyes reflect our love or sadness over her dying. Embodied reactions that are openly discussed may foster intimacy; alleviate the loneliness that loss, separation, and death create; and contribute to enriched narratives. However, self-disclosure must be used with caution and sensitivity, and always with the intent to benefit the other person. Yalom (2008) stresses that we should disclose information about ourselves only when such revelations will be of value to the other person, and when the purpose is to facilitate the therapeutic work. When personal disclosure takes place too early in the accompanying process, it runs the risk of frightening the dying or bereaved person, who needs time to ascertain that the relationship is safe. The proper timing and degree of self-disclosure come with experience and require a maturity that allows the care provider to avoid imposing personal needs or allowing personal disclosures to become the central focus in the caring relationship.

Another common way in which we incorporate a body narrative is through physical touch. In the traditional practice of medicine and nursing, touching in ways that do not involve the provision of clinical care is largely avoided and treated as taboo. Looking at and touching a naked body are acts of intimacy that clinicians strive to counteract by adopting a formal, distant, or impersonal approach in our encounters with patients. In palliative care, in contrast, the use of touch (e.g., holding hands, caressing the person, giving a hug) is perceived as an acceptable form of communication that is encouraged. In bereavement care, the use of touch varies, according to the professional's therapeutic approach. For example, the psychodynamic approach expects the care provider to remain neutral (a tabula rasa) and forbids physical touch or any form of personal disclosure. In contrast, the humanistic and existential approach draws attention to the professional's physical presence by encouraging touch and disclosure when appropriate, genuine, and authentic.

How touch is used depends on personal, interpersonal, situational, professional, and particularly cultural factors. Excluding it altogether from our encounters as a dangerous thing fraught with hazards prevents us from being fully present in our accompaniment. Touch can be empowering when it conveys a message such as "I'm standing by you," but it can also be disempowering when it communicates messages like "I feel sorry for you" or "You need me." Occasionally it becomes traumatizing, as when it is experienced as an intrusion or forced upon the other person in an attempt to project an inauthentic image of niceness. Equally harmful can be the total lack of touch, since it is often experienced by the dying and the bereaved as a sign of repulsion, abandonment, or rejection. In sum, physical touch should be practiced with caution to avoid any adverse effects and to maximize the positives that come with the humanization of care.

Psychological Presence

Being psychologically present requires commitment to the dying and bereaved, who often feel very vulnerable or torn apart. It suggests an ability to be attentive to their needs and concerns and to bear witness to their suffering without rushing to alleviate or fix their psychological or spiritual pain because it hurts or renders us anxious and uncomfortable. While it is imperative to immediately address and strive to control a person's physical pain, such an approach may be harmful in the case of psychosocial or spiritual pain. Why? Because it deprives people of the opportunity to grieve their impending death or the death of their loved ones and, therefore, prepare for and adjust to an altered reality, which is accepted and integrated into their life stories. One of the biggest challenges of being psychologically present is containing the unavoidable and normal suffering that people experience in death situations. What does it mean to contain suffering? It means creating a holding space or environment in which the person feels *safely overwhelmed* by events and situations, and where the person is unconditionally accepted and understood by a caring companion who is not threatened by his or her suffering. Containment enables people to express powerful, ambivalent emotions and disorganized or irrational thoughts without the fear that they will be criticized or rejected. Under such conditions, the person is more likely to explore his or her distressing experience and progressively integrate it into his or her life story, which is then reconstructed to accommodate it. Through containment, suffering can be endured, tempered, or transformed.

How is suffering transformed in the care provider–versus–care seeker relationship? In several ways, two of which are described here: (1) the sharing of personal stories in which distressing experiences are integrated into a meaningful and coherent narrative and (2) the sharing of present moments that enrich the caring relationship and are conducive to change.

Transforming suffering through the sharing of personal stories. The therapeutic value of translating a personally traumatic or upsetting experience into language has been overstressed by several psychologists.

Through a series of studies, Pennebaker (1995) discovered that when people put their emotional upheavals into words, their physical and mental health improves remarkably. The effects upon their well-being are positive regardless of whether they verbally share or write about their traumatic experiences. Through words, they organize what is lived; they reflect on and work through their feelings, thoughts, beliefs, and perceptions; and they integrate their experiences into a story. A story that is logically arranged into a comprehensive whole enables them to organize both the emotional effects of their experience and the experience itself. Thus it contributes to self-understanding. Once a complex experience is put into a story format, it is simplified. The mind doesn't need to work as hard to bring structure and meaning to it. Any gaps are filled in over time to make the story more coherent and complete. Told over and over again, the story becomes shorter and more compact. It is changed and, ultimately, integrated into one's life story, which is reconstructed so as to accommodate it. Pennebaker (2000) asserts that, ironically, good narratives can be beneficial in making a complex or traumatic illness or loss experience simpler and more understandable; however, one's perception and recollection of the experience can become distorted. Through organized and coherent narratives people put traumatic or distressing experiences behind them and move forward.

Narrative failure can be regarded as a symptom that reflects a fragmentary experience that thwarts narrative integration. It can also reflect the lack of a safe space or the absence of a care provider who is willing to listen to, accept, and contain the person's experience.

While narratives are important in our work with the dying and the bereaved, we should avoid focusing exclusively on language and be attentive to the benefits of alternative forms of self-expression, such as dance, art, music, or bodily movement. Some bereaved people, for example, are best able to express their thoughts and feelings through the melody of a song, poetry, painting, or the creation of a piece of art that helps them give shape to a distressing and traumatic experience. The paintings of Frida Kahlo, who lived with a serious disability, are a powerful example of how she put into art rather than words both her suffering and her hope. The multiple self-portraits she created at different periods in her life reflect her ongoing quest to redefine her self, which was often threatened by loss and infirmity.

Artists like Frida Kahlo, Edvard Munch, Salvador Dali, and Käthe Kollwitz and writers such as C. S. Lewis, Jean-Dominique Bauby, Simone de Beauvoir, and Primo Levi attempted to communicate through words, images, symbols, and colors their personal experiences, for example, as a patient with a life-threatening illness (Bauby, 1997), as a prisoner in a concentration camp (Levi, 1969), as the companion of a dying relative (de Beauvoir, 1964), and as a devastated widower (Lewis, 1961). Most of them were guided by a need to tell their story as it was, in its rawness, without trying to embellish any of its painful aspects or minimizing the love that transcends relationships in the face of loss. At the core of such narratives is a need to transmit to an abstract or imaginary audience a very powerful experience of which one is, simultaneously, the protagonist and a witness. The works of these individuals illuminate the human experiences that unfold at the limits of life and introduce us into an extraordinary space between life and death that invites self-exploration (Oppenheim, 2007).

By being psychologically present, we establish a safe space where dying and bereaved people can confide and create stories. Their narratives do not emerge ex nihilo. They stem from and are about experiences that are shared only with a person who is fully present and genuinely cares. Therefore, a key aspect of our psychological presence is that we listen to these stories while concurrently attending to the narrator without judging or telling him or her what to do and how to feel. Listening is not a passive activity but a dynamic process that invites reflection over life-and-death experiences and encourages the articulation of fears, concerns, and aspirations; the creation of representations of what is unknown, confusing, or desired; and the attribution of personal meaning to existential questions such as: "Who am I?" "What is important in life?" "What have I accomplished?" "Who did I want to be and will never become?" "What meaning does my life have for me and for others?" "How do I want to be remembered?" "How do I want to remember my loved one?"

Our task is not to offer answers to these questions, but to find a way to help people discover their own answers by facilitating a reflective process. We invite them to take a closer look at their lived experiences, and we join them in viewing and understanding themselves and their situations in a new light. We focus less on the account of events and center mostly upon the feelings and thoughts that arise from, and the meanings that are attributed to such events both in the here and now and in association with the person's life trajectory. The outcomes of a reflective process become evident in changes in how one perceives oneself, relates to others, and copes with challenges. Not infrequently, the individual's assumptive world is reconstructed, and his or her life story is re-storied and enriched by new values, priorities, and meanings.

It would be wrong to assume that every dying or bereaved person engages into a reflective process. Many people lack the stamina either because they are absorbed by their pain, which saps away all their energy, or because the journey is too risky or painful. Some have already undertaken a review of their values, priorities, and choices in life and do not need the presence of a professional to facilitate such a process. Still others are so deeply trapped in their suffering that they seek only to emotionally survive; several months or years after the illness or loss ordeal, they may feel safe enough to revisit their experiences and construct a meaningful or coherent story.

Our ability to be psychologically present should not be limited to those situations in which dying and bereaved people produce stories that are meaningful and comprehensive. Our presence is most needed in relationships that are characterized by the absence of narratives or by the chaos of inarticulate cries, raw grief, shrieks, or disjointed accounts. Bearing witness to the underlying anxiety, terror, and despair and accepting being temporarily lost in a no-man's-land may prove challenging and frightening for us, but most therapeutic for the other, who ceases to be alone in the darkness and wilderness of his or her experience. Eventually this enables people to abandon their isolation in order to connect to us and to other people. In this way, stillness and chaos are replaced by movement. Movement involves hope for a change, and change encompasses the creation of an altered reality that is bearable, because it is shared.

Transforming suffering through the sharing of present moments. While accompanying people through dying and bereavement, most of us occasionally experience something very profound that we dismiss because we do not know how to explain it. Such out-of-the-ordinary experiences usually occur unexpectedly, when the other person is in deep suffering or confronted with a novel, unfamiliar, or crisis situation. It lasts for few seconds (even though it is subjectively perceived as having a longer duration) and is emotionally so rich that it leaves a lasting imprint on both us and the other person. Stern (2004) names this phenomenon a "present moment" (pp. 31–40, 245). During a present moment (see Box 4.1), we become acutely conscious of our own and the other person's cognitions, behaviors, sensations, and perceptions as they are being experienced in the here and now. There is a reciprocal understanding of

Box 4.1

A PRESENT MOMENT

- It occurs unexpectedly and unfolds in unpredictable ways.
- It is of short duration, lasting only a few seconds (even though it is subjectively experienced as lasting a long time).
- It is experienced as a holistic, subjective experience, a gestalt.
- It is not a verbal account, but an experience that is lived in the here and now and felt by both the person and the care provider, who are mutually aware of their personal feelings, thoughts, desires, and subjective experiences, as well as those of the other person.
- It has a strong emotional impact upon the person, the care provider, and their relationship, which may be altered or transformed as a result.
- It contains all the basic elements of a lived story that is extremely rich and dense in subjective experiences and meanings. This story remains in verbalized but is lived in the present with intensity.

each person's subjective world, which contains elements of a lived story that is not verbalized yet is extremely dense with subjective experiences and meanings.

Months or years later, we may forget the name of that person and the details of his or her life story yet recall a look, a gesture, a shared silence, a particular intonation, or a caring act that created a deep connection that altered the experience of suffering and changed the quality of our relationship. Interestingly, these changes result not from a long reflective or meaning-reconstruction process, but from a brief, nonlinear experience that is short lived and opens up opportunities for insights, explorations, and transformations.

Helen was a very reserved 7-year-old girl living in a small village in central Greece. When she was diagnosed with acute myeloblastic leukemia, she was told that she had a serious disease that required long-term treatment and occasional hospitalizations. She was not very talkative but loved to paint, which she did with extraordinary skill. A few days after her diagnosis, I asked her to paint a story with a beginning, a middle, and an end. Her story, which consisted of six scenes, begins with a seed that grows and becomes a tree that blooms prematurely in spring; gives fruit in the summer; and, when a cloud hides the sun, fades away and dies (see Papadatou, 1991 for drawing). When she completed the drawing, I asked her to give it a title. She paused for a long time and I patiently waited until she finally said: "The Life of the Almond Tree." I then invited her to tell me the story of this almond tree, but she smiled shyly and was silent. So I encouraged her to describe a dialogue between the sun and the tree. She chose to focus on the end of her story, and told me: "Here the sun says good-bye to the almond tree, because a cloud will appear and will hide the sun, and the tree will die." Was she communicating an intuitive awareness of her premature "bloom" and shortened life trajectory, or was she projecting her fears and apprehensions about dying? The answer came a year later. One day, during one of her regular visits at the outpatient clinic, I saw her painting a picture of a little girl with a cloud—similar to the one that hid the sun in the story of the almond tree—hanging over her head. As I tried to initiate a discussion with her about her drawing, the physicians interrupted us to inform her that she had experienced a relapse that would require immediate hospitalization. Within a few days, her condition had deteriorated dramatically. Helen was dying in spite of the team's efforts to control her disease and achieve remission. I visited her daily and she always asked me to come back with paint and paper, which kept us engaged in prolonged silent yet shared activities. Through the co-creation of drawings, we found a way to maintain a rich communication.

One morning, I found Helen in great pain. Her stomach was hurting due to internal bleeding. Intuitively, I felt a need to do something physical, and I asked for her permission to lay my hands on her stomach, which she permitted. I had never done that before with any child, and even though I had read some articles about the value of touch, I did not practice any specific technique or intervention. With my hands on her stomach, we both looked straight into each other's eyes. This gaze lasted several minutes; at least it seemed so. Nothing was said, yet the exchange was extremely intense. Her parents and sister, who were present in the room, kept silent as they observed our encounter, and a physician who entered the room to examine Helen paused and quietly left without interrupting our nonverbal exchange.

Something happened during this brief exchange that was respected by all who were present. We were experiencing a present moment that encompassed a clear awareness of our personal experiences and those of the other, along with a reciprocal understanding. In a nonverbal way I was communicating to her: "I know that you know you are dying, and that you realize I am aware of it." Simultaneously, she was communicating to me: "I know that you know that I am aware of my dying, and that you are accepting it."

There was sadness in her eyes; there was also fear about the physical pain, the unfamiliarity of the situation, the unknown that lay ahead, and the separation. But there was also love. I reciprocated love, affection, and my sadness for her dying. I still remember encouraging her, with no words, to trust a process that entailed I knew not what, and reassuring her that I would stand by her side. During those seconds, we were co-creating a lived story about loving and about parting. In spite of the sadness, we both experienced an affective vitality that was profound. An entire world of experiences, meanings, and changes was contained in that present moment, and encompassed in what Stern (2004) describes as "a grain of sand" (p. xiv). This moment came to an end when Helen broke the silence to declare that she was not hurting anymore in her tummy. We both smiled and embraced. That night she died in peace.

It was only later that I reflected upon what had happened, wrote about it in my diary, discussed it with colleagues, and gradually realized its impact. This brief encounter changed my view of seriously ill children, whom I now perceived as possessing an inner wisdom that could be discovered if we looked far beyond verbal interactions; it changed my view of myself, as I began, as a novice psychologist, to have more trust in my intuition and develop an openness to the unknown, the unfamiliar, and the inexplicable; and, finally, it changed my view of the companionship process, which I came to understand as a reciprocal experience that holds the potential for changes in both care seekers and care providers during a moment of meeting. A "moment of meeting," according to Stern (2004),

> is an authentic and well-fitted response to the crisis created by the now moment. It is a moment that implicitly reorganizes the intersubjective field so that it becomes more coherent, and the two people sense an opening to the relationship, which permits them to explore new areas together implicitly or explicitly. The moment of meeting need not be verbalized to effectuate change. A now moment followed by a moment of meeting is a nodal event that can dramatically change a relationship or the course of therapy. (p. 220)

The example of Helen illustrates that when we are fully present in our encounter, we can provoke changes that may not result solely from reflection and verbal sharing or from the reconstruction of coherent and comprehensive narratives but rather from the sharing of lived moments in the here and now in which a story is lived without ever being verbalized. The impact of a lived story that is never narrated can be profound in various ways:

- It creates intimacy and becomes engraved in memory.
- It triggers movement by opening up the relationship to new opportunities, new explorations, and new transformations.
- It transforms suffering in ways that enhance growth.
- It affects third parties who witness the unfolding of a present moment.
- It enlarges the intersubjective space in which care is offered, received, and valued by all participants.

One of the many rewards of caregiving in this field is the poignancy and frequency of present moments that are shared in the face of death. It is often difficult to describe them because they do not correspond to measurable outcomes, yet they have a vitalizing impact that makes the reality of loss and death livable, meaningful, and sometimes extraordinary.

While theories of narrative reconstruction provide enlightenment as to how experiences are rendered explicit, coherent, and meaningful, I believe that we must develop new constructs that acknowledge the experiential aspect of being with the other in order to better understand its power to bring about change. When being with the other creates a sense of being together, then both care seeker and care provider experience being in the world (belonging) in a new and more enhancing way. Being fully present, in my view, means relating first as human being to human being, and subsequently as professional to patient. This form of connection enables the dying and bereaved to abandon his or her role as a patient or client and appear as a person who suffers, hopes, and is capable of growth in the face of death and adversity.

Presence versus absence. Can we be fully present in all our encounters? There is no doubt that from time to time we all experience cycles of psychological presence and psychological absence in our relations with others (Kahn, 1992). We choose when to be fully present and when to maintain some distance. Sometimes our choice is affected by situational or circumstantial factors. For example, being pregnant, experiencing an illness in the family, attending to a personal crisis, or becoming vicariously traumatized by the experience of a dying or bereaved person may render us temporarily psychologically absent. This is natural and healthy. Problems occur when we choose to be persistently absent and disengaged from the people we serve as a result of personal attachment difficulties and fears of being engulfed, abandoned, or rejected by them. These problems are further aggravated if the work setting overemphasizes task achievement, prohibits involvement with patients, and criticizes or isolates those of us who develop intimate bonds. Under those circumstances we display what is often described as psychological absenteeism and perform our role and tasks in an uninvolved, detached, and mechanical manner without ever being able to accompany people on their trajectory.

Some professionals, particularly physicians, argue that they have no time to invest in relationships and be fully present for the individuals they serve. This is true when they assume a heavy, almost superhuman workload that precludes any opportunity for accompaniment. However, sometimes the lack of time and busy schedule are used as a reason to avoid involvement or a sustained presence alongside people who struggle with death issues. Underlying our psychological or physical absence lies a fear of death, loss, and separation; a terror of failing to cope with the emotional impact of intimate encounters; or a desire to turn away from an examination of existential issues and concerns.

Our choice to accompany people through dying and bereavement is not determined by our workload, but rather by our choice, commitment, and competence to assume such a task. As suggested above, deep connections can unfold within seconds (e.g., a present moment). When these are associated with a sincere desire and commitment to be there *for* and *with* the other, then the dying or bereaved may carry within him- or herself our presence, which is perceived as comforting, encouraging, and validating, *even in our absence.* This becomes evident in comments such as "I could clearly see how you would respond and imagined what you would have told me if you had been here," or "If only you'd seen how I handled the situation, I'm sure you'd be proud of me!" or "I knew that you were thinking of me." Such comments indicate that sometimes the accompanying process can transcend the boundaries of space, time, and physical presence.

CONDITION 3

Being Vulnerable Enough

Being fully present also requires an ability to be vulnerable enough. The question is whether vulnerability is something to strive for. According to the *Oxford Advanced Learner's Dictionary,* a person who is vulnerable is someone who is "weak and easily hurt physically or emotionally" (2005, p.). Such a definition implies that vulnerability is a sign of weakness or a condition that we should avoid at any cost because it makes us uncomfortable and reveals our shortcomings. Most of us have been taught since childhood to strive to be invulnerable, strong, hardy, self-reliant, in control, on top of a situation, and able to resist suffering and to avoid being affected by death, separation, and other distressing experiences. Is such a goal realistic? Or do we need to redefine vulnerability in terms that can help us better understand its beneficial effects as well as its destructive effects?

Vulnerability is not a trait that we possess or lack. It is a lived experience that unfolds in novel, stressful, or threatening situations and exists on a continuum. We experience ourselves as more or less vulnerable when we accompany people through loss, separation, and bereavement (Figure 4.1). The factors that determine our vulnerability at a given time and its effects upon caregiving are many: personal, interpersonal, work related, and social. In what follows, I describe how vulnerability can affect our relationships with dying and bereaved people as well as with ourselves.

The Overwhelmed Care Provider	**The Unaffected Care Provider**
◄——————————————	——————————————►
Highly vulnerable	**Invulnerable**
Relation to others	**Relation to others**
High permeability	Low or no permeability
Lack of or diffused boundaries	Rigid boundaries
Symbiotic relationships	Distant relationships
Total identification	No engagement
Compulsive care giving	Display of chronic niceness
Relation to self	**Relation to self**
Overwhelmed by experience	Avoidance or suppression of feelings
Lack of elaboration of work-related experiences and personal loss issues	Lack of elaboration of work-related experiences and personal loss issues

Figure 4.1 Highly vulnerable and invulnerable care providers

The Experience of Being Highly Vulnerable

When we experience increased vulnerability, we maintain no boundaries in our relations with others. As a result, we tend to identify with the people we serve and become unable to differentiate which aspects of our experience belong to us and to the other. The other's experience becomes our personal affair. We own it. We are submerged in and preoccupied by it. We think constantly about the person and organize our professional and personal lives (even our days off and holidays) around his or her experience.

Carolyn, a physician, perceived herself as highly vulnerable. This became obvious in her description of her professional trajectory through pediatric oncology. "I've given my soul to this job. It became an integral part of me.... I offered myself unconditionally to children," she confessed. She offered examples of how she maintained no boundaries and assumed inappropriate roles by becoming a surrogate mother to dying children, or the best friend or surrogate partner of distressed parents. With no supervision or opportunities to step back, reflect, and process her experiences, Carolyn immersed herself in the lives and problems of patients and families. She spent more hours at work than at home, which her spouse and children resented. They, in turn, became jealous of her love for patients, to whom she referred as her "little angels." The needs of her little angels always came first, and no family member could compete with them for her attention. In the early years of her career, Carolyn derived great satisfaction from such intimate encounters; however, with time, she began to experience her job as suffocating, depleting her physical and emotional resources, and leaving her empty and depressed, as she confided to me:

> I think that I have aged quickly, both biologically and psychologically, as a result of this work.... Now, I experience a pressure upon my heart, a constant weight that does not allow me to breathe.... Now, I don't want to be close to any dying child or family. I cannot handle their suffering or my pain anymore. I cannot even sit by their side. Silence is very heavy.... I have nothing left to offer.... Words don't come out.... I cannot even give the special and tender look I once gave to my patients. If ever I give it, it's filled with despair.

Feeling guilty and ashamed for her feelings and behavior, Carolyn described how she progressively alienated herself from patients, families, and colleagues and moved to the other extreme of the vulnerability continuum. She became unavailable and impermeable at an emotional level yet remained highly skilled in her medical interventions, which she performed almost mechanically.

I saw her again few years later, and she told me that our interview had been an awakening experience that motivated her to seek psychotherapy. "Now I have a life that I own," she said with a smile, "and, as a result, I am doing a better job with my patients."

When we are highly vulnerable, we develop relationships in which the *I* (the care provider) and the *other* (the dying or bereaved person) become totally undifferentiated. We form an enmeshed relationship that is characterized by fusion and a lack of boundaries. The self and the other are not distinct. There is neither differentiation nor individuation. Both people exist in a form of symbiosis. This enmeshment serves various purposes. Most often it mitigates terror over separation and death and protects both the other and the self from reflecting upon experiences that are perceived as too threatening.

It is important to distinguish between the experience of increased vulnerability that is situational and vulnerability that is permanent, and part of a pattern by which we relate to others and they relate to us.

Usually situational vulnerability is triggered by a sudden or traumatic event or a series of events that overwhelm our resources and evoke a sense of powerlessness, helplessness, and hopelessness. For example, exposure to several deaths within a short period of time can be emotionally very taxing. An encounter with a particular person, event, or situation can render us highly vulnerable, as it may revive a past or current personal issue that has been repressed and is diligently avoided. The grief of a bereaved man who reminds us of our father, for example, may evoke the same sense of helplessness and hopelessness that we experienced in early childhood when we tried desperately and in vain to make our dad happy after the death of his beloved sister. When we acknowledge our responses and address these tender spots through reflection, supervision, or consultation, we are likely to experience a temporarily overwhelming sense of vulnerability, which offers an opportunity to discover new aspects of ourselves and alternative ways of relating to others.

Problems occur when increased vulnerability permeates all our relationships with dying and bereaved people and is permanent. This situation is indicative of a possible terror of death, or personal difficulties with loss or attachment. We become unable to accompany people and tend to depersonalize care or become engaged in compulsive caregiving.

In the latter situation, we use the professional relationship to attend to personal needs that have long remained unaddressed and seek to solve personal issues through dependant/ambivalent attachments to dying and bereaved people.

The Experience of Being Invulnerable

Being invulnerable is an illusion. All of us are more or less vulnerable in the face of loss and suffering. However, we often sustain the illusion of invulnerability, build rigid boundaries around us, and become impermeable to the experiences of others. How? By being distant and very formal in our interactions with them; by concentrating on bodies, diseases, and psychological disorders; by focusing on tasks and goals because they offer a sense of direction, control, and achievement through observable outcomes; or by projecting a false image of care and concern that is inauthentic. In summary, we strive to prove to ourselves and to others that we are the best or the most caring professional who fixes, solves, and manages *everything* without being threatened by *anything*. Through predetermined interventions we strive to ensure a good—if not perfect—death for the dying, and a full recovery for the bereft.

The World Health Organization (2002) reinforces our striving for control and perfection by asserting in its definition of palliative care the need to prevent and relieve suffering "by means of early identification and *impeccable assessment and treatment* of pain and other *problems*, physical, psychosocial and spiritual" (p. 84, emphasis added). This definition raises a number of questions: How impeccable can we be at assessing "problems" rather than the normal responses and concerns of people who are dying or grieving? Do the terminally ill and the bereaved experience "problems" when confronted with loss and mortality? Are their natural yet painful psychosocial and spiritual responses treatable? Do we seek to medicalize or pathologize their needs and concerns in order to control their condition and make it manageable?

Speck (2006a) suggests that the field of palliative and bereavement care attracts professionals with high ideals who risk falling prey to the desire to be perfect. They seek perfection and control through over-specialization and over-professionalization and hide behind a facade of invulnerability and impersonal expertise. Some impose well-defined models of intervention or adopt a step-by-step-by-the-book approach and therefore neglect people's individual needs, desires, and preferences. They prescribe a package of clinical, psychosocial, spiritual, or bereavement services and make people fit their theories or models of care. Probably one of the reasons that Kübler-Ross' model has been so popular for so long is its descriptive nature, which has been distorted and is often viewed as prescriptive by highly anxious and vulnerable professionals, who make responses fit into concrete stages and do not risk exploring the patients' and their own personal responses in the face of death. There is no doubt that theories and models of care can help us understand, structure, and organize our interventions. However, when they are used to *control* our anxiety and to hide the increased vulnerability that is evoked by death, then the quality of services we provide is seriously compromised.

A more subtle pattern by which we seek to appear invulnerable is the display of "chronic niceness" (Speck, 2000, p. 97). We put on a mask and project an image of always being empathic, always understanding, unconditionally loving toward *all* our patients and their families, whom we perceive and approach in exactly the same way. Through a stereotypical set of behaviors, we strive to convey that we are concerned and interested in them. Such behaviors are reinforced by a collective fantasy that we are nice professionals who care for really nice people in the nice environment that we provide for them. In return for being so nice, we expect them to reward us with a nice dignified death or a nice uncomplicated bereavement for which we take credit!

Chronic niceness is superficial, often manipulative, and far from genuine. It precludes companionship, since it denies that relationships with dying or bereaved people "can often arouse very primitive and powerful feelings which are disturbingly *not nice*" (Speck, 2000, p. 97). We may experience, for example, anger, anxiety, dislike, resentment, hatred, and disgust that we do not dare admit feeling to ourselves. Underlying our chronic niceness lies a chronic detachment from people, who are perceived as threatening due to their dying or mourning condition, and from ourselves.

Through chronic niceness and impersonal expertise we develop relationships between the *I*, who is perceived as *it* (the expert or nice professional), and the other, who is also viewed as *it* (a body, a disease, a case, a psychological diagnosis), upon whom a task is performed or a model of care is imposed. The person as a holistic entity is absent from the relationship and replaced by a task, a goal of intervention, or a theory.

The Experience of Being Vulnerable Enough

Somewhere between the experiences of being highly vulnerable and being completely invulnerable, we experience a vulnerability that is good enough and has beneficial effects on us and on others (Figure 4.2). It is not necessarily the degree but the nature of such vulnerability that determines its positive impact upon relationships. When we are vulnerable enough, we are open and permeable to experiences and to people, and flexible in our response to their individual needs. We do not force or impose ourselves upon others, nor do we intrude uninvited into their worlds. Sensitive to their concerns, needs, hopes, and desires, we establish a relationship that is comfortable to them and to us. In other words, we share an embodied encounter in which we display empathy and compassion. According to Maeve (1998), embodiment should not be confused with empathy, since empathy is the imaginative projection of a subjective state of another person, while embodiment refers to the immersion in a relationship that we experience through the physical body.

Empathy involves being able to imagine, sense, and appreciate another person's reality and communicate that understanding sensitively (Parkes et al., 1996). As noted by Carl Rogers (1957, 1961), it means

Highly vulnerable ⟷ **Vulnerable enough** ⟷ Invulnerable

Relation to others
Permeability and openness
Flexible boundaries
Embodied experiences
Relating with empathy and compassion
Openness to intimate encounters
Being fully present
Being good enough

Relation to self
Openness to self-awareness
Elaboration of work-related experiences
and personal loss issues
Confrontation with own mortality
Acknowledgment of strengths and limitations

Figure 4.2 The vulnerable-enough care provider

temporarily living in another's life, moving in it delicately without making judgments, and conveying the message "I am with you, I've been listening carefully to what you've been sharing, and I'm checking to see if my understanding is accurate."

Through empathy, we temporarily live in another person's private world. We do not conflate his or her world with our own. Instead, with a genuine curiosity and concern, we strive to understand it as if it were our own. *As if* is a critical element that helps us maintain two separate perspectives: the other's perspective and our own perspective of the same reality. We relate as two separate human beings as *I* (a subject—not a professional title or role) relates to *you* (a subject—not a patient or a client). While empathy is usually limited to the person's lived experiences, sometimes it extends to his or her life condition. This broader form of empathy requires a deep acquaintance with the individual's private and social world, which is brought into the intersubjective space of a shared relationship.

Compassion derives from the Latin root *com + pati*, which means "to bear, to suffer with," and is used primarily by Eastern philosophies and religions. It is a broader concept than embodiment and empathy but is not well defined. It involves a process through which we are open to the suffering of others in a non-defensive and nonjudgmental way and attempt to understand and relieve it (Gilbert, 2005). Compassion refers to the healing power of emotional connectedness and love (an unpopular word among Western scientists) as ways to relieve suffering. It is only recently that the concept of compassion has triggered debates among Western psychologists who seek alternative ways to address human suffering and its transcendence (Davidson & Harrington, 2002; Gilbert, 2005; Lee & Kwan, 2006; Neff, 2003).

Embodiment, empathy, and compassion are indicative of our ability to be open, sensitive, permeable, and available to the people we accompany. None of these characteristics makes us experts; they help us to be human and *good enough*. What does being good enough entail?

Winnicott was the first to use this concept to describe the qualities of a good-enough parent who contributes to the healthy psychosocial development of his or her infant. Such a parent is highly sensitive and capable of responding to the baby's needs by reinforcing the illusion that all needs can be met by a benevolent and generous world put at the infant's service. Progressively, however, this parent helps the child become disillusioned in order to move from a state of total dependence to relative dependence before he or she becomes independent. By adapting in a less-than-perfect way to the child's needs, he or she becomes good enough. His or her role involves introducing the external world to the child in small doses and helping him or her assimilate aspects of it and adapt to its demands. Through this process, the child develops the capacity to be alone in the presence of a concerned other. This aloneness helps the youngster to play, dream, become creative and explorative, and discover him- or herself as distinct from others, yet in relation to them.

As good-enough care providers, we display a similar vulnerability to that of good-enough parents. Alert to the changing needs of dying and bereaved people, we respond with sensitivity to the best of our ability, and empower them to use their resources. We introduce the reality of the dying and bereavement trajectory in small doses and provide a safe base from which people can explore present and future challenges. By not overprotecting, overproviding, or overstimulating them with information, interventions, and services, we strive to create a safe space where they can stand alone as they review their lives and confront their mortality. Standing alone without being devastated can be facilitated in the presence of a companion who—by being good enough—encourages such a process.

The myth at the beginning of this chapter vividly illustrates how Ariadne's love and companionship enabled Theseus to stand alone and face the Minotaur. She did not offer to help or save him from danger but provided him with the means to feel safe to enter the darkness of the labyrinth and confront both the terror of death and his own existence. Alone, Theseus was able to think through, plan for, and cope with the threats that loomed in each corner of the labyrinth. In silence, without distractions from the outer world, he was able to manage the ultimate threat of self-annihilation. However, his success was possible as a result of Ariadne's presence, love, and commitment to him. Through the *miton,* he was able to carry with him her caring presence.

Being vulnerable enough facilitates the formation of secure attachment bonds and the experience of intimate encounters. Kelly, a 7-year-old girl, was dying of cancer in a complex family environment. She had been raised by her mother, who had psychiatric problems that were aggravated by the diagnosis and rapid deterioration of her child's health. Kelly had never met her father, who abandoned his spouse the day Kelly was born. Mother and child lived on a small island, secluded in a dyadic world with limited support. Kelly flourished in the hospital and developed relationships with several members of the hospital personnel. Her bond with me was particularly strong, because I was looking after her highly distraught mother, whom Kelly—despite her young age—tried to support. A year following the diagnosis, when physicians had exhausted all available treatment procedures, they informed her mother of Kelly's impending death. Overwhelmed by terror, this fragile woman accused the physicians of medical abandonment and threatened to leave the hospital in order to save her child with the help of religious healers who promised a cure to those who were faithful to God. The risk of this little girl dying alone with a highly distressed mother in a foreign monastery was of great concern to our team. Kelly, who felt protective of her mother, did not openly object to her impulsive decision but expressed her desires in a drawing that she handed to me.

In her drawing, she depicted a house and printed the following words: "The name of this house is Danai." (Danai is my first name.) There were no people in this house. There was only a fireplace, from which warmth and light emanated into the room, and a colorful curtain that covered the house's front door. Outside the house, Kelly painted rain and snow, upon which she printed the words "The Wild Jungle." Above the house, which resembled a crèche, she placed a big, bright star. Her drawing clearly communicated a desire for a warm, safe relationship similar to the one she had seen depicted in the icons of Jesus and the Virgin Mary that hung on the wall next to her bed.

Sensitive to her needs, I assumed a mothering role toward Kelly and modeled some attending and caring behaviors, which her mother began to imitate. Along with the nurses who belonged to our team, we created a safe haven for both mother and daughter, who never left the hospital but found refuge in a room that became their own crèche. Kelly died peacefully in the arms of her mother, who was held and supported by our team.

It is important to note that being vulnerable enough does not mean that we develop an intimate bond with every person and family. A distance that feels right with one person at a given time may be uncomfortable at another time with the same or a different person. According to David Barnard (1995), intimacy in death situations comes about by surprise. It occurs when we truly connect with the other person as a human being, not solely as a professional with a patient or client.

I remember my surprise in discovering this unexpected form of intimacy with Haralambos, a 15-year-old with kidney failure, almost 30 years ago (Papadatou, 1991). Following the death of a patient named Maria on the dialysis unit, he was told that she had gone to the United States to receive a kidney transplant. He soon realized that the nurses and physicians avoided talking about Maria. One day, Haralambos found refuge in my office and, with no warning, asked me if Maria was dead.

"Yes, I am very sad to say that Maria died," I replied, after deciding in a split second that it was more important to be honest with this adolescent than loyal to my colleagues who had concealed the truth.

"I knew it!" he replied in a triumphant tone.

"How did you know?"

"I phoned her home, and when I asked to speak to her, her mother began to sob."

Assured that I was willing to talk about Maria's death, he bombarded me with questions. I invited him to talk about his feelings over Maria's death, his anger about not being told the truth, and his fear of dying too. In the middle of his account, he suddenly stopped talking, grew silent, and looked straight into my eyes. In deep sadness, he asked me: "Why do children die?" I felt extremely helpless to answer his question and empathized with his agony, despair, and quest.

"I do not know. . . . I really do not know," I replied. I did not fall into the common trap of changing the subject (e.g., "This is a tough question, let's talk about something else") or offering a religious explanation (e.g., "It's God's will"), and I avoided paraphrasing his question, as I was taught to do (e.g., "You seem to have difficulty making sense of death when it comes to children"). Instead, I admitted my inability to make sense of a very harsh reality and shared with him the pain of not knowing.

At that moment an intimate bond was established with this adolescent who was experiencing an acute loneliness and existential crisis. For awhile we stood in silence and shared a sense of unparallel solidarity and intimacy. Then Haralambos talked extensively about the unknown of death, the uncertainty of life, and his priorities and hopes for the future. We spent the rest of that morning together, and he followed me around in the wards as I visited other hospitalized children. He was the most expressive that I had ever seen him. We parted in joy, knowing that we had connected in a very intimate way. "I'll see you tomorrow," he said with anticipation as he accompanied me to my car after the end of my shift. But unfortunately there was no tomorrow, because Haralambos died that night due to a health complication, leaving me in acute grief.

This was my first experience with the death of a child. To this day I remember it vividly because it taught me three things that affected my subsequent work in palliative and bereavement care: first, that I am also vulnerable in the face of death; second, that the existential helplessness, meaninglessness, hopelessness, and loneliness caused by dying and death can be tempered or tolerated if shared in a trusting relationship in which both participants are willing to confront the transience of life and their mortality; and, third, that intimacy stems from relationships that are truly authentic and open to the unknown. In such relationships, suffering is transformed and we are changed, sometimes for a lifetime.

While connection and commitment are necessary for the development of trust in a relationship, it is openness and authenticity that enable intimacy. Barnard (1995) suggests that intimacy holds a promise and a fear. The promise relates to the rewards we derive from truly connecting with people who teach us about the value of human relationships and of life. The fear is associated with the risk of our undoing—in other words, the risk of falling apart, of being engulfed by the pain of the person, by the unknown of death, or by the perceived meaninglessness of a situation.

Our fear may also be related to a fantasy that the dying or the bereaved person has the power to carry us beyond the borders of life into death or into suffering. When we acknowledge this fantasy without being threatened by it, we are able to sustain it for the sake of the person who wishes to be accompanied all the way through the unknown. However, our ability to sustain it depends on our willingness to confront the threat of self-annihilation, to address issues related to our existence, to tolerate the anxiety they evoke, and to recognize that we may be changed by this process.

This self-confrontation enables the dying and bereaved to accept us as being both competent and limited in our role as companions. Such an acceptance frees us from the need to be perfect, omnipotent, and in total control and allows us to relate to another person first as a human being, and then as a professional.

When we accompany people through dying or grief, we cannot promise a perfect cure, a perfect death, or a perfect recovery from bereavement. All we can promise is a committed, trusting, and authentic relationship that may become intimate, and a source of potential growth for all parties involved.

CONDITION 4

Developing a Holding Environment for Ourselves and Co-Workers

To be effective in our role as companions, we all need a holding environment that functions as a safe haven in times of distress, and as a secure base from which to explore new knowledge, experiment with novel initiatives and collaborations, and move forward into unknown territories. It is only when we are well supported that we can efficiently support others and maintain an image as good-enough professionals.

In the field of palliative and bereavement care there is a tacit acceptance that we must look after ourselves and receive appropriate support (International Work Group on Death, Dying, and Bereavement, 1979, 1993a, 1993b, 2002, 2006). In practice, however, most of us are left to manage our distress alone. We seek support only when we are totally burned out or in an acute crisis. Our tendency to neglect our needs and disregard the importance of self-care is often related to our lifestyle. In our fast-paced culture we value efficiency and speed above effectiveness. This prevents us from slowing down to review the services we provide, reflect upon how they affect us, and attend to our own needs. Whenever we acknowledge our needs, we rely on our own resources to take care of them. Self-reliance is a key value of Western societies that reinforces individualism and alienates us from others when we are in need of support.

Rare are those work settings that recognize the importance of establishing a holding environment for their employees. Nurses, physicians, psychologists, social workers, and chaplains learn through basic education that, armed with the appropriate knowledge and skills, they must be able to do a good job and do it right. Specialization and ongoing training have been overemphasized. They also learn that working with death and trauma situations involves several hazards, and they come to believe that burnout, compassion fatigue, and vicarious traumatization are inevitable. So they develop strategies to control, manage, or treat their distress symptoms that are often similar to the strategies they use to control, manage, or treat the symptoms of the people they serve. Believing that caring for people who are suffering is a dangerous job, they disregard the rewards and benefits of caregiving.

It is my belief that self-care cannot be limited to a prescribed set of self-help guidelines and stress management techniques. Self-care requires time for the self, as well as the active presence of caring others in a safe environment. Such an environment does not function solely as a safe haven where we deposit our raw suffering or painful feelings and thoughts but also becomes a place where we can elaborate on our personal attitudes about dying and bereavement, and a basis for the development of our personal and team resources.

When I conducted individual interviews with nurses who worked in oncology, I invited them to tell me what they perceived to be the most distressing experience in providing care to people with cancer. The vast majority referred to the death of their patients. However, further probing revealed that death was perceived as intolerable only when they were left alone to care for a terminally ill patient or to support a bereaved family during the night shift. These nurses were competent in coping with the clinical demands of such situations but expressed a desire for the presence of a colleague who could share the emotional burden of their encounters with death. When colleagues were available, nurses felt accompanied in their coping with death and mortality. Bonds among coworkers were described as life binding.

In summary, to promote a culture of companioning for the dying and the bereaved, we must ensure a culture of companioning for care providers through peer support and ongoing supervision. Our job is so challenging that it is most effective if and when our experiences are shared. Through sharing, we offer and receive feedback, guidance, and support that enable us to move beyond our distress, limitations, and shortcomings in order to expand our caregiving and care-receiving abilities.

WORKING IN PRIVATE PRACTICE

What about care providers who live in remote communities and have no colleagues with whom to share and process their experiences? For them, solo practice is the only option. They go to great lengths to establish a network of support via the Internet, telephone, or professional meetings. For other professionals, particularly counselors, psychologists, and psychiatrists, solo practice is a matter of choice. While it can be argued that private practice protects them from witnessing the ravages of a diseased body, the actual dying of a person, or the trauma of the bereaved, it does not spare them from being affected by the reality of death. People who come to counseling or therapy with a desire to manage their suffering are confronted during the therapeutic process with existential issues related to death and the value of life (Sourkes, 1982). These issues leave *no* professional unaffected. How are they addressed when one is working alone? Bound by the rules of confidentiality, caregivers avoid discussing their responses with colleagues and become defensive or ashamed of being affected. With limited or no training, they doubt the effectiveness of their interventions and are unsure of how to support a dying or bereaved person, who is usually referred to an "expert" therapist who specializes in grief work.

Burton (1962) compared the results of a survey of a randomly selected sample of 300 members of the American Psychoanalytic Association who worked in private practice to those of a control group of recent graduates. He noted that the therapists' responses to questions such as "Is death a beginning or an end?" and "Do you believe that discussion about death should be avoided with your patients?" were brief and often hostile. While therapists reported that discussions should not be avoided, they also admitted that death rarely came up as an issue in their practices. Twenty years later, Clarke (1981) assessed whether the analysts' views had changed. Findings revealed a tendency to deny that they were being affected by death issues brought into therapy, and the researcher questioned whether such a tendency compromised the therapeutic process.

Challenges are compounded when the person who is in counseling or therapy suffers from a life-threatening illness or is actually dying. A report of the Working Group on Assisted Suicide and End-of-Life Decisions of the American Psychological Association (2000) suggests that "there is little evidence that organized psychology has played an important role in discussing quality of care for dying persons, producing a body of research concerning end-of-life decision-making, engaging in the national discourse on end-of-life care and public policy, or in educating its own members regarding this important final stage of life" (p. 17). This is also true for counselors, psychologists, and psychiatrists, who, according to Yalom (2008), avoid working directly with people's death anxiety, either because they are reluctant to face their own mortality or because professional schools offer little or no training in how to address death issues in therapy.

Only recently has the role of psychologists and psychiatrists been recognized in end-of-life care (Chochinov & Breitbart, 2000; Haley, Kasl-Godley, Neimeyer, & Kwilosz, 2003; Werth, Anderson, & Blevins, 2005). However, the focus of debates has remained limited to practical issues concerning the care of dying people: Should home or hospital visits be allowed when a patient is dying? Should interaction between the therapist and grieving relatives be encouraged? Can sessions be conducted by phone when a person is unable to travel to the therapist's office? How should the therapist respond to the dying person's need for more frequent sessions? How does irregularity in the frequency of sessions get handled? Can 50-minute sessions be adapted to the needs of dying clients?

Roose (1969) challenged some of the psychoanalytic rules and discussed issues such as becoming more active in sessions when the person is less able to talk, touching the hands of patients who are in bed, attending the funeral, or offering to make burial arrangements when family members are unable to do so. Roose advocated that therapists must be less preoccupied by the content and timing of interpretations, and more concerned with being present for the person who is dying or the relative who is grieving. Similarly, Norton (1963) emphasized the importance of making oneself available by assuming the role of companion. Mayer (1994), in contrast, argued that the focus should be placed more on the patient's self-understanding through the use of appropriate interpretations, and less on the therapist's presence. Death, according to the author, is perceived as a co-therapist who motivates the person and the analyst to work more productively, given time limitations.

For her doctoral dissertation, Karen Redding (1999) interviewed and analyzed the experiences of eight psychoanalysts whose clients had died. She found that in order to effectively respond to their needs, therapists used a flexible frame of work that allowed for telephone sessions, home or hospital visits, a readjustment of policies about missed appointments, referral to community resources that would enhance patients' welfare, and a greater use of physical touch during critical phases in the people's illnesses. Most analysts maintained a high frequency of contact until death that seemed to meet the person's needs, as well as their own, and reported to have greatly benefited from accompanying their clients until the very end of life. Redding's findings shed light not only upon the feelings of sadness, anger, helplessness, fear, guilt but also upon the love, fascination, and gratitude that therapists who work in private practice often experience in the face of death.

> It took the patient a long time to trust that I was really interested in her . . . and cared for her. Once that happened, I think her love for me became even stronger. And ultimately, I loved her. . . . She had never been close to anyone. At the end, all I could do was to be there for her in whatever way that she needed me and to give her whatever I could to make it better. Why worry about keeping a frame at a time like this with the analysis? For what? It felt important to be a person there for her, who cared for her, and listened to her. That's the greatest gift, I think that you can give someone. (Qtd. in Redding, 1999, p. 87)

The accompaniment of a seriously ill or dying person is an emotionally taxing experience for the professional. Who, then, supports him or her? Sometimes a peer group of counselors or therapists who meet regularly once or twice a month to review cases and discuss concerns and successes. Other times, a supervisor or a consultant. Schaverien (2002), a Jungian analyst, makes a strong call for supervision in her book *The Dying Patient in Psychotherapy.* She describes how it helped her to process feelings of love and hate that she and her client experienced when death became imminent and contributed to making her a wiser and more competent analyst. There is no doubt that supervision and/or peer-group review are imperative when one works alone; these are an ethical responsibility for every provider who offers services to dying and bereaved people.

No other work implicates professionals so personally in the care they provide. It is a work that is extremely personal in nature, and as such, it demands that we be aware of what we bring into our relationships with others and how we are affected in return. Yet it is also a work that is extremely social in nature and that can be safely carried out in the company, and with the guidance and support, of others.

Although the existence of a holding environment in one's setting is a prerequisite for working with the dying and the bereaved, it is also important that such holding be available in our personal lives. Having a private and social life and spending time with partners, children, friends, or community fellows who provide opportunities to turn our attention away from work can help us recharge our physical and emotional batteries through restful, fun, and creative activities and experiences (e.g., a weekend excursion, participating in a social activity, reading a novel, cooking). This may prove to be a real challenge for some care providers who devote their lives to doing the right thing by helping others; as a result, they remain unable to enjoy the pleasures of life and focus on their own needs.

WHEN THE CARE PROVIDER IS SERIOUSLY ILL OR DYING

What happens when the care provider is seriously ill or dying? There is some debate among analysts who work in private practice as to whether (and, if so, how) therapists should inform patients of their illness. The example of two analysts who were ill and handled the issue quite differently is enlightening. While Dewald (1982) disclosed his illness to his clients, the amount of factual information he gave each was determined through careful consideration and assessment of each patient's condition. In fact, he found that patients who were doing poorly needed more factual information, whereas higher-functioning patients were better off with less information. Abend (1982), on the other hand, chose to provide no information about his absence from work, because he believed that such information would invite patients' sympathy and impede the process of transference.

Morrison (1997), who suffered from cancer, described her moral dilemmas when she was confronted with the decision to take on new patients, to disclose her illness to them, and to terminate therapy with those who were highly vulnerable due to their history of traumatic or repeated losses. She dealt with each dilemma by adopting a case-by-case approach and discussed the ramifications of self-disclosure. She supported that disclosure allows an individual to choose whether to enter into or continue therapy. Conversely, nondisclosure increases the risk that the person feels excluded, unimportant, or betrayed, when she or he later learns of the therapist's major life experience.

While a few of her patients (who had also happened to lose a previous therapist to cancer) terminated within months after disclosure, for the majority the therapy deepened as well as their relationship with her.

> To me, the main positive effect of occasional, ordinary self-disclosure, is in its *humanizing of the relationship*. In an extraordinary situation, such as the serious illness of the therapist, which has ultimate ramifications for the patient, the main effect, I think, is in the therapist's offering of authenticity and honesty, in what I consider a real relationship, beyond the transference. (Morisson, 1997, p. 236, emphasis added)

While clinicians have a choice to disclose or hide a serious illness from their clients when no signs of disease are apparent, the situation is quite different when the symptoms are obvious. One has no choice but to acknowledge and talk about it. The illness experience becomes the elephant in the room that neither the person nor the professional can ignore or deny. Therefore, rather than treating the illness as insignificant, the professional is challenged to find creative ways to integrate it into the therapeutic process.

Whether to disclose, what and how to share personal information, how to assess its impact upon the analytic process, and when to terminate the therapy are crucial issues that have no clear answers. Sometimes the disclosure leads to therapeutic progress, while for others, information is misperceived and raises anxieties in patients, who relive loss, trauma, or abandonment that must be addressed during a critical period when the termination of analysis is often in sight (Feinsilver, 1998). The ramifications are complex also for care providers who are faced with the misperceptions, rumors, and stigma that a life-threatening illness engenders in their clients and colleagues.

It is generally recommended that the referral of patients to other clinicians when the analyst is seriously ill or dying must be undertaken with great caution; otherwise, it can impede upon the therapeutic work, complicate the mourning, harm the well-being of patients (Alexander, Kolodziejski, Sanville, & Shaw, 1989; Halpert, 1982; Philip & Stevens, 1992), and negatively affect care providers. Some clinicians recommend the establishment of a peer group of senior colleagues who serve as consultants and help the dying care provider process his or her own personal anxieties and feelings and prepare patients to terminate therapy while he or she is still able to concentrate on the therapeutic work (Philip & Stevens, 1992).

THE END OF ACCOMPANIMENT

In closing this chapter, I wish to return to the myth of Theseus and Ariadne. When Theseus killed the Minotaur and freed Athenians from their debt to King Minos, he left Crete and took Ariadne with him. According to one variant of the myth, he was ordered by the goddess Athena to leave Ariadne on the island of Naxos, where she was found by the god Dionysus, whom she wedded and with whom she had numerous children. According to another version, Ariadne was deserted by Theseus and died in despair. Dionysus placed her crown in the sky, where it formed a constellation of stars known as Corona Borealis.

In both versions, Ariadne was left behind by Theseus. Something similar happens when we accompany dying and bereaved people during a critical period in their lives. Even though we may form intimate and privileged bonds with them, there comes a time when we are left behind as a result of the person's death or the bereaved person's desire to move on with life by setting new goals, priorities, and aspirations.

How do we experience being left behind by someone with whom we may form a privileged bond? Our responses vary. Some may feel bitter, betrayed, and deserted, as Ariadne felt in one variant of the myth. In despair, they decide not to form new bonds or accompany dying and bereaved people through their trajectory anymore. Others grieve over the loss of a person whom they have come to intimately know and carry their acquired wisdom and love into the development of new bonds with other dying and bereaved people, like Ariadne, who gave birth to several children in the alternative variant of the myth.

We have different ways of bringing closure to a shared journey. Our coping with loss and separation stems from personal experiences but is also affected by cultural, institutional, and work-related factors. Accompanying people through dying and bereavement teaches us not only about the essence of connecting to others, but also about the importance of coping with endings. In the same way that a river threads its way into the sea, our relationship to dying and bereaved people threads its way through the twists and turns of life, which acquire new meanings in the presence of loss, separation, and death.

SECTION II

The Care Provider in Death Situations

5 The Wounded Healer

In Greek mythology the great healer of suffering was a wounded healer named Chiron. Chiron was a centaur who had the head and torso of a human, and the legs of a horse. Chiron was born to Cronus (a god) and Philyra (a nymph) and as a result was half immortal. At the time of his conception, his parents, who were having an illicit love affair, were transformed into horses, which explains his odd appearance. When his mother realized that her newborn son was not a perfect human being, she begged the Olympian gods for help. The gods took pity and transformed her into a linden tree. So Chiron was left an orphan until he was found by Apollo, the god of music, light, and poetry, who became his foster parent. Under the guidance of Apollo, Chiron developed into a charismatic centaur, very unique and different from the other centaurs, who were forceful, unruly, aggressive, and violent, representing the wild forces of nature in Greek mythology. Unlike them, Chiron was wise, kind, fair, and highly respected by humans. He became the mentor of several mythological heroes, to whom he taught the arts of medicine, ethics, music, hunting, and fighting (Kakridis, 1986). One of his students was Hercules.

According to the myth, one day Hercules went to visit Pholos, a centaur friend of his. Being a good host, Pholos offered Hercules wine, the scent of which attracted other centaurs who lived in the region. They all gathered, got drunk, and began to fight with one another. Hercules used his poisonous arrows to ward off the wild, aggressive centaurs and to protect himself from the violence. However, by mistake, one of his arrows wounded Chiron in the knee. Hercules immediately tended to the wound by following his teacher's instructions, but the wound proved to be incurable and Chiron had to live with deep suffering.

Motivated to find a way to alleviate his suffering, Chiron became very knowledgeable about the healing powers of plants, which he used in the care of the sick. His wounded knee forced him to slow down and pay attention to the horse part of his body, which was the cause of an earlier psychic wound that occurred when he was abandoned at birth by his mother. So, both physical and psychic wounds allowed Chiron to turn inward and face his limitations. He, the renowned mentor and educator, learned to befriend the experience of being wounded and less than perfect. Along with this came increased wisdom, which allowed him to be receptive and empathic to the suffering of others. In fact, his reputation as a great healer was related not only to his ability to use herbs and plants for curative purposes, but also to his ability to be empathic and compassionate toward the wounds of others (Kearney, 1996).

According to the legend, Chiron taught Aesculapius, the god of medicine and healing, that every healer carries within him a wound to remind him that he is vulnerable, limited, and finite. While the wound causes suffering, it also holds the potential for wisdom and growth. To transform suffering into wisdom, the healer must first come to terms with the realization that he is not all powerful, all knowing, and invincible in the face of illness, pain, suffering, and death. Healing does not ensure immunity, nor does it spare the healer from suffering. In fact, when the healer acknowledges his own limitations and personal suffering, he is able to empathize with the suffering of others and care for them with greater competence, sensitivity, and compassion. Chiron's personal experience made him a great healer of those in suffering, and a greater teacher of those learning the art of caregiving.

What do we learn from this myth that is relevant to our role in the care of seriously ill, dying, and bereaved people?

First, we learn that we are not immune to suffering. Even though we may possess expertise, this does not prevent us from being vulnerable in the face of pain, loss, and death. Second, we learn that to become competent healers, we must turn our gaze inward and address our personal wounds. This introspective process challenges the illusion of omnipotence and confronts us with our limitations. It offers us an opportunity to examine our fears, anxieties, and personal experiences with regard to illness, loss, suffering, and death, as a result of which we gain a broader perspective of our role and contribution in the care of others. It also allows us to discover our talents, strengths, and creativity through caregiving, and to foster our connectedness to the people we serve. Finally, the myth of the wounded healer teaches that wisdom and growth can stem from accepting our strengths and limitations, and from relating to others with a sense of humility and respect. Last but not least, it incites us to step down from a pedestal upon which we occasionally place ourselves and enhances our sense of belonging to the human community.

FROM MYTH TO REALITY: THE SUFFERING OF THE CARE PROVIDER

What about our suffering? As has already been suggested, caring for individuals who are dying, and listening to painful, chaotic, or traumatic accounts of the bereaved, is a profound experience that affects most of us and elicits suffering, aspects of which are unavoidable. Only when we acknowledge our suffering can we begin to cope with it in appropriate ways. However, such an acknowledgment is uncommon in modern societies, which perceive suffering as something that is invariably bad, affecting only the "victims" of illness and death, not the "experts" who help and support them. In addition to the suffering we experience in our work, we are often stigmatized or marginalized as a result of our work in death situations. Think for a moment about how people react when you tell them that you provide services to dying and/or bereaved people. Some may react with curiosity or sympathy, asking questions such as "How can you do that job?" What is left unsaid is that this job is perceived as terrible, horrific, weird, macabre. Others, on the other hand, respond with admiration and put you on a pedestal by distancing themselves from you (e.g., "You are a hero.... I could never work in that field"). Finally, there are also those who react with disdain or aversion (e.g., "What a job! It must be very depressing," "What's wrong with you?").

Quite often people perceive us as different because we offer services that are socially unappealing. As a result, we end up feeling alienated and discriminated against. This social discrimination, which can be subtle or overt, appears in different forms:

First, it is experienced as a dismissal of our services, which are viewed as unimportant or even unnecessary. We are not experts who treat and cure people and demonstrate through observable and measurable outcomes the positive effects of our interventions. Rather, we are perceived as second-class professionals whose task accompanying people through dying and bereavement is not understood and is therefore considered insignificant.

Second, it is experienced as a dismissal or negation of our personal experiences. Our family members, friends, and even colleagues who work in different work settings are not interested in listening to stories about loss, dying, and bereavement or cannot stand doing so for too long. Sometimes they admit feeling traumatized by our accounts, which are too painful for them to bear. Even though they care for us, they tend to interrupt our stories with remarks such as "That's enough! Let's talk about something happy," "You should take your mind off this," and "Let's not discuss such topics while we are eating." In extreme situations, we are entirely avoided by people who perceive us as death "contaminators" or carriers of the stigma of death.

Third, social discrimination is experienced as an overt or subtle form of aggression directed at us or at our team because our work elicits anxiety over death and reminds people that we are *all* mortal.

Finally, social discrimination occurs when we, in addition to the work we do, are idealized. Invested with heroic, extraordinary, or superhuman abilities and qualities, we are set apart from the rest of society. Being placed on a pedestal may temporarily seduce us; however, such a position fosters feelings of alienation and loneliness and exerts an immense pressure upon us to conform with certain social expectations. These expectations are as follows:

- We must be knowledgeable and skillful in fixing and relieving suffering.
- We must prevent suffering by not addressing death matters; discussions about death and loss issues can cause more harm than good and can foster despair by taking away hope.
- We must display concern yet remain detached from dying and bereaved people in order to ascertain an objective and scientific approach.
- We must protect ourselves by being strong and immune to the suffering of others; death is a reality that we must get used to.

Unfortunately, these expectations are reinforced during our formal education in medicine, nursing, psychology, and other health sciences.

We are trained to view physical and emotional suffering as a problem to be fixed, treated, and alleviated at any cost and are expected to prevent suffering in others and in ourselves.

The reality is that we cannot effectively care for dying and bereaved people unless we challenge the above expectations and obstructive beliefs and develop a space in which the suffering of others, as well as our own, is fully acknowledged, accepted, tempered, and occasionally transformed.

To this date, no adequate theory explaining human suffering exists, even though descriptive—rather than explanatory—models have been proposed in the health care field. Most of these models describe the suffering of patients with chronic or life-threatening diseases and illuminate various aspects of their private world. The use of these models to explain the suffering of care providers has not yielded convincing results, mostly because the suffering of a person who is actually dying or grieving is distinct from the suffering we experience as a result of accompanying him or her.

Rowe (2003) relies on Cassell's definition of patient suffering and defines the professional's suffering as "the severe distress associated with events that threaten the intactness of the healer in the role of healer" (p. 17). In an analogous way, Rushton (2004) draws upon Reich's definition of suffering and describes our suffering as

> an anguish experienced as a threat to our composure and our integrity, the fulfillment of our intentions, and more deeply as a frustration to the concrete meaning that we have found in our personal experience. It is the anguish over the injury or threat of injury to the self, and thus the meaning of the self that is at the core of suffering. (p. 225)

She further argues that we experience various threats that affect our sense of integrity, which may lead to disintegration of the self, which is displayed in psychopathology, maladaptive coping, dysfunctional relationships, or disruptions in our spiritual integrity.

Such definitions are vague and sometimes confusing. They imply that suffering is invariably bad. Suffering is neither invariably evil nor invariably good (i.e., always leading to growth or some desired end). Suffering just is; it is painful, yet integral to our human existence. When we associate our suffering with dysfunction or psychopathology and argue that it invariably impairs our capacity to connect with others, we dismiss the natural and unavoidable aspects of a pain that is inevitable as a result of our ability to maintain bonds and share the reality of loss and death with the dying and the bereaved.

ASPECTS OF CARE PROVIDERS' SUFFERING

What is the nature of our suffering? Is our suffering a psychological state? Is it a process? Is it the outcome of encounters with death and loss situations? There are no definite answers to these questions; however, by offering some personal reflections, I hope to contribute to the beginning of a fruitful debate.

Experiencing suffering when we are confronted with death situations is natural, and often unavoidable. It is integral to the process of developing secure and intimate bonds, which are severed by death. Our suffering may or may not threaten our intactness or integrity; it does not always lead to major reorganizations in how we perceive ourselves, others, and life, yet it almost unfailingly affects the care we provide and the relationships we develop with the people we serve or collaborate with.

I believe that in order to understand our suffering, we must first situate it in the context of relationships. It is our relationships with ourselves, with others, and with the world (and our sense of belonging in it) that suffer. Our suffering not only stems from relationships but is increased, relieved, or transformed by them. I perceive suffering as both a personal and interpersonal process that stems from and affects our sense of community and connectedness with others, as well as our connectedness to ourselves. While it may alienate us from others and from ourselves, it may concurrently bring us closer and prompt us to develop renewed and more enriching relationships.

Kleinman (1992) suggests that suffering is best understood when situated within the "local world" of the sufferer, which is illuminated by the wider context of knowledge, practices, and experiences of one's family, workplace, and community. When we tell a story about the suffering we experience in this field of work, it usually involves encounters with patients and families; with co-workers, superiors, and administration representatives; or with community members or political leaders. Our suffering always has a psychosocial component; almost unfailingly it has also a spiritual component that stems from the realization that we are mortal, and that all valued and cherished relationships come to an end. We find ourselves experiencing existential concerns similar to those of dying and bereaved people: "Is my life fulfilling?" "Is it meaningful?"

"If not, why?" "If I were to die tomorrow or lose my loved ones, would I feel that I've led a life worth living or one that has slipped away?" "Have I realized or stifled my dreams for happiness and fulfillment?" "What would make my dying appropriate?" "Is there a higher power or cosmic plan?" "Is there life after death?"

Exploring these existential issues may eventually render life more poignant, precious, and meaningful and may affect the quality of care we provide in positive ways.

My purpose is to briefly describe some concepts that are used to illuminate how we are affected by the caregiving process in general, and by our encounters with the dying and the bereaved in particular. The concepts of countertransference, burnout, compassion fatigue, vicarious traumatization, and grief will be analyzed in an attempt to understand some of our responses in the face of death.

Countertransference

Some of the first attempts to describe how care providers are affected by people who experience physical or psychic pain were undertaken by psychoanalysts. Freud proposed the concept of countertransference to describe the process by which the therapist develops a distorted view of the patient that is far different from the way others see that person. Through this distortion, the clinician sees in the other person aspects of him- or herself and strives to meet his or her personal needs or to address unresolved conflicts through the client. For example, a care provider may grow angry and impatient with a bereaved person for his tendency to ruminate over past losses; she may even become judgmental of her client for not getting his act together and moving on with his life. Exploring her personal responses in supervision, the professional may recognize that underneath her reaction to the bereaved person lies her unaddressed experience of being burdened and stifled in her development by the chronic grief of her mother over the death of her sister. Thus the responses of this therapist to her client reveal a deeper suffering that is triggered by the therapeutic process.

Freud urged therapists to explore and work through their conscious and unconscious responses to patient transference, which he regarded as obstacles to the quality of care. While the concept had a negative connotation in Freud's definition, several publications over the past decade contributed to a review of the concept of countertransference, which was extended to include the totality of feelings experienced by the clinician toward a person, regardless of whether these feelings are triggered by the individual's or the therapist's issues (Gabbard, 1999; Gold & Nemiah, 1993; Wilson & Lindy, 1994). Today, countertransference is regarded as a natural, appropriate, and inevitable response that helps professionals understand intrapersonal and interpersonal processes that unfold between a person and a therapist (Katz & Johnson, 2006a).

Because the concept of countertransference is widely misunderstood, it is rarely used in the clinical practice of palliative and bereavement care. Only a few thanatologists succeed in introducing it without the associated psychoanalytic jargon and help illuminate some of our emotional, cognitive, and behavioral responses to death (Katz & Johnson, 2006b; Sourkes, 1982).

Burnout

Burnout is a very popular concept in health care that describes the cumulative effects of caring for people in need. Maslach (1982) describes it as a syndrome that involves an increased sense of emotional exhaustion, the loss of compassion that results in a depersonalized approach to people and a reduced sense of personal accomplishments that lead to impaired job performance. In quite similar terms, Pines and Aronson (1988) define burnout as "a state of physical, emotional, and mental exhaustion caused by long term involvement in emotionally demanding situations" (p. 9). While burnout is described as a state, it is often presented as a process that develops gradually among care providers who set unrealistic goals and overinvest in their relationships with people in their care. Confronted with multiple job stressors, they progressively experience an erosion of their idealism and become resentful that work does not meet their personal and professionals needs and aspirations. Dissatisfied, they become apathetic and derive no satisfaction from a job that has lost its meaning.

Skovholt (2001) distinguishes between two types of burnout: caring burnout and meaning burnout. He argues that *caring burnout* is caused by the long-term effects of a caring cycle that involves "empathic attachment," "active involvement," and "felt separation" between the caregiver and the person in need. When too many losses occur and the practitioner experiences no gains from caregiving, then he or she feels depleted, disengages him- or herself from the caring cycle, and experiences caring burnout. In contrast, *meaning burnout* occurs when the process of caring for others loses its purpose and meaning, either because it becomes routine, boring, or insignificant for the practitioner, or because the practitioner has doubts about the effectiveness of his or her work.

Studies show a high prevalence of burnout among American nurses who work in hospital settings (Aiken, Clarke, Sloane, Sochalski, & Silber, 2002), while findings on physician burnout are more conflicting, according to recent reviews (Gundersen, 2001; Spickard, Gabbe, & Christensen, 2002). What about the prevalence of burnout in palliative and bereavement care? Researchers have hypothesized that providers who are repeatedly exposed to death encounters are more at risk of manifesting high levels of burnout than care providers who are not involved in death situations. This hypothesis is based on findings suggesting that the death of a patient (particularly of a young one) is perceived as the most stressful event in the hierarchy of work-related stressors. Research evidence, however, does not support this hypothesis (Bené & Foxall, 1991; Foxall, Zimmerman, Standley, & Bené, 1990; Jenkins & Ostchega, 1986; Oehler & Davidson, 1992; Papadatou, Anagnostopoulos, & Monos, 1994; Van Servellen & Leake, 1993; Yasko, 1983). Findings show that even though care providers experience increased distress in their encounters with death, they concurrently derive significant rewards from caring for dying people (Bram & Katz, 1989; Chiriboga, Jenkins, & Bailey, 1983; Eifried, 2003; Gray-Toft & Anderson, 1986–1987; Maeve, 1998; Woolley, Stein, Forrest, & Baum, 1989). Rewarding experiences with dying and bereaved people, along with an increased awareness of the value of life, seem to counteract the suffering they experience as a result of repeated exposure to death. Vachon (1997) suggests that the low prevalence of burnout among these care providers can also be explained by the fact that they benefit from supportive services, which are usually available for team members of palliative, hospice, and home care programs.

Even though the concept of burnout has generated several studies, it is often used in a generic way to describe multiple forms of occupational distress. This usage has unfortunately led to simplifications of the subtle effects of our responses to dying and bereaved people.

Compassion Stress and Compassion Fatigue

With the development of the field of traumatology, new concepts emerged. Figley (1995) used the concept of secondary traumatic stress to describe the responses of frontline care providers who are directly exposed to traumatized people (primary crisis workers) or indirectly exposed as a result of listening to their clients' traumatic accounts (secondary crisis workers). Secondary traumatic stress is defined as "the natural consequent behaviours and emotions... resulting from helping or wanting to help a traumatized or suffering person" (p. 10). In other words, it is perceived as a natural byproduct of exposure to work-related trauma that is not pathological. Figley argued that care providers who are most vulnerable to secondary traumatic stress are, ironically, those who do a better job of being empathic to traumatized people. Motivated to act and reduce suffering, they engage in various helping behaviors and caring acts. When they are satisfied with the help they provide, they experience a sense of achievement and self-efficacy. In contrast, when they fail to reduce the suffering of traumatized people, they experience secondary traumatic stress, or what has also been referred to as *compassion stress*.

Whenever such stress is ignored and left unattended, it develops into a disorder known as secondary traumatic stress disorder, which involves symptoms nearly identical to those of posttraumatic stress disorder, except that exposure to a traumatizing event experienced by one person (the trauma victim) becomes a traumatizing event for the other person (the care provider). Figley used the more user-friendly term *compassion fatigue* in an attempt to minimize the pathological or derogatory connotation often associated with mental disorders. However, he never denied that caring for people in traumatic situations may result in a psychic disorganization among some care providers. Stamm (1999) went a step further by suggesting that compassion fatigue may reflect only one of the possible idioms of distress, others being dissociation, depression, substance abuse, and somatic reactions.

Even though the concepts of compassion stress and compassion fatigue are under study, there is wide consensus among researchers and clinicians that these phenomena stem from professionals' exposure to the trauma of people with whom they engage empathically. While empathy helps a provider understand someone who is traumatized, it can also be traumatizing.

Who are the professionals who are most vulnerable to compassion stress or compassion fatigue? According to Figley (1999), they are those who harbor unresolved traumatic experiences that are reactivated by direct or indirect exposure to similar trauma in the victims, and those who work with vulnerable populations (e.g., traumatized children). Moreover, they are care providers who tend "to view themselves as saviors, or at least as rescuers" (Figley, 1989, pp.144–145).

Most studies of compassion stress and compassion fatigue explore the responses of firefighters, police officers, and mental health professionals who work with physically and sexually abused people. We know little about care providers who care for seriously ill and bereaved people. The concept of compassion fatigue has only been used loosely to describe the responses of nurses, who often overextend themselves by thinking, "I can always give a little bit more" (Joinson, 1992), and of physicians, who engage with their patients but take no time to appreciate the love, respect, and appreciation they seek to share with them (Pfifferling & Gilley, 2000).

Recently attention has been drawn to the coexistence of compassion fatigue and compassion satisfaction, which mitigates the negative impact of trauma (Stamm, 1997), and new tools have been developed to assess both aspects of care providers' responses to people who experience traumatic situations, including death.

Vicarious Traumatization

The symptoms of vicarious traumatization are quite similar to what has been described as secondary traumatic stress. However, McCann and Pearlman (1990) used a constructivist theoretical approach to illuminate the disruptions in cognitive schemas, or beliefs that care providers experience about themselves and others, as a result of exposure to client victimization. They argued that disruptions to one's frame of reference affect three domains: one's identity (e.g., as a person, as a care provider), one's worldview (e.g., life philosophy, moral principles and values), and one's spirituality (e.g., meaning and hope).

Vicarious traumatization is described as "the transformation in the therapist's inner experience that comes about as a result of the empathic engagement with a client's 'trauma material'" (Pearlman & Saakvitne, 1995, p. 151). This transformation may be highly distressing when the clinician experiences intrusive imagery related to the client's traumatic material, anxiety, depression, exhaustion, and severe disruptions to his or her basic needs for safety, trust, esteem, intimacy, and control. Vicarious traumatization develops either suddenly, following exposure to a person's trauma, or gradually as a result of the cumulative effects of witnessing or listening to too many tragic stories. The professional displays similar vulnerabilities with trauma survivors (e.g., viewing the world as an unsafe place, relationships as not trustworthy, him- or herself as powerless or hopeless) and often shares his or her clients' anger, resentment, or despair. When traumatized vicariously, one loses hope and the ability to help and care for others.

Can vicarious traumatization be avoided or prevented? Following her return from Rwanda, Laurie Anne Pearlman (1999), who helped people heal in the aftermath of the 1994 genocide, made an important point: "We are not the masters of our vicarious traumatization. We must learn to live with it; and that means honouring and acknowledging it, treating it with respect, and working with it" (p. l). She described vicarious traumatization as an ongoing process, not as an event, a diagnosis, or even an experience: "It is fluid, ever-changing, always shadowing us.... As long as we are engaging empathically with trauma survivors and feeling responsible to help in some way, we are going to experience vicarious traumatization" (p. xlix).

Such a definition makes the study of vicarious traumatization extremely difficult but also highlights the need for self-care on an ongoing basis. To minimize and alleviate the ill effects of vicarious traumatization, according to the author, care providers must balance work, play, and rest and engage in an examination of their cognitive distortions, which prevent a process of reconnecting with themselves, others, and life (Saakvitne & Pearlman, 1998).

Commonalities and Differences

In what ways do these concepts differ? First, they differ in terms of the theoretical and research backgrounds of those who proposed them. Vicarious traumatization and compassion fatigue are concepts derived from studies conducted with care providers who work in traumatic situations. Exposure to sudden and tragic death, abuse, suicide attempts, terrorism, and disasters is perceived and interpreted through the lens of trauma and defined according to a related terminology (e.g., "trauma workers," "trauma victims," "trauma survivors"). It is argued that such exposure consumes the energy of care providers, who are left feeling helpless, powerless, and traumatized by the intensity and magnitude of the trauma.

In contrast, the concept of burnout derives from studies that focus on accumulated distress resulting in exhaustion and the impairment of one's ability to care. Research on burnout has not been limited to the individual care provider but has also explored organizational and work-related stressors that contribute to burnout and affect the well-being of practitioners.

Each of the above concepts illuminates different aspects of our responses to death-related situations. The study of secondary traumatic stress, along with its associated disorder (secondary traumatic stress disorder), clarify the acute responses that occur suddenly, with no warning in situations that we experience as traumatic. Vicarious traumatization sheds light on the qualitative changes and disruptions that we experience in our identity, relations, and worldview. Burnout illuminates the long-term effects of caregiving that overwhelm our capacity to cope with distress, deplete our resources, and lead to disillusionment and apathy.

There is consensus among clinicians and researchers that these expressions of caregivers' suffering are occupational hazards that are emotionally painful, unavoidable, cumulative, permanent if unacknowledged, and modifiable if appropriate action is undertaken.

Strategies that have been proposed to prevent and cope with these phenomena are strikingly similar. They can be grouped in two major categories: *self-care strategies* and *organizational interventions*.

1 Self-care strategies involve the acknowledgment and management of stress responses and burnout symptoms; the cognitive restructuring of disrupted beliefs and assumptions; the review of our goals and expectations regarding work; opportunities for rest, play, leisure activities, and physical exercise; and the development of a balance between work and home life.
2 Organizational interventions comprise clinical supervision, peer support, ongoing training, monitoring of one's workload, rest and recreation, variety in work tasks, opportunities for advancement, provision of human and material resources, and the like.

It is important to note that dying and bereaved people do *not* cause our burnout, compassion fatigue, or vicarious traumatization. It is not something they do to us. We are burned out or vicariously traumatized as a result of our *relationships* with them, ourselves, our co-workers, and a work context, which is perceived as unsafe or uncaring. In other words, to fully understand burnout, compassion stress, and vicarious traumatization, we need to go beyond the assessment of a diagnosis, the description of symptoms, or the identification of specific stress management techniques. We must explore the dynamic interplay among personal, interpersonal, and work-related factors that affect our responses and develop a supportive environment that acknowledges and creatively addresses our distress and suffering in death situations, while preventing the long-term damage of vicarious trauma and burnout.

These concepts illuminate only some aspects of our responses in death situations, especially those that are extreme and erode our desire to care for others. In my view, they do not take into account some more common responses that reflect aspects of suffering that is inherent to the process of accompanying people through dying and bereavement. These natural responses do not need to be eradicated through stress management techniques, but rather understood and accepted as integral to the process of caregiving in death situations.

GRIEF: A HEALTHY RESPONSE TO DEATH SITUATIONS

We are not always exposed to death events that are sudden, tragic, horrific, and perceived as traumatic. Some deaths are anticipated and occur in the context of a long-term relationship with the sick person and his or her family. Under those circumstances we are often deeply affected, but not necessarily traumatized or burned out. We display a wide array of healthy, normal, and unavoidable responses that reflect what Jeanne Quint Benoliel (1974) described as "grief responses." She was the first to observe that both nurses and physicians who develop close relationships with their patients grieve over the anticipated and actual deaths of these individuals. Since then, various clinicians have recorded similar observations, most of which are descriptive or anecdotal (Brunelli, 2005; Chalifour, 1998; Eakes, 1984; Hinds et al., 1994; Larson, 2000; Lerea & LiMauro, 1982; Lev, 1989; Plante, Dumas, & Houle, 1993; Rawnsley, 1990; Rushton, 2004; Saunders & Valente, 1994; Shanfield, 1981; Shread, 1984; Slater, 1988; Stowers, 1983; Waldman, 1990).

To this day, professionals' grief remains largely disenfranchised. According to Doka (1989) disenfranchised grief is experienced when people cannot openly acknowledge their loss because the importance of the relationship is not socially recognized, they cannot publicly mourn it, and consequently they are deprived of social support. The social negation of loss and the subsequent lack of support alienates care providers, who are alone in bearing the burden of a hidden suffering (Lev, 1989; Rawnsley, 1990).

The disenfranchisement of care providers' grief may explain the surprising lack of research on this topic. Its effects are not as disturbing or incapacitating as those caused by burnout and traumatic disorders.

Only a few qualitative studies conducted with samples of pediatricians, nurses, and school counselors illuminated their grief responses, probably as a result of the profound effect that childhood death has upon them (Behnke, Reiss, Neimeyer, & Bandstra, 1987; Davies et al., 1996; Donnelly, 2006; Kaplan, 2000; Papadatou, Bellali, Papazoglou, & Petraki, 2002; Papadatou, Martinson, & Chung, 2001; Rashotte, Fothergrill-Bourbonnais, & Chamberlain, 1997).

In these studies, grief is described as a distressing experience that is unavoidable when professionals care for dying people. Davies and her colleagues (1996) described two aspects in nurses' experiences of caring for children with cancer: *grief distress,* which was managed effectively when nurses acknowledged and expressed their emotions over the dying process or death of a child, and *moral distress,* which occurred when they were faced with the dilemma of whether to follow cure-oriented orders or to provide a comfortable death.

In similar terms, Kaplan (2000) referred to the *"emotional tension"* that pediatric nurses experience in their struggle to find a balance between the intense feelings of grief evoked by the dying process of children and their professional responsibility to provide competent care. Achieving such balance enables them to continue offering services in pediatric palliative care and investing their work with positive meaning.

Grief responses are typical not only among care providers who maintain long-term relationships with sick children, but also among those who provide critical care to children who die from an acute or sudden condition, as demonstrated by Rashotte and her colleagues (1997).

My own research efforts elicited similar findings. In collaboration with Ida Martinson, a professor of nursing known for her seminal work in pediatric palliative care, and the help of our graduate students, we conducted a transcultural study in Greece and Hong Kong and invited nurses who work in pediatric oncology and acute care units to share their experiences of caring for dying children and their families (Papadatou et al., 2001). The qualitative methodology and grounded theory approach that we used to analyze the data yielded interesting results that motivated us to expand our initial study to include physicians (Papadatou et al., 2002). In a series of personal in-depth interviews, care providers were encouraged to describe how they handled the care of terminally ill patients and how they were affected by the death of their patients. Our goal was to identify similarities and differences between care providers' responses to death and compare their experiences in terms of cultural background (Greece versus Hong Kong), professional expertise (physicians versus nurses), and work settings (oncology versus critical care). We did not assume that care providers were grieving, traumatized, or burned out and avoided phrasing our questions in ways that would prompt such responses.

I was privileged to conduct in-depth interviews with more than 70 nurses and physicians. I knew a few of them personally, since we belonged to the same team 15 years before, and others were aware of my work in the field. This facilitated the establishment of a trusting relationship and the disclosure of personal stories. The interviews gave professionals an opportunity to take some distance and reflect upon the impact that the care of dying children and grieving families had upon their professional and personal lives. For some, it was the first time they shared their stories, while for others it was an opportunity to integrate their experiences into a narrative that made sense. A few were surprised by the emotionality of their narratives and admitted to reliving some experiences of loss that had gone unacknowledged for many years, or even decades. The narratives were extremely rich in insights with regard to the costs and rewards of caregiving. Suffering and dimensions of personal growth were pervasive in most accounts. The care providers' suffering was expressed through their choice of words, the plot of their stories, their tears, their silences, and their feelings, which ranged from relief to anxiety and rage about deaths that were perceived as unjust or meaningless. However, they also spoke about the rewards of palliative work, the opportunities for self-actualization, and the value of life. In their accounts, I occasionally recognized aspects of wisdom similar to that of the wounded healer.

Findings from our studies led to the formulation of a model that is presented in the following chapter. This model can serve as a beginning in our understanding of the unavoidable suffering we often experience when we accompany people through dying and bereavement.

6 A Model for Professionals' Grieving Process

Most models and theories of grief derive from clinical observations or studies with samples of people mourning the loss of a significant person in their lives. These models and theories propose a set of assumptions that enable scholars and clinicians to understand the experiences of bereaved people and support them in appropriate ways. Let's briefly consider the key assumptions that these models and theories propose with regard to grief.

Based on his clinical observations, Freud (1917/1957) was the first to formulate some basic assumptions with regard to the grief process in humans. His main suggestion was that bereaved people actively engage in a psychological process, which he referred to as the work of grief or the work of mourning (nowadays referred to as *grief work*). This process, which is both conscious and unconscious, helps them process the loss and adjust to the absence of a loved one. How? By allowing them to gradually withdraw their psychological investment in the deceased, thus making it possible for such investments to be transferred into new relationships. Freud hypothesized that if people do not actively engage in grief work, they are likely to experience psychological difficulties at a later point in time.

Based on Freud's assumptions about grief, Lindemann (1944), who interviewed 101 bereaved individuals, was able to distinguish between what he described as "symptoms of normal grief" and abnormal or pathological grief reactions. He identified two major categories of pathological reactions to loss: delayed grief, which is characteristic of an absence of normal grief responses, and distorted grief, which involves overactivity without a sense of loss, hostility, and agitated depression and is indicative of an unresolved grief reaction.

Bowlby's (1980) studies on separation contributed to a further elaboration of the grief process, which he described as a series of stages that people experience when their attachment bond to a loved one has been severed by death.

The idea that grief occurs in a series of predictable and sequential stages or phases was reinforced by other clinicians, who proposed various models to account for people's responses in loss situations (Kübler-Ross, 1969; Sanders, 1999). These stages or phases can be grouped in three major periods: (1) an initial period of shock and disbelief, (2) a period of acute mourning and disorientation, (3) and a period of reorganization and adjustment to a life from which the deceased is missing.

Worden (2008) described the grief process in terms of tasks to be accomplished by the bereaved, which involve (1) to accept the reality of the loss, (2) to process the pain of grief, (3) to adjust to a world without the deceased, and (4) to find an enduring connection with the deceased in the midst of embarking on a new life. Along similar lines, Rando (1993) referred to six processes that enable the bereaved, without forgetting loved ones, to adapt to a new world and invest in new relationships, goals, and pursuits.

Of particular interest is Parkes' (1971, 1988) description of grief as a psychosocial transition that occurs with major life difficulties, including the loss of a loved one. Central to this transition is the invalidation of a person's "assumptive world." According to Parkes (1988), the assumptive world refers to the internal model that each individual constructs early in life and against which he or she matches incoming data in order to orient him- or herself, recognize what is happening, and plan future behavior. It offers order and coherence with regard to our past and present experiences and helps us predict the future by giving direction to our lives. The diagnosis of a serious illness, the certainty of an impending death, and the death of a loved one oftentimes disconfirm our assumptive worlds and trigger a grieving process that involves the rebuilding of damaged assumptions. Along similar lines, Neimeyer (1998) suggests that central to grieving is a process through which one reconstructs a world of meaning that has been disrupted by the threat or reality of loss.

Today, alternative models are being proposed by those who conduct research in this field that are not all that different from earlier descriptions, but highlight various aspects of the grieving process. These focus on the stressors associated with loss, and on the coping patterns or level of functioning of bereaved people (e.g., Bonnano, 2004; Bonnano et al., 2002; Rubin, 1981; Stroebe & Schut, 1999). Stroebe and Schut (1999, 2001), for example, describe mourning as a "dual process" in which the bereaved experiences various stressors and copes by oscillating between two contrasting modes of functioning: a loss orientation, which involves an active grieving process over the loss of a loved one in an attempt to come to terms with what happened and attribute meaning to experiences, and a restoration orientation, which involves a striving to meet the challenges and accomplish the tasks that one must perform in order to adjust to the new reality created by the loss. A comprehensive compilation of current models and theories on bereavement and of the research advances in this field is included in Stroebe, Hansson, Stroebe, and Schut's (2007) *Handbook of Bereavement Research: Consequences, Coping, and Care.*

In light of the above theories and models, how can we better understand our grief? Do these theories reflect the grieving process that we experience in our encounters with dying and bereaved people? Applying the available models to our experiences is arbitrary and unscientific. We should never forget that our exposure to loss and death usually stems from a choice to work with the seriously ill and bereaved, to whom we have something of value to offer. Sometimes, affected by their death or loss, we grieve. Our grief, however, does not always involve the rebuilding of shattered assumptions, nor major reorganizations of our worldview or identity. We do not have to adjust to an altered reality every time a patient dies or a family is bereaved.

Our own grief presents unique features. These are described here in a model that resulted from my own qualitative studies. Even though the model derives from the experiences of care providers who work with children in a Western country (Greece) and an Eastern country (Hong Kong), preliminary findings and observations suggest that its basic propositions also reflect the grieving process that is experienced by care providers who work with adults in different workplaces and cultural settings. However, it has yet to be validated through extensive research.

My purpose here is to advance seven propositions (Box 6.1) in an attempt to illuminate aspects of our grief when we are directly exposed to death and accompany families through terminal care. Note that the

Box 6.1

BASIC PROPOSITIONS REGARDING THE GRIEVING PROCESS OF CARE PROVIDERS

Proposition 1: Professionals who experience death as a personal loss are likely to grieve.

Proposition 2: Grieving involves a fluctuation between experiencing and avoiding loss and grief.

Proposition 3: Through grieving, meanings are attributed to death, dying, and caregiving.

Proposition 4: Personal meanings are affected by meanings that are shared by co-workers, and vice versa.

Proposition 5: Grief overload and grief complications occur when there is no fluctuation between experiencing and avoiding loss and grief.

Proposition 6: Grief offers opportunities for personal growth.

Proposition 7: The professional's grieving process is affected by several interacting variables.

proposed model does not reflect the experiences of clinicians who work in disaster situations and are frequently exposed to the deaths of people who are unknown to them.

PROPOSITION 1

Professionals who experience the death of a person as a personal loss are likely to grieve

Not every death is experienced as a loss. Our responses largely depend on how we relate to others, which goals we strive to achieve, and which meanings we attribute to death-related experiences, given our personal history and philosophy of care as well as our team's.

Death does not hold a universal meaning, nor does the loss of life affect all of us in the same way. Even when the dying process and death of a person are experienced as a loss by several practitioners who belong to the same team, that loss is unique and has different meanings for each care provider. Our research findings suggest that the losses we experience can be grouped into six broad categories (see Box 6.2).

Box 6.2

NATURE OF LOSS EVENTS THAT TRIGGER A GRIEVING PROCESS

- The loss of a personal bond with the person who dies
- The loss of valued relationships through an identification with the bereaved
- The non-realization of our professional goals and expectations
- The loss of our assumptions about ourselves, others, and life
- The emergence of past unaddressed or traumatic personal losses
- Awareness of our mortality

The Loss of a Personal Bond With the Person Who Dies

We do not develop an attachment bond with every person and therefore do not grieve over the death of all the people we serve. However, the dying process and death of some patients with whom we share a special bond affect us deeply. Sometimes grief is evoked by the realization that the death of a specific patient is not just probable, but inevitable or imminent. This is evidenced in the following account of a nurse:

> I cry and cry for a week before the death… and after the death, I sometimes dream of the patient and light a candle, especially if I have not attended the funeral. At home, I withdraw and I do not want to talk to anybody… not even to my children.

Other times, it is the actual death of a patient that triggers a grieving process, which was previously inhibited or avoided in our striving to address the needs of the dying person and grieving family.

The Loss of Valued Relationships Through an Identification With the Bereaved

Sometimes we grieve not the death of a person but rather the loss of valued relationships by those who are bereft. Consider the following account: "I do not grieve for that child. I've accepted her death and feel at peace. What I'm grieving for is the pain that these parents experience." She adds later on, "Losing a child evokes an unconceivable pain." This care provider, who is also a parent, grieves over the "unconceivable pain" that these parents experience when they are deprived of their beloved daughter.

Identification with family members is more likely to occur when we are the same age or gender as the person who dies, or when we have a similar family condition or type of relationship. Through the losses of others, we grieve losses we have experienced in the past or losses we anticipate encountering in the future, as evidenced in the following account:

> This always happens to me when a patient dies.... I think of the deaths of significant people in my own life. It's someone from my home: my mother, my father, my brother. Sometimes it is even the husband I will someday marry or my unborn children. In every death, I imagine the funeral of my own loved ones.

Grieving in this case is about the realization that all valued relationships come to an end, because we are mortal and human.

The Non-Realization of Our Professional Goals and Expectations

Within the traditional practice of medicine, the death of a patient is perceived as a personal failure and is often associated with the loss of power, control, or meaning, as reflected in the account of the medical director of an adult ICU: "What makes me angry and depressed is not the death of *this* patient, which was, for that matter, inevitable, but the fact that he died suddenly, before we were able to understand what caused his death."

In this account it is obvious that the experience of loss is associated with the physician's failure to achieve his goals, these being the resolution of the "riddle of the disease" through the achievement of a correct diagnosis, the selection of an appropriate treatment, and the assessment of an accurate prognosis.

Unrealistic expectations become a major source of disappointment and frustration even in the most caring environments. For example, the failure to achieve a "good" death for all patients may be experienced as a major disruption to one's perception of oneself and the team's competence and may become a source of ongoing grief. Some deaths, however, are indeed painful, and we grieve over our inability to prevent them or to have a positive effect upon the lives of the people we serve.

> He had a terrible death. His pain was not physical; it was psychological. He wanted his two children to visit him, and none of them came. Moreover, he did not want any of us to stand by his side. I tried to approach him, but

> he was verbally abusive. I gave up on him. He left this world alone and bitter with several unfinished issues. I was sad, angry, guilty, depressed, thinking of him constantly, and haunted by a sense of failure. I totally failed to ensure a dignified death for this man.... I failed in my role.... We failed as a team.... We failed as a service. For me, this situation was more painful than the death itself.

Death for this care provider—and for many others—is not the most painful experience. Failure to meet ambitious goals and maintain a positive or idealized image of oneself can elicit intense grief.

The Loss of Assumptions About Ourselves, Others, and Life

For those who provide palliative services, death is usually accepted and perceived as inevitable and natural. It does not invalidate our personal assumptions or disconfirm our goals, practices, and professional identity. For example, the "appropriate" death of an elderly person who has lived a full life, the inevitable death of a patient who has suffered a prolonged illness, and the natural anticipatory grief of a bereaved relative are congruent with our expectations and assumptions about life. These experiences are therefore smoothly integrated into our cognitive frame, despite the suffering they may elicit. However, some deaths (particularly of children or young people, of individuals who have suffered unduly, or of patients who were victims of medical errors) challenge the familiar and cherished assumptions through which we make sense of the world, organize our experiences, and attribute meaning to our daily work and lives. Other times, it is not specific deaths that challenge our assumptive world, but rather the repeated exposure to multiple encounters with dying, death, and bereavement that invalidates our view of the world, which ceases to have order, meaning, or coherence. The shattering of our assumptive worlds engenders losses that we grieve, sometimes even over the span of several years. In the following account, an experienced care provider describes how her worldview and professional role changed as a result of her exposure to multiple losses.

> Over the years I've been exposed to several sudden, violent, meaningless deaths.... I've gone through a period of anger, despair, and utter helplessness. Some deaths did not make any sense, and I felt I could do nothing about it. I was convinced that we are all left to the whims of serendipity... that there is no order in the universe, no God in charge, no divine plan. It took me a long time to come to terms with the realization that there is no

> such thing as a good death. Death is death. It is an irreversible end that does not always occur in a peaceful, nice, tidy, controlled, or predictable manner. If anything good can be attached to death, it is the positive things that can stem from the suffering it creates. I have seen people who, confronted with impending death, learned to love themselves and show love for others for the first time in their entire lives!…I view my role as one of helping them cope with their suffering and turn it into something that can be of value to them and to those around them. When this is achieved, I feel I have contributed, in my own humble way, to making the world a better place to live and to die in.

The Emergence of Past Unaddressed or Traumatic Personal Losses

Sometimes the death or bereavement of another person brings to the surface personal, often traumatic, losses that we experienced earlier in life and that have affected our choices and life trajectories. When we revisit these losses, a grief that was sanctioned or disenfranchised may come to the surface. In fact, for many care providers, a personal traumatic loss becomes the primary—and often unconscious—motivation for choosing to work with people in life-and-death situations, in the hope that they will come to terms with an illness, injury, or death-related experience that has not been processed or grieved.

Bion (1961) calls people's tendency to be drawn to a particular work setting because it offers opportunities to work through their own losses "valency." He argues that such settings attract professionals with similar needs and defenses, which are used to fulfill the institution's goals and primary task. Collective defenses against common anxieties (e.g., death, loss, and separation) affect task performance, and one is often drawn unconsciously into certain roles on behalf of the institution as a whole.

Awareness of Our Mortality

Death confrontations evoke anxiety in all of us, and sometimes an anticipatory grief over the fact that our lives will inevitably come to an end. At the same time, it elicits a striving to give purpose to our lives and live meaningfully, as evidenced in the following account:

> I think of death very often because I want to be prepared when my time comes. I do not mean physically, but spiritually.…I prepare my soul.…I go to confession. I offer my services to people who suffer. I do the right thing.…Through my services to others, I prepare myself for my own death.

Grieving is most acute for care providers who are themselves diagnosed with a life-threatening disease and live with an uncertain future. They tend to identify with patients, whose frail bodies waste away before their eyes, and see themselves in the dying process of each patient. Anxiety—sometimes even terror—stems from the realization that dying and death happen not only to others, but also to us. Death is not perceived as an abstract possibility, or as a natural phenomenon; it is lived as a real, imminent, and poignant threat.

In summary, the death of a person to whom we have provided services is often experienced as a loss, which may have different sources. These losses evoke a natural grieving process that presents unique characteristics distinct from the traditional grief models, which describe a series of stages, phases, or specific grief tasks to be accomplished by the bereaved person.

PROPOSITION 2

Grieving involves a fluctuation between experiencing and avoiding loss and grief

Grieving is not something that is happening to us, or something we experience passively, waiting for time to heal our pain. Grieving is an active process filled with choices. We choose how to perceive and cope with the challenges that result from our loss. We choose whether to avoid or confront death and the losses it engenders; we choose when and how to express our grief. We choose the meanings that we attach to our experiences. We choose how to use time to address or disregard the changes that occur as a result of loss in our lives.

The grieving process we experience as a result of job-related losses involves an ongoing fluctuation between grief responses resulting from a focus on the loss and avoidance or repression of grief responses, which occurs when we move away from it (Figure 6.1). This fluctuation from one pole to the other is necessary, adaptive, and healthy. It is eloquently described in the following account of a nurse who experienced the death of a child he had been caring for during his shift:

> Even though I have tears when a child is dying, I hold them back because I am aware that the child understands everything. However, the moment the patient expires, I cry a great deal.... I don't know why.... It's a form of intense release...over having been there all night, over the fact that this

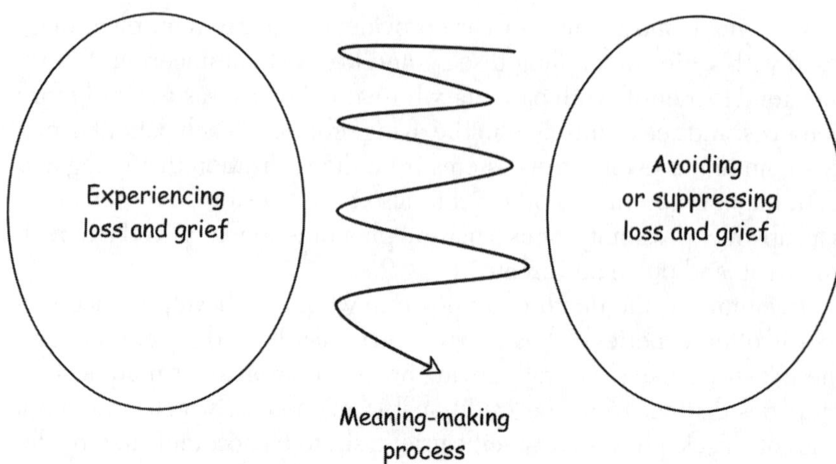

Figure 6.1 Care providers' grieving process

> child has just died. . . . I don't know. This emotional release liberates me from a heavy burden, and then I can think: "What next?" I am then able to collect myself and get into another mood: that of my role as a nurse. I then become a leader—a leader who must bring everything back to order, who must see to the parents, to the dead child, to the unit, and to all the duties that need to be carried out before dawn. . . . Grief does not stop the day after the child's death and is not limited to the confines of the unit. We will always remember some of the things a particular patient did, or some other child will bring back memories of our favorite one. It is as if there is an ongoing relocation of the loss . . . a stirring that never stops.

This nurse's account illustrates how fluctuation unfolds within a few moments or hours and suggests that grieving is ongoing. Care providers tend to rethink and reconstruct their experiences of loss, attach meanings to them, and progressively integrate them into their private worlds and the team's history.

Another care provider, aware of her need to grieve over patients' deaths, described how she focuses and de-focuses on her losses and grief in the following account:

> I need my own space and time to grieve for my patients. I have to get it out, to write it down, to put it on paper, to paint it, to express it through music. Sometimes I even dance my pain in commemoration of a patient who has been important to me. . . . Whenever my workload is too demanding or whenever family issues require my attention, I put my pain away in a

> small drawer and open it again when I am alone...quiet...when the world around me is silent. Whenever I don't find this space and time to grieve, I suffer a pain that is unsettling, and long lasting. It may not be apparent to others, but it colors every aspect of my life.

In what follows, I wish to explore in greater depth how we experience and suppress grief (Papadatou, 2001, 2006).

The Experience of Grief and Loss

When we grieve, we display a wide range of affective, cognitive, and behavioral responses; physical symptoms; and existential concerns. What are some of the common responses that reflect a process of active grieving?

At a *cognitive level,* responses vary. They may include a sense of shock and temporary disbelief or confusion, especially if the loss was unexpected or we felt emotionally unprepared for the death of a particular patient. Most common, however, is a preoccupation with the dying conditions, the event of the death, or the bereavement process of a family member; it absorbs our thinking and energy. Recurrent (positive or negative) thoughts are common. These are not involuntary thought-intrusions reflective of a traumatic response; on the contrary, they result from a purposeful review of our experiences in an attempt to understand, accept, and attribute meaning to them. Such a review may lead to an array of emotions and cognitions. Considerations such as "If only I had done or said this or that" often evoke guilt. Sometimes guilt results from relief that a particular person died, or from surviving the deceased and being alive and happy. The latter is evident in the following account:

> Sometimes when I drive home and listen to music, I am overwhelmed by guilt because I find myself singing shortly after a patient has died. I feel guilty for being able to listen to music and sing a tune....I feel guilty for eagerly anticipating returning home and hugging my children and spouse....I feel guilty for enjoying a full life when my patient and his family have just lost everything...everything...and I have it all!

When we are preoccupied by a patient's dying process or death, we often have dreams that are indicative of how effectively we are coping with our loss and grief. Whereas dreams keep us asleep, nightmares awaken us as a result of their highly anxious content. Nightmares reflect our personal difficulties and the anxiety that results from caring for dying and bereaved people.

Grief responses at an *emotional level* vary in intensity and means of expression. A profound sense of sadness or temporary signs of depression are common when we encounter several losses within a short period of time. Moments of despair are often related to a sense of helplessness or to hopelessness when we doubt the value of our interventions. Questions such as "Is it worth it?" "What's the purpose?" and "What's the point?" incite us to review and evaluate our services, address ethical and moral issues, and attribute meaning to the care we provide.

Anger, another natural grief response, is illustrated in the following account of a young psychologist who was repeatedly confronted with death:

> If only I could cry today, I would find an outlet [for] my pain. But my pain is not sorrow. . . . It is anger. I feel rage. It's like a storm that turns everything upside down in me and leaves nothing intact. . . . *nothing.* Death seems so unfair! (Papadatou, 1991, p. 287)

In the privacy of her room, another nurse allowed herself to express her anger and resentment over the death of a beloved patient:

> It's terrible. . . . When I go home, I sit on my bed and stare at an armchair in front of me. . . . I often feel like throwing it out the window. . . . I will throw it someday. . . . I sit there with a cup of coffee, and I think, think, think of the child [who died], of what happened. . . . I sit all by myself for hours.

Sometimes we are angry because death annulled our efforts to save a person's life or alleviate suffering. Other times our anger is directed at God, who did not respond to our prayers. Still other times, it is directed at the patient, who did not try hard enough to fight the disease or achieve a dignified death by fulfilling his or her wishes. Statements such as "He died on me," "He gave up fighting," and "She withdrew and refused our help" reflect resentment at dying and bereaved people for denying us the opportunity to meet professional expectations or ideals.

Anxiety is another common response triggered by loss and separation. We experience various fears that affect how we act toward others. Out of fear of losing our loved ones to death, we seek them out to affirm our love and bonds with them, we become dependent and overprotective, or we distance ourselves to avoid the pain of being deprived of them one day.

Grieving does not involve only painful feelings, as is widely assumed. It is often associated with the experience and expression of love, care, and affection, emotions that are equally powerful. It is not uncommon to experience both pain and love, sadness and relief, at the end of a long and painful dying process, as well as total exhaustion, and deep satisfaction over having offered the best possible care.

At a *behavioral and interpersonal level,* responses vary greatly and are often affected by work-related rules and expectations that determine the appropriate professional conduct in death situations. For some care providers, the act of being present at the bedside of a person who is dying elicits a sense of closure. In a similar way, attending a funeral or giving a eulogy upon the family's request and participating in rituals that commemorate the deceased are behavioral expressions of a grief that is shared.

Crying is another common response that has a cathartic effect for some care providers, and a distressing effect for others, who misperceive their response as unprofessional or a sign of weakness. Along with crying, our grief is often expressed through physical responses such as a lack of energy, frequent sighing, breathlessness, a hollow feeling in the stomach, and a tightness in the chest and throat.

At an *interpersonal level,* grieving may be experienced as a private affair or a social process that is shared with others. We seek the support of our co-workers, supervisors, and loved ones. When they are unavailable or unwilling to share our grief, we may be burdened, as evidenced in the following account:

> Nobody in my personal life can *really* understand what I am going through.... They ask, "How was your day?" but they do not want to hear about the deaths of my patients or any of my feelings. So I have learned to hide my pain and protect my spouse and children from it.... I spare them from the burden of supporting me. They see me as the strong, brave, courageous one who cures sick people and faithfully stands by them when treatment fails. I'm seduced by how they view me, and in one way or another, I cultivate this heroic image. However, the price I pay for such a noble image is pretty high, because I end up feeling very lonely. I am alone with no one to share my pain.

Not only is it important to acknowledge that these responses are expressions of our grief, but it is equally necessary to explore how we cope with them. Do we interpret them as natural responses or as a threat to our mental health? Do we embrace them or discard them? Do we project them upon others, or do we blame others for our pain? Do we use our grief to approach our patients, colleagues, and loved ones, or to pull them away from them and hide? Do we somatize our grief or do we find constructive ways to express it?

The Avoidance or Suppression of Grief

As has already been suggested, we fluctuate between experiencing and avoiding our grief responses. Avoidance and suppression are not necessarily dysfunctional strategies when used temporarily to ward off the impact of loss and grief and manage work tasks. They are different from denial. When we deny the reality of the loss, we do not allow any aspect of reality to become conscious and therefore do not grieve. Most often, however, we selectively suppress or avoid aspects of a reality that is perceived as threatening and anxiety provoking in order to protect ourselves and meet professional duties and tasks.

One common avoidance response is numbness or the shutting down of our emotional responses in order to cope with the challenges of terminal or bereavement care. Statements such as "I feel nothing" and "I am in limbo" are common. We try to control our thoughts and emotions by telling ourselves, "I must be strong," "I must control my tears, because I wear a uniform," "I must hide my pain or grief," and "Patients' needs have priority over my own." This form of self-talk is effective when used temporarily and as long as we do not disregard and neglect our feelings and need to grieve.

Another avoidance response involves the use of distancing tactics that increase the gap between ourselves and dying and grieving individuals. Sometimes we become totally immersed in clinical duties and practical tasks that keep us busy, unavailable to them, and distracted from our grief and suffering. Other times we become overactive to save their lives and pursue futile cure-oriented goals in order to counteract the anxiety we experience over death, loss, and grief, as evidenced in the following account: "I do anything in my power to keep the child alive. I even do useless things and go to extremes so that he does not die before my shift is over."

Frequently we impose a specific plan of care by taking for granted, instead of exploring, the needs of dying and bereaved people and therefore prevent surprises and unexpected situations that may trigger emotional responses we strive to avoid. Avoidance is also achieved through dissociation, which allows us to extract ourselves from a situation by rendering ourselves absent. One nurse described how she avoided a bereaved family with whom she was intimately connected by removing herself from the situation: "I pass by them as if I do not exist, as if I am not there, not present." Other care providers go to extremes and render the dying individual and family invisible by forgetting the person, or by not seeing the relatives, whose needs are neglected.

Depersonalization is another common response that allows us to avoid loss and grief. For example, we divest a comatose patient of all human qualities and perceive him or her as a doll that is fed, changed, and cared for. Conversely, we humanize a deceased person, who is perceived as alive yet asleep, in order to manage the care of his or her dead body.

When exposure to death and dying evokes terror, avoidance patterns are massive. Through them we transform an extraordinary event such as death into a banal, everyday event that is not invested with feelings or particular meaning. This is expressed in the following account of a critical care nurse:

> I'm ashamed because I feel nothing. It's as if I'm washing dishes.... That's the way I manage the cleaning of a dead body.... That moment I must be cool and collected... but when the shift is over, I go away and cry for my patient.

The image of death as something dirty that needs cleaning, and the transformation of a caring act into a daily activity or chore, reflects how this particular care provider was able to temporarily disconnect from a situation that was highly distressing. Only when she was physically distant from the death scene was she able to put her experience into perspective, get in touch with her pain, and grieve over the loss of a person with whom she shared a special bond.

Like her, other professionals create a geographical distance between work and home (which is occasionally increased by vacations, a leave of absence, or a sabbatical). This enables them to safely revisit their work-related experiences and grieve over losses that they have avoided thinking about or suppressed. We need to be aware that avoidance of loss and grief does not solely involve responses that distract us or distort our view of reality. These can also involve life-oriented responses that generate a sense of being alive and living, far from dying and death. We engage in intimate, passionate, or erotic relationships that give us a sense of being loved and in love, or we engage in various activities (such as playing, gardening, cooking, exercising, reading, creating art) through which we lose our sense of self. We find refuge in a space in which we disconnect from work and reconnect with ourselves and others.

Life-oriented responses help us affirm and validate our bonds with others and cultivate a subjective sense of wholeness. They enable us to develop a renewed sense of ourselves that goes beyond our professional role and experiences of loss.

What is important to remember is that avoidance responses are normal as long as they are not used systematically to avoid loss and regulate grief. In summary, the fluctuation between experiencing and avoiding loss and grief is a basic feature of the grieving process that we experience when caring for dying people and their grieving families. Each of us, however, has a distinct way of fluctuating between these two conditions. Our research findings on Greek physicians and nurses who care for dying children revealed that even though all professionals experienced the dying process and death of a child as highly distressing, each had a different way of perceiving and coping with that reality. Physicians were more likely to perceive the death of a child as a failure to achieve their professional goals and to grieve over unmet goals and expectations, while nurses grieved with greater frequency over the loss of the personal relationship they developed with a specific child and family (Papadatou et al., 2002).

Differences were also apparent in the fluctuation process between experiencing and avoiding grief responses. Physicians reported increased avoidance responses and a privatization of their grief, while nurses tended to be more social about it and sought each other out in order to share their experiences and offer or receive support.

Similar findings were found by Smith (2005), who interviewed 30 physicians, nurses, chaplains, and social workers in order to explore how their spiritual and religious beliefs affect the care they provide to dying patients and grieving families. He found that while nurses talked to each other and valued peer support, physicians avoided sharing their grief and disappointments and tended to remain alone in coping with death-related issues. If they ever shared their experiences, it was usually with their spouses.

PROPOSITION 3

Through grieving, meanings are attributed to death, dying, and caregiving

As has already been suggested, the fluctuations that characterize our grief help us acknowledge our losses and set them aside in order to function appropriately without being overwhelmed. Moving in and out of grief, looking closely but also from a distance at the uniqueness of each death, enables us to accomplish a basic function of grieving: attributing meaning to death-related experiences and perceived losses.

Meaning making is a subjective experience through which we perceive and make sense of reality. Reality is always construed through meanings we attach to our experiences. These meanings are in accordance to our worldview and beliefs about how such events should occur in life. If a particular death threatens our view of ourselves or of the world, then we experience a sense of danger, anxiety, confusion, injustice, unfairness, betrayal, or guilt. To temper and cope with these feelings, we seek to redefine ourselves and rebuild our worldview in ways that make sense to us. Thus, through meaning making we work through our losses, temper our pain, and facilitate integration of loss-related experiences into our life scheme or assumptive world (Neimeyer, 2001). This process is integral to grieving, and vital when we are exposed to multiple deaths.

It is important to clarify that meaning making is distinct from cognitive appraisal[1] and similar to what has often been described as a process of 'working through' experiences. According to Taylor (1983), through meaning making we strive to determine the significance of an event by identifying why it happened and what impact it had upon our life.

In the present model, meaning making appears to be both a process and the outcome of grieving. It helps us make sense of why a particular patient died, how death occurred, and how our services contributed to the care of that person and family.

Every time we are confronted with death and loss, we tend to attribute *situational meanings* to our experience; these are compared and contrasted with *global meanings* that we hold about life and death in general, and about the value and purpose of our work. When situational meanings and global meanings converge, then our experience of loss is integrated into our private world, while global meanings are reinforced and validated. In contrast, when situational and global meanings diverge, we experience increased distress and attempt to reconstruct our meaning systems. What we often define as a bad or unacceptable death is usually one that does not fit neatly into a subjective view of the world that we find sensible and comprehensive. For example, we may have great difficulty accepting that nice people die and that the not-so-nice survive, or that young children die while older people go on living for a very long time.

Meanings vary greatly both in terms of *content* and in terms of the *process* through which they are created. With regard to the process, our research findings identified four distinct patterns by which we make sense of death-related events.

- *A linear pattern.* We seek clear-cut causal explanations that identify a cause and an outcome, for example, "Patients die because science cannot cure all diseases," "Patients die because it was meant to happen," and "Patients die because we failed to save them."
- *An interactive correlational pattern.* We seek to explain death through a number of interacting variables. For example, we make statements such as "Death is due to a number of genetic, environmental, and psychological factors."
- *A teleological pattern.* We seek to attribute a purpose to events. This pattern is reflected in statements such as "Each life has a purpose, which is determined by a higher power," "When we complete the purpose for which we were born, we die," and "Death happens for a reason: to test the family's faith, to teach them lessons of love, and so forth."
- *An agnostic pattern.* We accept that death is a big unknown, to which meanings cannot be attached, and argue, for example, that death is neither meaningless nor meaningful. It just is.

With regard to the content of meanings, these are associated with three basic aspects of our experiences—death, the dying process, and caregiving in death situations as depicted in Figure 6.2 and further analyzed.

Making Sense of Death

We strive to make sense of a person's death by raising questions such as "Why do people die?" "Why did this particular person die?" "How do I make sense of this death compared to other deaths I have experienced?" "How do my scientific, spiritual, or religious beliefs assist me in making sense of this loss?"

Such questions incite us to construct a system of meanings that is coherent enough to facilitate an integration of our death-related experiences in a philosophy and approach to end-of-life care. Alternative meanings include scientific or biological meanings, philosophical or spiritual meanings, religious meanings, and meanings in light of one's life trajectory. Sometimes we attribute no meaning at all or combine multiple meanings.

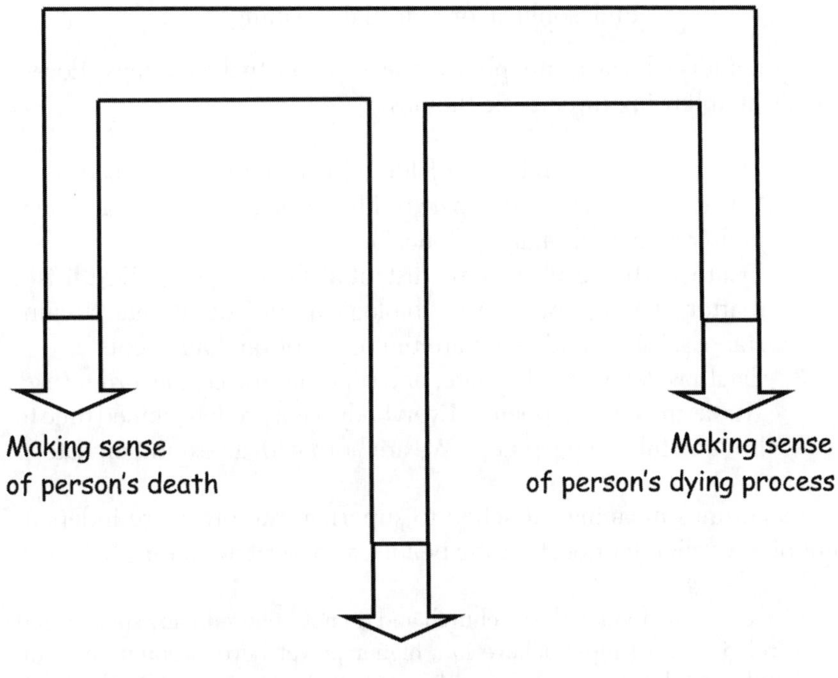

Figure 6.2 Meaning making in end-of-life care

Scientific or Biological Meanings

Care providers who attribute death to biological or scientific causes often refer to the fatal nature of a disease, to the limited control of science, or to the natural disintegration of a diseased body, for example, "The only explanation I can give to death is a biological one. For some reason the body and its various organs fail to function," "It's a matter of biological predisposition. Man is genetically programmed. We are vulnerable to diseases that cannot be cured by science," and "Death exists because we have bodies that are perishable." Such explanations rely on scientific knowledge and biological facts.

Philosophical or Spiritual Meanings

Care providers who attribute philosophical or spiritual meanings address one of the following three basic themes.

1. Death is an integral part of life and of human existence (e.g., "Death is natural," "It is part of life's cycle," "Death is an inevitable reality of human existence").
2. Death is the result of circumstantial factors (e.g., "Death is a matter of temporal, spatial, biological, and situational circumstances," "Life and death are the result of random events").
3. Death is determined by fate, or a supernatural cosmic order (e.g., "It was meant to happen," "Everybody has a predetermined time to live and fulfill a purpose," "We are born with an expiration date").

Sometimes meanings attached to supernatural forces are independent of any religion or ecclesiastic beliefs, as described here:

> I have no affiliation with the church and do not believe in any specific god or religion. . . . I simply believe in a higher power beyond comprehension that doesn't deprive, test, or punish people with diseases and death. It neither interferes with nor determines our life and death. It simply exists, and its existence helps me accept our non-being in death.

Religious Meanings

Some care providers resort to religious explanations and make sense of death by attributing it to God's will, or to karma, or to the master plan of a deity who puts the dying and the bereaved to the test, for example, "I believe in a higher power—whether this is God, the Virgin Mary, or Christ—who decides what our purpose and destination in life are and when it all comes to an end."

Religious meanings provide a context for understanding not only death but also life after death, as expressed in the following belief: "Death is not the end; it is the beginning of another life for the deceased."

Meanings in Light of One's Life Trajectory

Death is accepted and invested with positive meaning when a person's life is perceived as meaningful, fulfilling, or purposeful. "He died because he completed his purpose in life by offering his loved ones so many opportunities to learn and grow. . . . He did not die in vain."

No Meaning

For some care providers, making sense of death is a highly distressing experience, and as a result they avoid it altogether.

> I do not make any sense [of death]. I do not consider myself mature enough to plunge into deep waters, and therefore, I do not seek answers because the process is emotionally draining.... You see, I tend to avoid whatever causes me distress.

For others, what they perceive as death's meaninglessness becomes a source of anger and resentment.

> There is no meaning in death. I curse the moment a patient dies and then I do not think about it anymore. I have no explanation. I once tried to make sense of death but concluded that there is no logic to it.... It's meaningless, absurd, and senseless.

Finally, some practitioners accept their inability to attribute any meaning to death and are at peace with not knowing or making sense of a person's death:

> Every time I'm confronted with the death of a patient, I am faced with the realization that there is no sense to be made of it. And that's OK with me. I've learned to live with no answers, no explanations, no religious beliefs or philosophies. What has meaning for me is what I can do to help a person live till he dies...to comfort and to care, to make life easier for him and his relatives.

Multiple Meanings

The attribution of multiple meanings to death reflects either a temporary state of confusion or an advanced level of maturity and an understanding of the complexity of reality. In response to the question "How do you make sense of death?" the following care provider offered a statement that lacked clarity or coherence.

> It's a question of bad luck. It may be caused by unpredictable and circumstantial factors, but it may also be caused by a vicious disease that we were unable to cure. Sometimes I believe that the person's psychology may play a part, but then again, I am not sure.... The only thing I am certain about is that death is *not* God's will and *not* part of a divine plan.

To transcend the confusion evoked by these divergent meanings, this care provider resorted to explanations of what death is not. Winchester-Nadeau (1998), who studied meaning making in bereaved families, describes "not statements" as helping to define death in terms of what it is not. She suggests that they occur in the early phases of the meaning-making process, when one is struggling with alternative meanings to provide answers to existential concerns. "Not statements" change in the advanced stages of meaning making, when care providers integrate divergent and conflicting meanings into a representation of a reality that is characterized by a higher order of coherence.

Making Sense of the Dying Process

We seek to make sense by reflecting on not only why patients die, but also how they die. In other words, we strive to answer questions such as "How was the dying process for this person?" "Why did he or she die in this way?" "Was dying foreseeable, preventable, pain-free, and peaceful, or was it unexpected, filled with physical and emotional suffering?" "Was the death appropriate and dignified?"

We make sense of a person's dying by evaluating whether it led to a good or a bad death, according to our goals of care. For some care providers, dignified dying conditions are associated with a terminal period that is free of pain for a person who is aware and prepared to die, and surrounded by loved ones who respect his or her needs, wishes, and preferences. For others, it is associated with an extremely brief dying trajectory that prevents suffering and the realization of one's critical condition. Still others find meaning in a dying process that occurs in a cocoon-like environment that protects the person from coming to an awareness of his or her terminal condition and spares the family from the anguish of death.

The ongoing debate between proponents and opponents of euthanasia is another indication of how we, the professionals, strive to make sense of how people die and our responsibility to ensure that dying is meaningful to them and to us. For example, for proponents of euthanasia, conditions that lead to a dignified death involve the respect of a person's fundamental right to end his or her life when suffering is intolerable. Through the act of euthanasia, biological death is hastened so that social death can be avoided. For opponents of euthanasia and legislation permitting it, dying is invested with positive meanings when physical pain is under control, and the person's and family's suffering is mitigated through communication and the provision of psychosocial and spiritual support by an interdisciplinary team of skilled professionals.

Making Sense of Our Contribution to and Role in the Care of Others

Not every care provider develops a coherent and consistent system of meanings to account for death and dying. However, all of us strive to make sense of the services we provide. We attach various appraisal meanings to them by seeking to answer questions such as "Were my services effective, meaningful, and worthwhile?" "How do I know that I did a good job?" "How did I contribute to the quality of life of this person or family?" "How have I been helpful or unhelpful to them?" "How was I affected by this person's death?" "What did I learn that will help me assist others more efficiently?" "What contribution am I making?"

By attributing positive meaning to our role and interventions, we succeed in integrating losses into our personal and professional worlds. In so doing, we achieve two important tasks: first, we put the care of the dying and the bereaved in a broader contextual framework, and second, we derive satisfaction from being engaged in important and relevant work.

Some care providers consider their number one priority the striving to cure disease or to prolong life. As a result, they attach *biological-related meanings* to the care they provide, as well as to all attempts that aim to prevent death, prolong life, and eradicate physical suffering. Death acquires meaning because of their actions and interventions to prevent or control it. They think: "At least I've tried all sorts of interventions to save his life" or "I did my best to alleviate her physical pain." These statements are indicative of an appraisal that is focused on task-oriented interventions. These are placed in a meaningful context that associates caregiving with *doing to* or *acting upon* a person's physical condition. Specialized knowledge, expertise, and competence in managing the threat of death through scientific means are overemphasized.

Other professionals consider palliation their number one priority and attach meanings to *being with* and *accompanying* a person and family through terminal illness by offering a supportive presence and secure bond.

> He had the best death ever, with family, physicians, and nurses—even the lab technician—at his bedside. He left this world in glory and honor. . . . and I was satisfied with the care we were able to provide to him.

Such *relationship-related meanings* derive from an approach that reinforces the development of an accompaniment approach that fosters intimate bonds and assists the dying and his or her family with the challenges of terminal care.

Finally, some professionals attach meanings to their role and contribution only in the context of a broader framework that fosters teamwork and interdisciplinary collaboration. Meanings are associated with the orchestration of various services and collaboration among co-workers in an attempt to *do* to and *be with* people who are dying and grieving.

In summary, grieving involves the construction of meanings about death, about the process of dying, and about our contribution to the care of others. Are specific meanings more appropriate than others? For example, do religious meanings facilitate the acceptance of death, or the integration of our losses into our life and work, any more or less than scientific ones? How is loss integration affected by biological- versus relationship-related meanings that we attach to our contribution to and role in the care of others? Are there positive and negative meanings that can be objectively determined? These are questions for which we do not yet have clear answers and that demand extensive research.

It is my belief that meanings are simply meanings. We cannot objectively classify them as positive or negative. Some of them are more emotionally charged than others or have a distinct importance in one's view of life. As a result, they affect grieving in different ways. The belief that death is God's will, for example, may help one care provider integrate loss-related experiences into a religious framework that accepts death as a reality that cannot be prevented, controlled, or understood by humans, but it may hinder integration in another provider who holds ambivalent feelings about God, whom he or she resents for causing suffering. Thus, a particular meaning may facilitate or hinder the grieving process in different care providers. Conversely, different—even divergent—meanings may have similar effects and facilitate loss integration. For example, care providers who believe that they did their best by engaging in extreme curative interventions to save a person's life and care providers who did their best by developing an intimate relationship with the person and family they accompanied through dying hold divergent systems of meanings with regard to how they appraise their services and value their work; however, in spite of their differences, both have systems of meanings that help them integrate patient death into their assumptive worlds and professional modes of operation.

What is therefore important to consider is how meanings associated with dying, death, and caregiving confirm or disconfirm our assumptive worlds, facilitate or hinder grieving and loss integration, and fit with or oppose the collective meanings that are held by our team.

PROPOSITION 4

Personal meanings are affected by meanings that are shared by co-workers, and vice versa

Meaning making is not solely an individual intrapsychic process, but also a social process. Winchester-Nadeau (1998) asserts that "meanings are the products of interactions with others... and symbolically represent various elements of reality" (p. 159). Therefore, the meanings we attach to death, dying, and caregiving are not only representations of our subjective reality but also the result of interactions with others, particularly with our co-workers, who are exposed to the same death situations and caring conditions.

When our team engages in a collective process of meaning making, we distance ourselves from our lived experiences and compare our personal meanings to those of our co-workers and/or supervisors. Along with them, we develop collective or shared meanings that offer us an opportunity to construct a new reality. These collective or shared meanings may affect our perception and experience of reality.

How are collective meanings created? In at least two ways: through the sharing of narratives and experiences, and through participation in collective rituals.

Sharing experiences with colleagues and co-workers contributes to the construction of collective meanings. We tell and listen to stories that explain someone's illness, suffering, and death, and the value of specific practices over others. Through these shared accounts, certain themes arise that contribute to the creation of collective constructs associated with death, dying, and caregiving in death situations. In some teams, death is discussed only in scientific terms focusing on the person's disease, lab tests, and interventions. In other teams, discussions illuminate multiple aspects of end-of-life care and encourage co-workers to recount their personal experiences. Sometimes conflicts among team members over moral dilemmas (e.g., truth telling, advanced directives, pain control) incite them to reflect upon aspects of their work that are invested with divergent meanings, yet accepted as integral to the team's mode of functioning.

Talking, according to Seale (1998), is a ritual. Few teams opt to remain silent in the face of death and carry on as if nothing happened.

What is said, as well as what is left unsaid, contributes to the creation of collective meanings.

Sometimes sharing goes beyond mere narration and involves the sharing of experiences through action. Think for a moment when you last observed a colleague doing something different that led you to reconsider your role and approach or review the meanings you attach to death, dying, or caregiving in loss situations. Without always being aware of it, we compare and contrast our personal values, feelings, thoughts, and behaviors to those of our co-workers and often adopt identical ideas and behaviors in the care of dying and bereaved people. In that way, we develop collective patterns that are invested with collective meanings that remain unverbalized.

Development of and participation in collective rituals becomes another way by which we create collective meanings. These rituals may involve the commemoration of deceased patients, a day of remembrance that is attended by bereaved families and care providers, and social or other activities dedicated to team building. Through planned rituals, we grieve over the loss of our patients but also affirm our own social belonging among the living. Even though most teams do not develop formal rituals, they often engage in behaviors or activities that serve as rituals.

In an oncology unit, for example, physicians who accompanied their patients through the dying process perceived the closing of a patient's file as a ritual that marked the end of the person's life as well as their relationship to him or her. Nurses who washed and dressed the corpse of a beloved patient also engaged in a ritual activity of love and farewell; this shared ritual helped them attribute positive meaning to both the person's death and their contribution to his or her care. Mental health professionals found the recording of detailed notes of their encounters with dying and bereaved people an opportunity to process and attribute meaning to their experiences, which were subsequently shared with other team members and integrated into the patients' files.

In summary, shared meanings validate the goals, values, and practices of a team regarding the care of dying and bereaved people. They are formed within team boundaries but also serve to maintain them. They enable us to integrate our loss-related experiences into a meaningful narrative and fill the gaps whenever we cannot make sense of a situation.

Occasionally, the death of a person disconfirms collective meanings. This can create a personal or team crisis, as eloquently described in the following account.

> I had never given serious thought to death, probably because I had not experienced any losses besides the deaths of my grandparents. So when I was hired, I willingly adopted the unit's belief that death should be prevented at any cost, even when this causes physical and mental suffering. Fighting death by every possible means became seductive! Fighting was *all* that mattered. Death was justified only if we had exhausted *all* our sophisticated high-tech interventions.... This is how we all perceived our work with seriously ill patients, until we met Mr. Pappas. He was an older man in his mid-70s. He had several heart complications and was brought to the unit by a neighbor, who was relieved to transfer the responsibility for his care to us. During his hospitalization Mr. Pappas begged us to let him die. He objected to all our "barbaric interventions"—that's how he referred to them—and looked forward to being reunited with his son and wife, who had died in a car accident several years before. With them gone, his life had come to an end. He perceived his heart complications as his "passport" to rejoin his family. We totally ignored his protests, avoided all discussions about dying, and carried on with interventions that were unduly life sustaining, thus postponing his unavoidable death. I will never forget the day that our medical director announced triumphantly to Mr. Pappas that we had managed, one more time, to save his life. Mr. Pappas looked at him sadly and said: "You have only saved a frail body, not my life.... You deprived me of the hope of joining my son and wife, because you never listened when I told you that I am prepared and willing to die. Instead, you were busy with your self-serving interventions." That was the last time we saw Mr. Pappas. His words haunted me for a long time. It forced me to think about death and about my work in cardiology. I had doubts about the effectiveness of our services, and I seriously questioned the ideology that supported our actions. I began to seek my own answers to a number of issues. This hasn't been an easy process. Saving lives still remains a priority, but today I do not consider death something invariably bad, nor do I view it as my worst enemy. Conversely, I do not perceive life as invariably good and valuable. Things are not black and white, and our job demands that we cope with a reality that has various shades of gray. In this gray zone we do not have clear-cut answers about what is in the best interest of our patients. *They* have the answers. And all we have to do is to listen carefully and work closely with them, to make the passage from life to death bearable and acceptable.

This account illustrates how meaning making is an ongoing process that is both personal and interpersonal. It is true that we all find comfort in knowing that our colleagues share similar beliefs and attribute similar meanings to death, but in order for collective meanings to be functional and help us make sense of our experiences, they must meet three basic criteria. They must have (1) *internal coherence* (they must have an internal logic), (2) *practical utility* (they must determine concrete ways in which delivered services are effective and meaningful in the face of death), and (3) a high degree of *consensual validation by others* (they must be accepted by colleagues, patients, families, and society).

What happens when the process of collective meaning making leads to divergent meanings? In reality, team consensus (defined as agreement among all team members) is rare. Most often, care providers form subgroups that adopt different values and meanings. Therefore, a team may contain two or three clusters of shared meanings. These may be complementary, different, or divergent. They represent various aspects of the team's reality and experience of death. What is critical to consider is how the team manages divergent meanings, which in turn affects how care providers cope with grief and other responses in the face of death.

Consider the example of a palliative care team whose members refrained from openly sharing beliefs that differed from the "official" beliefs of the team in order to avoid conflict and disorder. Care providers were expected to strive to ensure a good and dignified death, which was often romanticized. Such a death was to be achieved through the bypassing of aggressive treatments and the development of intimate relationships with patients and family members, in which open communication was the golden rule for quality care. Euthanasia was not an option. Everyone had to abide by this philosophy of care and its associated beliefs. There was no tolerance for diversity. Alternative ideas of what constitutes a good or appropriate death and ways to achieve it were expressed only in small groups. Care providers' grief remained private, and personal beliefs were not shared. This led to a major split among team members, who developed opposing views and practices that eventually compromised the quality of care.

In another critical care team, conflicting beliefs were brought out in the open, which gave rise to lively debates, strong oppositions, and conflicts, especially with regard to the issue of euthanasia. Everyone's views and personal meanings were heard and respected, and no one was forced to engage in practices that were in direct opposition to his or her personal philosophy of care and beliefs about life and death. With the support of the leader, the team was engaged in an ongoing dialogue, displayed high tolerance for cognitive confusion and emotional tension, and allowed new beliefs to emerge, new roles and responsibilities to be assumed, and alternative ways of coping with death-related experiences to be practiced. Team members gradually developed refined approaches toward individuals and families who voiced requests for euthanasia, palliative care, or treatments aimed at prolonging life. In this team, learning to respect individual and collective meanings and work in collaboration became more important than reaching a consensus among team members. Out of temporary disorder, a new order of divergent beliefs emerged that allowed loss integration into team members' modes of functioning and enriched the team's approach to end-of-life care.

PROPOSITION 5

Grief overload and grief complications occur when there is no fluctuation between experiencing and avoiding loss and grief

We experience grief overload and grief complications when there is discontinuity or an absence of fluctuation between experiencing and avoiding loss and grief. Under these conditions, we become overwhelmed and consumed by grief; unable to set it aside to effectively manage the care of others, we end up suppressing it and avoiding all thoughts and feelings that relate to our experiences of loss. Grief overload is distinct from grief complications, which have a long and pervasive negative impact upon our functioning and well-being.

Grief overload has a temporary effect on our daily functioning and is more or less transitory. It usually occurs when we are exposed to multiple losses or deaths within a short period of time or relive a personal loss triggered by work-related experiences. Under those circumstances, we feel overwhelmed by grief that we have difficulty managing. "Only this month, six of my little friends died," a young psychologist who was working with terminally ill children wrote in her diary. "I don't want to face any more death. Death is like a sun. It may illuminate deeper levels of awareness and enhance both meaning and purpose in my life, but it may also hurt my eyes and blind my soul when I'm exposed repeatedly."

For some time this psychologist avoided entering the rooms of seriously ill people, discussing their health conditions, and supporting family members and was absent minded and disengaged during staff meetings. For a few weeks she distanced herself from death situations and focused solely upon patients who were responsive to treatment and had a good prognosis. Through supervision she explored her grief over her patients' deaths and recognized a parallel grief over the loss of beliefs that were important to her. Beliefs such as "Giving the best of oneself in a caring relationship can ensure a good death," "I must protect the young and the disadvantaged from suffering," and "Only good things happen to good people" were disconfirmed; this led to the gradual development of more realistic ones.

Cook and Oltjenbrun (1998) use the term "incremental grief" to describe the additive effect of related losses that are grieved and re-grieved over time. These losses comprise not only death, but also the loss of one's goals and ideals, as well as the changes experienced in one's constructions and assumptive worlds. When grief over several losses is disenfranchised, it oftentime surfaces when one least expects it, as reported by one nurse:

> Sometimes it happens when I least expect it. While I am crying for something personal, I include in my sorrow a second grief for a patient who died in our unit, and I cry also for those other patients who died and with whom I shared a special bond.

Grief complications occur when the absence of a fluctuation between experiencing and avoiding loss and grief becomes chronic and compromises our well-being as well as the quality of care we provide. We know very little about grief complications in care providers, probably because they are often confused or coexist with depression, anxiety disorders, compassion fatigue, burnout, and chronic psychosomatic conditions that impair one's physical and mental health. Sometimes they coexist with alcoholism and drug abuse, or are hidden behind violent patterns of interaction with patients, their families, and colleagues.

In an attempt to illuminate grief complications, I wish to describe three forms that are common in clinical practice: chronic and compounded grief, inhibited grief, and grief in coexistence with trauma responses.

Chronic and Compounded Grief

In the description of her long career trajectory through oncology, Elisabeth, an experienced physician who was loved by patients, their families, and colleagues, described how she changed over the years. The bonds she developed with patients, which were initially a source of significant gratification, progressively came to be an unbearable burden. She admitted having developed a superficial closeness with patients in order to avoid what she referred to as "an intimacy that kills me" and described her life as "inundated by death and ongoing grief," which she experienced only in private. She recognized her difficulty addressing and processing her experiences, as well as her inability to keep them at a distance from her family life. Unable to differentiate her own pain from that of her patients, she said: "I don't laugh anymore. . . . I feel totally overwhelmed by my own pain, which seems endless. . . . I am trapped in a suffering from which I cannot escape."

Feldstein and Buschman-Gemma (1995), who conducted a study on the grief of oncology nurses who were repeatedly exposed to the deaths of their adult patients, found that professionals to whom they administered the Grief Experience Inventory experienced increased levels of despair, social isolation, and somatization. The researchers identified and described a phenomenon, referred to as chronic compounded grief, among nurses who worked in oncology, as well as among nurses who had resigned or transferred to other work settings.

Chronic grief is ongoing and affects one's entire life. Sometimes it is somatized; other times it is kept private and hidden from public view; still other times, it is idealized and used to gain attention or meet other personal needs. Let's consider these three patterns.

When somatized, our grief is displayed through chronic pains, physical symptoms, and health problems or disorders that occur in the absence of emotional suffering. We feel unwell. Our attention is displaced from the chronic pain of grief to the physical management of symptoms, which is less threatening and invites concern and sympathy from others.

When chronic grief becomes a private affair, we spend our energy masking a suffering of which we feel ashamed. We fear that if we openly express it, we will let loose hidden dragons that will burden our loved ones or will bring us into conflict with colleagues or our team. As a result, we cultivate emotional restraint that disallows expression. Utterly lonely and alone, we are deprived of a holding environment in which we can safely process our experiences. In the interviews I conducted with care providers, several admitted that for the first time in their lives, they abandoned their professional facades in order to openly share a grief that they described as "ever present," "ongoing," and "profound" for several years.

Finally, sometimes we idealize our grief and thus render it chronic. We perceive it as a virtue that brings us closer to patients and families, with whom we develop enmeshed relationships. We endure suffering, which is often dramatized, and adopt a martyr role that gives purpose and meaning to our work. Our accounts are filled with pride over our ability to experience the suffering of patients and their families to whom we are unconditionally dedicated and attached. Giving up our suffering would deprive us of a valued purpose and disrupt our conviction that we sacrifice our happiness for a higher or noble cause. Chronic grief becomes our trophy.

Inhibited Grief

Grief that is systematically inhibited leaves us estranged from ourselves and others. We either deny or systematically suppress our grief responses, as described in the following account:

> [When death occurs] I carry on as if nothing happened. My days are scheduled with so many activities and responsibilities that I do not have time to think or feel. I have a busy life: responsibilities at work, lectures I have to prepare for conferences, looking after the needs of my children, being involved with the parents' association at their school, accompanying my husband to business dinners. Even though such a life seems hectic, I must admit that it suits me. It normalizes things. It fills life with action and distracts me from the pain and the stillness of death.

Keeping busy becomes a refuge that helps many professionals systematically avoid grief. Instead of taking action, others mobilize cognitive and emotional processes to suppress their feelings and thoughts and project an image of overcompetence. "I put my pain in a little drawer and do not allow myself to think or feel.... I've learned to simply switch off and avoid all visual images of what I've witnessed." This physician was proud that during the two decades she worked in oncology, she had managed to avoid being present at her patients' deaths. Still others resort to symbolic acts that give them permission to move forward and forget about their loss. "After a patient dies, I want to be the one to sign the death certificate. Signing helps me to close the parentheses... and switch off everything."

What does the signing a death certificate mean for this particular care provider? What does she put in parentheses—the patient's life? the patient's death? her grief? her services?

When a work setting is threatened by the suffering of its members, it adopts rules that overregulate emotional expression and encourage grief inhibition (see principle 2 in chapter 9). Under those conditions, care providers acknowledge yet suppress or deny their grief. This phenomenon is described by Eyetsemitan (1998) as "stifled grief." When stifled grief becomes chronic, it leads to dysfunctional patterns that increase the suffering of care providers.

Grief in Coexistence With Trauma Responses

It is often assumed that grief cannot coexist with acute trauma. Clinical experience, however, shows that some deaths that are perceived as traumatic may elicit both grief and acute trauma responses. As a result, one day we may be grieving over an anticipated or actual loss, and the next, we may be struggling with traumatic responses displayed through flashbacks, intrusive thoughts and feelings, or an overwhelming sense of guilt over missed opportunities to prevent death. Grieving is thus complicated by trauma, which triggers an involuntary intrusion-avoidance oscillation that fragments our experience.

In summary, grief complications delay or prevent our ability to integrate death and loss into our work and personal lives. As a result, we often experience a sense of immobilization, of being trapped or stuck in an emotional impasse from which we cannot escape. Our sense of time is suspended. There is no movement or growth. We remain silent or ruminate over experiences over which we feel anxiety and despair. We hardly ever learn from our experience, since we avoid addressing our grief. Our ability to benefit and grow through suffering is seriously compromised.

There is no doubt that extensive research is warranted to allow us to better understand which care providers are most vulnerable to grief complications, and which factors contribute to their increased suffering that may extend over several years.

PROPOSITION 6

Grief offers opportunities for personal growth

While grieving can lead to complications, it also holds the potential for growth. It is only during the past decade that attention has been drawn to the positive changes that can result from the struggle of coping with major losses or traumatic experiences (e.g., Tedeschi & Calhoun, 1995; Calhoun & Tedeschi, 1998). Yet even more recently, studies have been conducted to assess the growth that is experienced by care providers who offer services to dying and bereaved people (e.g., Clarke-Steffen, 1998;

Eifried, 2003; Maeve, 1998). These studies acknowledge the personal and professional benefits that we derive from our confrontations with death.

Nevertheless, coming to terms with death and grief proves to be a major challenge for some care providers. Not all of us are willing to face death and accept the pain of loss that is associated with such confrontations. Death denial and grief avoidance narrow our inner lives, blur our vision, and prevent us from helping others face their mortality and grief. By becoming oblivious to death, loss, and grief, we end up developing relationships characterized by a conspiracy of silence surrounding death and the suffering that such experiences elicit in ourselves and in others.

Unfortunately, many care providers enter the professions of medicine, psychology, nursing, and pastoral care with a strong desire to save people from death and suffering, and the expectation that they will always be able to alleviate physical, psychosocial, and spiritual pain while remaining unaffected by their losses. Such unrealistic goals prevent them from accepting the inevitability of death, the transience of life, and their pain over the severance of human bonds. Most importantly, these goals deprive them of the possibility of deriving an enduring sense of satisfaction from the services they provide and diminish opportunities for personal growth.

Based on his vast clinical experience and existential approach, Yalom (2008) describes how death confrontation can awaken us to a fuller life that makes us mindful of our existence. Not only death but also the inevitable experience of grief can be an awakening experience. Both realities render us more conscious of our ability to love, to bond, and to connect with people whom we accompany. Through companioning, we must develop realistic goals and accept that we cannot provide the dying and the bereaved with what they most desire. In other words, we cannot prevent death for a person who is dying, nor can we bring back the deceased in order to spare the bereaved from his or her suffering. At the same time, neither the dying nor the bereaved can gratify our desire to alleviate all their pain (Parkes, 1972). Thus, helping people who are dying and grieving requires an acceptance of mortality (including our own), of suffering, and the potential for growth.

Thus, when we accept death and grieve our losses, we also help others to do the same. In so doing, we are likely to experience changes that lead to a sense of personal and professional growth. Growth is associated with changes in our views of ourselves, others, life, and our ability to develop caring relationships. These are further elaborated below.

Growth Associated With Our Perception of Ourselves

I feel more whole as a person, with a clear orientation and purpose in life.

Examples of changes in our views and experience of ourselves include an altered, more positive self concept; an altered view of our ability to cope with stress and regulate affect and personal suffering; an altered view of our identity as professionals (e.g., more competent, empathic, compassionate); an acceptance of our strengths, vulnerabilities, and limitations; and the elaboration and working through of unaddressed personal issues that affect our encounters with loss and experience of grief.

We cease to view ourselves as omnipotent, striving to save the world, and able to eradicate all suffering. Rather, we experience ourselves as vulnerable and good enough, aware of our strengths and limitations. Paradoxically, vulnerability coexists with a positive view of self.

Growth Associated With Our Perception of and Connection to Others

All I have learned through this job is about love... loving others and giving myself permission to be loved in return.

Examples of changes in our relationships with others are the development of an empathic view of others, characterized by increased understanding and compassion; an enriched way of relating both in joy and in pain; an openness and desire to learn from others and from their experiences; and an ability to develop intimate relationships that sustain suffering and enhance growth.

We are less concerned with enacting a role and maintaining a professional position or title and become more involved with others. Genuine and expressive, we display greater warmth and caring and are willing to offer and receive support in times of trouble. We acknowledge the universality of suffering in the face of death but also recognize the value of connectedness, which tempers and alleviates the pain of loss and separation.

Growth Associated With Our View and Experience of Caregiving

I have come to the awareness that caring for patients who are terminally ill is not *a* significant job, but a job that is significant to *me*.

Examples of changes in our approaches to caregiving are the development of an appreciation of shared experiences with the individuals and families whom we care for; an increased sense of fulfillment at having facilitated the natural yet painful process of bonding, parting, and grieving in others and ourselves; an ability to incorporate the realities of dying and bereaved people into our understandings of our own lives; and an ability to pass along the wisdom that we acquire from accompanying people through dying and bereavement.

We value what we offer but also recognize what we gain in return. This enlarges our horizon, allowing us to engage in more altruistic actions, and enhances our sense of contribution to the community and to human welfare. Commitment, purpose, and meaningfulness become integral to the process of caregiving and help us transcend the hardships of a stressful and challenging job.

Growth Associated With Our Life Perspective

> I have learned to appreciate every day and have come to terms with the reality that death and suffering are part of the deal.

Changes in our philosophy and approach to life may involve a confrontation with mortality and acceptance of life's transience; an increased awareness of our goals, values, and priorities in life; an altered sense of time; an active striving to live a fuller life that is invested with positive meaning; and an increased sense of belonging to the world and to the human community.

Life is not perceived superficially, but valued and lived with increased awareness. The present is lived with greater clarity, and the future is imagined, anticipated, and invested in with goals and dreams, without being taken for granted. Some feel connected to something larger, transcendent, and all encompassing, whether this is God, a higher power, or a cosmic plan. We experience life as beautiful, precious, and unique, as well as full of challenges, adversities, and suffering. The dark side of life makes us value and treasure with greater awareness the little and big joys of life.

I wish to introduce a word of caution with regard to the concept of growth. Sometimes what is perceived as growth is merely a strategy of self-protection against the anxiety of death and threats to our worldview (Davis & McKearney, 2003). We exaggerate the meaningfulness of our work and of life in order to temper the threat of mortality and constrict our grief or suffering in loss situations. Viewing life and work as highly meaningful and idealizing the rewards of caregiving prevent us from working through our suffering and protect us from despair. It is therefore important to view growth as a *process* that stems from our struggle to cope with loss and suffering, rather than as the outcome of a challenging job or the direct effect of our experiences of loss. It is a process of becoming and evolving that requires time and a willingness to process experiences. According to Davis and McKearney (2003), "it is a process of finding new goals, new perspectives, new identities, and testing them and refining them against the data of life experience" (p. 490). Such a process is not restricted to the identification of meaningful goals but involves an active movement toward achieving these goals, which are interwoven in every aspect of life, personal and professional.

Not every care provider experiences growth. Even though many professionals report changes in their perception of themselves, others, life, and caregiving—usually after having experienced distressing experiences, losses, or traumas—these changes are often ephemeral. Moreover, when suffering and grief are overpowering, losses are accumulative, and care providers are overwhelmed by the demands of their work, then the possibility of growth diminishes or disappears.

In summary, when we acknowledge and address our grief, not only are we helped to integrate losses into our private and team worlds, but we allow these worlds to be enriched by transforming the pain of grief into a conscious living of a fuller life. Moreover, we become more able to help others temper their fear of death, accept their suffering, and allow themselves to be changed by it. Unlike many colleagues who work in other fields of health care, we are privileged to work with people who provide us with many opportunities to benefit from leading a more fulfilling life as a result of our confrontation with death and grief.

PROPOSITION 7

The professional's grieving process is affected by several interacting variables

The final proposition suggests that in order to fully understand our grief, we must explore it in the larger context within which it occurs and recognize the multiple variables that affect it. These variables, for descriptive purposes, are clustered in the following categories: personal, work-related, situational, education- and profession-related, and sociocultural variables (Papadatou, 2001).

Personal and Work-Related Variables

Each of us has a unique way of experiencing and coping with loss that is affected by several variables. Of these variables, the ones over which we can exert control are those that are personal and work related. In an attempt to understand them, we will explore how grief is affected by our lifestyle and by our team's style or mode of functioning.

Our *lifestyle*[2] comprises a system of basic assumptions, beliefs, and values about ourselves, others, and life that we develop early in childhood and that provides a consistent way of perceiving, interpreting, and behaving in everyday living, and of predicting the future (Adler, 1923/1971). We interpret, attribute meanings to, and cope with loss encounters according to our idiosyncratic system of beliefs, values, and assumptions. Our lifestyle offers a familiar cognitive map (which is biased and subjective) that guides us in understanding and coping with life events, making choices, and relating to others. Major loss and death events occurring in early childhood affect our beliefs about what to expect and strive for in loss situations. They orient our behavior and determine to a large degree our grief responses to loss later in life. Many of the ways in which we interpret and cope with daily losses at work can be understood in light of our lifestyle.

For example, a care provider who was affected during early childhood by the sudden death of his father perceived himself as weak and helpless, others as non-trusting, and life as unpredictable and full of unpleasant surprises. His movement in life was determined by the belief that he would be safe, valued, and appreciated in life only if he had absolute control over situations, over his feelings and experiences, and over others. Caring for dying individuals was a constant striving to prove by way of his specialized knowledge and expertise that he could master challenging situations and remain in control. As an overachiever, he also strove to gain the trust and respect of others. His work in an intensive care unit gave him the opportunity to perform heroic acts in order to save people's lives. Death, however, was experienced as a personal failure that elicited feelings of helplessness and worthlessness.

A *team's work style,* on the other hand, is a collective system of assumptions, beliefs, and values about care that govern the team's collective mode of functioning. The work style of a team provides care providers with an organized and consistent approach to care that determines—among other things—how they should feel and behave as well as how they should perceive and make sense of death-related experiences. Its collective mode of operation affects whether professionals acknowledge, suppress, or deny their suffering; whether they seek and receive support from co-workers; and how they regulate the fluctuation between experiencing and avoiding grief (see principle 2 in chapter 9).

In a pediatric oncology unit, for example, professionals made a clear distinction between "their" patients—those who were diagnosed and cared for exclusively by the team—and "foreign" patients, who were diagnosed in other institutions and were cared for only partially in that particular unit. As a result of this distinction, the team had different ways of investing in relationships and caregiving. Patients who "belonged" to the unit were "owned" by care providers ("our patients"). Their deaths affected team members who openly shared their grief in contrast to patients in transit, who were referred to as the "foreigners."

A team's work style can reinforce, complement, or be in conflict with a care provider's lifestyle (Papadatou, 2000). In that respect, it may facilitate or hinder the grieving process and the integration of work-related losses into one's assumptive world and mode of team functioning (see principles 2 and 3 in chapter 9). Both personal and work-related variables affect the kind of relationships we develop with others as well as our ability to form and maintain secure attachments with dying and bereaved people.

Situational Variables

Situational variables are related to specific circumstances that occur in our personal lives (e.g., a sudden illness, death, divorce). During these times, we experience an increased vulnerability that can lead to the development of enmeshed or avoidant relationships with the people we accompany.

However, situational variables are also related to specific circumstances we experience at work and strongly affect our responses to loss encounters. Consider, for example, a care provider who happens to be on vacation when her favorite patient suddenly dies. Her absence from the death scene, her lack of involvement in the death rituals, and her nonparticipation in staff meetings in which the patient's trajectory and professionals' experiences and feelings are reviewed seem to complicate her grief, which is affected by increased guilt and a sense that she has not attained closure. On her return to the unit, her grief remains unaddressed and resurfaces every time she is confronted with a sudden death.

Education- and Profession-Related Variables

Our grief is also affected by the expectations, beliefs, and values that are transmitted to us through our formal education and through the prevailing culture of our professional discipline, which determine what our role and professional responsibility are in death situations. During our formative years in medicine, nursing, psychology, or other allied disciplines, we are socialized into the world of death, dying, and bereavement by observing our instructors, clinical supervisors, and senior colleagues and using them as role models. This socialization process affects not only the nature of services we provide, but also our responses to the illness, dying, and bereavement processes of the people we serve.

Even though recent revisions to educational curricula in medicine, nursing, and psychology have attempted to integrate courses on palliative and bereavement care, it must be noted that such courses rarely provide an opportunity for self-exploration and understanding of personal and collective responses in the face of human loss. Educators and supervisors remain uncomfortable with the sharing of personal feelings and responses to dying and bereaved people, and graduates are left alone to make sense of their suffering, which they learn to disregard or repress when they enter the workplace.

Sociocultural Variables

Last but not least, our responses are also affected by the sociocultural contexts in which we live, work, and offer our services. Sociocultural values and norms affect at least three parameters: how we express grief, how we make sense of patients' deaths, and what types of supports we seek or receive when grieving the loss of our patients.

In the transcultural study we conducted, the large majority of nurses in Greece and Hong Kong acknowledged that they experienced grief over the death of children, but they had distinct ways of expressing it as a result of their cultural backgrounds. Greek professionals expressed their emotions more openly, cried more frequently, sought support from each other, and displayed their pain in their interactions with families as well as with the researcher who interviewed them. In contrast, Chinese professionals were more private about their suffering, which they suppressed by retreating into practical duties and tasks (Papadatou et al., 2001).

Moreover, the two groups of professionals attributed different meanings to death, which were affected by religious and cultural factors. These meanings sometimes facilitated and at other times aggravated their grief. While most Greek and Chinese nurses relied on their religious beliefs to make sense of childhood death, their religious meanings elicited distinct feelings. Greek nurses experienced a strong sense of injustice and were angry at God, who—according to their Orthodox Christian beliefs—is perceived as all powerful, loving, and protective of the innocent. The idea that the child's death was His will was met with ambivalence and resentment. In contrast, Chinese nurses, who believed in the law of karma, accepted death more readily and perceived it as a form of salvation from suffering or as a path toward reincarnation. Less expressive of their grief, they strove to ensure a peaceful passage that was believed to ascertain a good reincarnation.

Finally, sociocultural factors affect the types of supports that are available and upon which we rely when we offer end-of-life care. In Greek culture, mutual support among co-workers is highly valued and facilitates the display and sharing of grief, while in Chinese culture, grief is more private and rarely shared with others.

It is interesting to note that in individualistic and achievement-oriented cultures, professionals are expected to be self-reliant, autonomous high achievers and accountable for their behavior. These cultural values affect not only how they provide support to others, but also how they seek and receive support when they are under stress. A typical example of this is the current implementation of employee assistance programs in U.S. organizations. These worksite-based programs are designed to assist organizations in addressing productivity issues and help employees identify and resolve personal concerns and emotional issues that affect their job performance (McClure, 2004). Such programs use a variety of strategies to reduce the incidence, prevalence, and extent of psychopathology in the workplace and are considered suitable for addressing care providers' suffering, which is, unfortunately, viewed and treated as atypical. In contrast, in cultures that value interdependence, collaboration, and mutual support, care providers are more likely to rely on work-related and community sources of formal and informal supports in order to manage the challenges of caring, as well as their need to share grief with colleagues who are exposed to the same work conditions.

In an increasingly multicultural world, supportive services for care providers must be adjusted to individual and team preferences, and the organizational and sociocultural context in which professionals' grief occurs and unfolds must be taken into consideration. The complexity and synergy of the multiple factors described above illustrate why there is not one type of supportive intervention that can address all professionals who care for people in death situations. Huggard (2003) argues that nowadays, health care organizations are challenged more than ever before to respect and care for their employees in the same way they require their employees to care for patients. In so doing, organizations support and assist care providers in sustaining and further developing their humanism.

In conclusion, the proposed model of care providers' grieving process suggests that while we are providing care to dying and bereaved people, we are likely to experience a normal and healthy grieving process over the multiple losses we encounter as a result of our repeated exposure to death. Characteristic of our grief is the fluctuation between experiencing and suppressing our grief responses that enables us to attribute meaning to the deaths of our patients as well as to caregiving. Our responses to loss are affected by the interactions between several personal, work-related, situational, institutional, and sociocultural variables. These variables can contribute to the disenfranchisement of our grief and lead to shame, loneliness, and alienation, or they can facilitate loss integration and personal growth.

Do we maintain continuing bonds with the people we serve? We hold onto memories of patients who, through their experiences, provided us with opportunities to review our work, our practices, and our lives. Without always being aware of it, we internalize their presence and/or our relationships with them, which serves to guide our actions, the formulation of professional goals, and even some personal choices in life. Thus the bond that is being maintained with unforgettable patients serves as a symbol for the many forgotten bonds that affect the quality of services we provide to people at the end of life and through bereavement.

NOTES

1. *Meaning making* is often confounded with *cognitive appraisal*. While the first involves cognitive, emotional, and behavioral components in one's attempt to make

sense of a given situation, the latter refers to a cognitive process by which a person defines an event as positive, negative, or neutral.

2. Adler's concept of lifestyle is quite similar to concepts proposed by other theorists who used different terminologies. For example, Bowlby referred to our "internal working model," Parkes to our "assumptive worlds," and Neimeyer to a system of "internal constructs" against which we match any new information resulting from an experience of loss in order to recognize what is happening and plan future behavior.

7 The Rewards of Caregiving

Melanie was a very close friend of mine. We met at a jazz club, where we had both gone to listen to a favorite local pianist. We immediately connected and spent a very pleasant evening talking about life and academic challenges, since we were both students at the University of Arizona. To my surprise, a few weeks later, Melanie appeared in my class on death, dying, and bereavement. She had been invited as a guest speaker to share her experience of being diagnosed with a rare form of cancer and of living with an uncertain future and poor prognosis. She shared with clarity and humor her adventures with treatments, hospitalizations, and professionals who were oblivious to the needs of their patients, hiding their insecurities behind uniforms and professional titles.

I was impressed by her feisty spirit, positive attitude about life, and determination to use her experience to teach others about caring in a humane and sensitive way and respecting the rights of patients. At the end of class we reconnected, and from that day on we were best friends and soul sisters.

In the years that followed, Melanie spent most of her time in the hospital due to repeated relapses. During her long hospitalizations, my day would start with a visit to her room to share a fresh cup of coffee and end after the closing of the university library at night, when I stopped by to see her and chat. As we shared our daily experiences, we allowed each other to become acquainted with each other's world: on one hand, the hospital world, where illness and death served as daily reminders of the value of life, and on the other hand, the academic world, where information and knowledge aimed to prepare the young to become competent and skilled professionals. In both worlds, learning about life was distinct yet profound.

Melanie formed personal relationships with all the members of the oncology team, whom she addressed by surname. Outspoken, inquisitive, and assertive, she always made sure that her needs were met and demanded that her rights as a patient be respected. She expected to be informed about every aspect of her care and to receive detailed explanations and a rationale for proposed protocols, and she studied the side effects of each proposed treatment before she gave her consent or negotiated the administration of experimental drugs. This caused considerable distress for the medical professionals, who at times resented her need for such a degree of control. She had to have the last word on what was done to her body, a body that she insisted to "own."

Her treating physician was a young, bright, and competent physician known for his work in the treatment of her disease. Trained in a biomedical approach, he was stiff and formal in his interactions with patients. One morning, I happened to be present when he entered Melanie's room with a few residents. He stood at the edge of her bed and solemnly announced that the lab results were positive, indicating a new relapse. As soon as he began to present a new treatment protocol, Melanie interrupted him and gently said to him: "Do you know what I need *most,* right now?" There was silence in the room. Then she said in a calm voice, "I need you to sit on my bed, right here next to me, and give me a hug." Despite his discomfort, the physician reluctantly sat on her bed and, in front of the interns, who giggled to hide their own malaise, gave Melanie a big hug. They chatted for awhile in a friendly tone and decided to discuss the options for treatment at a later time. It was obvious that both of them were moved by this brief encounter.

There were many occasions when Melanie would surprise members of the team, do the unexpected, and challenge them but also show genuine care and concern for them as both individuals and professionals who had highly stressful jobs. She was encouraging to those who were compassionate and humane in their approach and gave them feedback on what they were doing that was helpful to her.

"You will become an excellent doctor," she once told a resident, "because when I complain about my suffering, I do not just feel *listened to,* but I am actually *heard* by you." Another time, she complimented a young nurse who felt helpless to assist her with some tough decisions by telling her, "What I like about you is that you can stand by me in this ordeal even though nothing makes sense to me or to you."

When Melanie died, several staff members of the unit attended her funeral. Among them was her treating physician, who admitted that this was the first time he had ever participated in a patient's funeral.

Ten years later, I flew back to Tucson to visit Phil, a beloved friend of mine whose wife had just died from a life-threatening disease. While we were talking, the phone rang and I heard Phil describe Joan's last days of life at home to the person at the other end of the receiver. They were peaceful and he was doing OK. When he hung up the phone, I was surprised to learn that it was her physician, who was calling to find out how Phil was doing after his spouse's death. Phil described him as a highly competent and a compassionate physician. During Joan's last visit to his office, he proposed a protocol, which she declined. Even though he admitted disagreeing with her decision, he showed total respect for her choice to receive palliative care services at home and promised to remain available to Joan and to Phil. When she was ready to leave his office, Phil recounted, he accompanied her to the door and gave her a hug, which she greatly appreciated.

I hurried to ask the name of this physician who respected Joan's choice, put her needs first over his scientific goals or preferences, and remained very caring for both his patient and bereaved spouse. It was Melanie's physician!

I use Melanie's example to illustrate that the rewards of caregiving stem from relationships. They have the potential to enrich our personal lives and subsequently allow us to further enrich the lives of others. Melanie's experience with cancer had a profound effect not only upon her physician (and possibly upon other staff members), but also upon me, as I learned the value of connecting and communicating by observing her interactions with the professionals who cared for her. Her experiences later affected my clinical work in pediatric palliative care and my role as an educator of future health care professionals.

For many decades, the literature on health care provider professionals has focused on the "hazards" of caregiving and neglected the potentially positive benefits and satisfaction that we can derive from caring for people in illness, loss, and trauma situations. It has mistakenly been assumed that listening to the suffering or witnessing the illness and death of another person is highly distressing and depressing and increases the risk of burnout with no benefits. Nevertheless, initial research with hospice care providers, emergency workers, and soldiers has shown that coping with death, trauma, and destruction can be positively related to benefit finding and rewarding experiences.

The question that is subsequently raised is: Who are the care providers who are most likely to derive greater rewards and benefit personally and professionally from the care they provide to dying and bereaved people? According to Britt, Adler, and Bartone (2001) these are professionals who are hardy[1] and tend to attribute positive meaning to their work. Tedeschi and Calhoun (1995) describe individuals who are extraverted, open to their subjective experiences, optimistic, and hardy. However, the authors suggest that people who cope well with adversity may have less to gain from confronting difficult or painful situations by comparison to those who perceive themselves as moderately capable (neither too competent and hardy nor too vulnerable and pessimistic about their coping abilities). It seems that the latter are likely to reap the most significant rewards from coping with stressful experiences and to experience personal growth. To this day, this question remains unanswered, and our knowledge limited.

In an attempt to address this unexplored issue, it would be helpful to focus first on the obstacles that prevent us from deriving rewards and then to consider the conditions that promote the ability to find benefits in our encounters with death situations.

OBSTACLES TO REWARDING EXPERIENCES

I have found through my clinical and teaching experience in palliative and bereavement care that some of the ways we perceive and cope with death situations prevent us from deriving rewards through caregiving. What makes our lives and work so difficult that we cannot experience any satisfaction when we accompany people through dying and bereavement?

- *A terror of death that paralyzes us when we relate to people whose lives are affected by loss.* Quite often, underlying this terror is an unwillingness to confront our mortality out of fear that we may discover that we have set futile goals, stifled our dreams, and led lives that are slipping away from us.
- *The denial or suppression of suffering that we cannot avoid experiencing in death situations.* We spend most of our energy protecting

ourselves from being affected by the dying and bereavement processes of others and avoiding addressing our own losses and grief. By not allowing ourselves to experience the pain of caring, we also deprive ourselves of the joys and rewards.

- *The fear of intimacy that is usually associated with the fear of being abandoned or rejected by others or of being engulfed by their suffering or death.* Behind our inability to form intimate relationships often lie personal attachment and loss issues that prevent us from being fully present for another person.
- *A striving for perfection that is associated with the pursuit of unrealistic goals.* Self-absorbed, we do things for others to acquire status, power, control, prestige, a position, or a title. We are unable to develop genuine and authentic relationships since our primary concern is our own image and performance. Occasionally, we derive satisfaction from personal achievements obtained through the care of others; however, the rewards are only ephemeral, since we remain absorbed by an endless striving to be perfect, do the "right" thing, save the world, and remain on the top, above others, whom we fear may surpass, judge, or criticize us.
- *A perceived lack of meaning in the roles we assume and the care we provide.* Our inability to derive rewards often stems from the perception that our jobs are worthless, and our roles meaningless. While meaning attribution is determined by both personal and work-related factors, it is important to remember that even in the most sterile work environment, we can experience rewards as long as we integrate both the positive and negative experiences into a broader contextual framework that values end-of-life and bereavement care. It is often the lack of such a framework that prevents us from valuing the services we provide and finding purpose in the care we provide.

CONDITIONS THAT PROMOTE REWARDING EXPERIENCES

To better understand the rewards of caregiving in death situations, let's consider five conditions that promote rewarding experiences and lead to significant benefits in our personal and professional lives:

- Acknowledgment of caregiving motives and needs
- Connection to others

- Openness to the experience and to self-understanding
- Rippling
- Acceptance of mortality and a willingness to address existential issues

These conditions enable us not solely to continue to work in this challenging field but also to thrive in situations that are highly stressful.

Acknowledgment of Caregiving Motives and Needs

To understand why and how we benefit from caring for the dying and the bereaved, we must reflect upon our trajectory in this field. What got us here? What were our motives? Why have we chosen to work in death situations? What attracted us to a job that focuses on death? What keeps us in this field of work?

Our motivation to help people in adverse situations is best understood if we seek to understand both our altruistic motives and the personal needs that each of us seeks to satisfy through the care of others (International Work Group on Death, Dying, and Bereavement, 2006). Personal needs vary and may change over the course of our careers. However, knowing them can help us identify some of the key sources of our distress and of the experiences that we find rewarding.

Outlined here are some common needs we seek to satisfy by assisting others in death situations. While addressing these personal needs can lead to rewarding experiences and enhance the care we provide, occasionally they overshadow our efforts to care for others and negatively affect the quality of our services.

- *The need to make a difference in the lives of others.* Striving to have a positive impact on the lives of others is healthy and normal. Seeing them grow and develop as a result of our interventions is deeply fulfilling. However, sometimes the need to make a difference in their lives is associated with idealistic goals (e.g., saving a life at any cost, ensuring a perfect death, eradicating all suffering) that are related to our ego and professional identity. In this field of work, lives are not always saved, suffering is rarely totally eradicated, and a good death cannot always be achieved. Unless we review our expectations and unrealistic ideals and accept that some people will be helped and changed by our interventions, and others not, we risk experiencing repeated frustrations and disappointments and depriving ourselves from the many rewards of caregiving.

- *The need to be needed, to be loved, and to be appreciated by others.* Caring for people in loss situations, when they are highly vulnerable, often leads to the development of intimate bonds and privileged relationships that are rewarding to them and to us. In such relationships we thrive when our services are deeply appreciated and valued. Sometimes, however, our need to be needed by others and to be loved is so profound that we end up using others to feel affirmed, appreciated, and valued. When our needs become more important than the needs of those we serve, we risk developing relationships that are highly dependent, enmeshed, and unrewarding.
- *The need to address personal loss or trauma issues or use them to benefit others.* Some of us choose a job in this field as a result of a significant loss we experienced in the past. Thus, our personal experience becomes the motivating factor for helping people who struggle with similar situations and concerns. As long as we understand how our own losses have affected our goals, values, and choices in life (including our choice to offer palliative or bereavement services), we can be effective in assisting dying and bereaved people. When we are unaware of our own experiences, we impose our personal agendas upon others, whose experiences we use to address and work through our losses.
- *The need to address existential concerns.* Sometimes our desire to care for people in death situations stems from a need to answer some existential questions related to human existence that are particularly important to us. By helping others cope with dying and grief, we seek to confront our mortality and prepare ourselves for our own dying or the loss of our loved ones. Other times, however, unable to tolerate the uncertainty that is associated with existential issues, we use others to discover or impose "absolute" truths.
- *The need to be unique and distinct from other professionals by working in death-related situations.* Doing a job that is out of the ordinary, highly challenging, and unique is very attractive to some. We feel special when we have the ability to offer services in extreme situations that are commonly avoided by other professionals. In so doing, we seek to be distinct and gain the respect of patients, families, colleagues, and society. Difficulties arise when

> our need to be different leads to an ongoing competition with our peers, a striving for superiority and for prestige. Under those circumstances, caregiving loses its social function and robs us of the potential rewards.

It is evident that seeking to help others and concurrently striving to meet some of our own personal needs is quite complex. In order to increase the likelihood of obtaining significant rewards from providing quality care, we must acknowledge and honor both their and our own needs and remain constantly aware of what we can offer, what to expect in return, and how to mutually benefit from a two-way process of giving and receiving.

Connection to Others

Rewarding experiences come in various shapes and forms. Some are associated with the outcomes of our interventions (e.g., achieving a desired goal, accomplishing a specific task), and others are associated with the process through which we reach our goals (e.g., developing secure bonds, collaborating effectively with colleagues, communicating effectively about difficult issues). When we are caring for dying and bereaved people, no goal is ever successfully achieved unless we empathically connect with those who strive to ensure a meaningful existence in the midst of loss and separation. Connectedness (which can range in form from a partnership to an attachment bond) is at the heart of companioning. It fosters belonging, which, in the face of death and separation, reduces or tempers a suffering that is shared. Belonging ascertains some sort of non-mortality at a collective level, but also an awareness of the inevitability of mortality at an individual level.

Connectedness allows the dying and bereaved to engage in two parallel processes: one of grieving over an impending separation or actual loss and another of investing in life, living, and seeking to connect with others (see chapter 3).

This process becomes obvious when the person who is dying and fading away suddenly fully reappears in the world and connects with others before he or she disappears forever (De M'Uzan, 1977). It is as if he or she suddenly awakens from a deep sleep or coma to share a few words, to describe a dream, to ask for a favorite food despite an inability to eat for days, to express loving words or a wish, or to engage in an activity that is significant to him or her. This process is possible only if there is someone to share death with—someone who is not terrorized by it; someone who is able to maintain, for the sake of the dying, the *illusion* that death can be shared.

The opposite happens with the bereaved individual, who disappears into the empty space left by his or her loved one before reappearing in the world and reconnecting with others. Again, this emotional disappearance becomes tolerable when there is someone with whom to connect and share the pain of loss without depriving the person of it—a companion who does not fear being destroyed by suffering.

When we respond to the call for connection, we often find ourselves in a dyadic relationship that resembles an early attachment bond. Whenever this attachment is secure enough to shift between the worlds of being and nonbeing, then we, along with the people we serve, are enriched by the connection. In contrast, when there is no connection or the attachment is insecure, we condemn the dying or bereaved individual to social isolation and exacerbate his or her existential loneliness. Worst of all, we are left with the terror that when our own time will come, we might be abandoned to bear the pain alone or die in despair.

Openness to the Experience and to Self-Understanding

We are open to experience when we are "vulnerable enough" in our encounters with others (see chapter 4). Openness involves three interrelated levels: (1) an openness to life, with all the pleasant or tragic events it contains; (2) an openness toward others and their experiences; and (3) an openness toward oneself, whom we come to know better and befriend. Openness permits us to meet the unknown in life, in others, or in ourselves without preconceived ideas or rigid theories and planned interventions. It allows us to welcome the unexpected without always trying to provide a logical explanation, and to work through the paradoxes that are inherent in death situations.

Openness does not necessarily imply an accumulation of experiences. Rather, it involves the creative use of information that is introduced by each novel, unfamiliar, conflicting, or even chaotic experience. This process demands time, energy, and commitment. When we are consumed by the everyday and rush from one activity, task, or crisis to the next, we do not engage in a deeper examination of our experiences and we restrict our capacity to provide effective care and to reap the rewards.

One thing I have realized over the years is that the experiences and people that cause us the greatest trouble are those who offer us the greatest opportunities to learn something about our vulnerabilities, limitations, and shortcomings, as well as about our inner resources. Positive and negative experiences associated with caregiving can be valuable to us as long as we strive to learn something through them. Clarke-Steffen (1998) describes them as peak and nadir experiences.

A *peak experience* is defined as "an intensely meaningful or highly significant and unforgettable experience that is often accompanied by feelings of awe, wonder, unity, fulfillment, or going beyond ordinary experience" (Clarke-Steffen, 1998, p. 26). For example, an intimate connection with a person or family, our contribution to an appropriate death, or the sense of pride in a job well done in difficult situations can be perceived as peak experiences.

A *nadir experience* is defined as "an intensely meaningful or highly significant and unforgettable negative experience that is often accompanied by feelings of agony, distress, pain, embarrassment, sorrow, or regret" (Clarke-Steffen, 1998, p. 26). For example, the sense of helplessness over our inability to reduce suffering, the guilt over a perceived error, or the terror associated with a particularly traumatic death, are all unfamiliar and painful experiences that may be perceived as nadir experiences.

While we all have peak and nadir experiences, it is the way we perceive and cope with them that determines whether we lose or gain something from them. Those who remain open to such experiences and take the time to reflect on and process them—alone or with others—are more likely to learn something new that may subsequently change and enrich their view of themselves, of others, of life, and of caregiving. Key experiences invite us to revise our goals, values, and interventions and enable us to invest our role and work with personal meaning. Most importantly, they help us build upon our strengths, accept our limitations, and learn how to transform nadir experiences into peak experiences and opportunities for the development of self-awareness and personal growth.

Rippling

When we are young and inexperienced, rewards are usually attached to our ability to be competent and skillful in the care we provide. Rewards arise from our capacity to effectively care for others and from our ability to find meaning in a work that is well done.

As we grow older and more experienced, rewards shift from the self and our immediate microcosmos to the larger community of humans. Thus, we experience deep satisfaction from passing on our wisdom, experience, skills, and knowledge to others; from contributing to their fulfillment and enhancement; and from making the world a better place to live in. Yalom (2008) describes this phenomenon as "rippling." This term refers

> to the fact that each of us creates—often without our conscious intent or knowledge—concentric circles of influence that may affect others for years, even for generations. That is, the effect we have on other people is in turn passed on to others, much as the ripples of a pond go on until they are no longer visible but continuing at a nano level. (p. 83)

Rippling is not necessarily associated with fame, nor with the establishment of a name or prestigious image. It is not limited to the microcosmos of the dying and the bereaved but encompasses our co-workers, students, friends, loved ones, and even people we do not know. Their lives are enlarged by our experience, which is directly or indirectly communicated to them.

Rippling is not a one-way but a two-way process. We create ripples of influence when we are less preoccupied with ourselves and with doing the right thing and allow dying and bereaved people to affect and change us at a personal and professional level. Thus, our patients become our most valued teachers, and—in the same way that Melanie's physician benefited from his challenging encounters with her—we pass on a wealth of wisdom that helps others transform suffering into growth, relate more meaningfully to others, and lead more satisfying lives. Teaching, publishing, initiating an innovative project, and engaging in social and community pursuits can all be significant reflections of rippling that persist when we retire or die. Being aware that our work, our guidance, and our wisdom (and not our persona) are and will continue to be of value to others is one of the most rewarding experiences that can result from caregiving.

Acceptance of Mortality and a Willingness to Address Existential Issues

Dying and bereaved people, through their own experiences with death, offer us an invaluable gift: the opportunity to confront our mortality and awaken to a fuller life. We rarely realize the value of this gift, because confronting death arouses anxiety. This is inevitable. While this anxiety cannot and should not be totally eliminated, it can nevertheless be tempered when we face death and accept our mortality. This is not an easy process.

Yalom (2008) wisely suggests that facing death and mortality is like staring at the sun: we can stand only so much of it. For some, it can be a terrifying experience, while for others it can be an awakening experience that enriches their lives. When does death confrontation become an awakening experience? When we review our lives, imagine our ultimate end, and contemplate the finality of all our valued relationships. Although painful at times, this process opens up possibilities and offers new choices and an incredible freedom to live differently. While some of us are threatened by this freedom, others benefit by developing a deeper awareness of who we are and how we want to live our lives. Such confrontations make us meaning makers (Kauffman, 1995) and resourceful in coping.

Sometimes we realize that we are leading unfulfilling lives and regret the paths we have chosen or the opportunities we have let slip by. Our anxiety may consequently increase; we may even grieve over a life that we never lived yet always desired. By addressing our disappointments, regrets, unrealized goals, or dreams—alone or with the help of a colleague, supervisor, therapist, or mentor—we can free ourselves and choose whether to feel sorry for ourselves, submerge ourselves in suffering, or learn from experience and move on to living more fully.

The lessons learned when we address our existential concerns are invariably rewarding. Not only can they change and enrich us, but they can help us assist dying and bereaved people to address their own concerns, value life, and love themselves and others with greater depth and clarity.

THE WISDOM OF THE WOUNDED HEALER

Let's imagine that we are given a choice to live forever or to die. How would life be if we were immortal in this physical world? It would probably be an experience of ultimate suffering, since everything we strive for, get attached to, love, or accomplish would have no beginning or end and would remain unchanged. With the absence of death, the lack of chronological boundaries, and an unlimited existence, we would probably be trapped in a repetitive, meaningless existence and lose all desire to change, grow, and hope for a future.

This was the unfortunate fate of Chiron, the wounded healer who, as the son of a god, was immortal. As the years went by, his immortality became unbearable. It deprived him of the hope for a future and the possibility of experiencing things differently, choosing alternative paths, and being changed and transformed.

It was then that Hercules reappeared in the myth and presented Chiron with the option of dying. He informed him that Zeus had decided that Prometheus (who had tricked Zeus by giving the precious gift of fire to humans) would be freed from his imprisonment only if an immortal being agreed to surrender his immortality and go to the underworld in Prometheus's place. Chiron saw in death a new opportunity and accepted it. He exchanged immortality for death. He welcomed with relief the prospect of being human and finite. With this choice he developed a new understanding of his suffering, along with an appreciation for a time-limited existence.

After his death, Chiron descended to Hades, the land of the underworld. There, he was not the great teacher of healing, but a novice apprentice who waited in the dark and listened to stories of the underworld and thus was initiated into new learning. Eventually, Zeus removed Chiron from Hades and set his image among the stars, forming the Centaurus constellation.

According to Kearney (1996), Chiron's shift in attention from the upper to the lower half of his body (his wounded knee) and his subsequent descent from the world of the living to the dark and mysterious underworld are a metaphor for transformation through suffering. This metaphor represents a movement from the world of consciousness to the depths of the unconscious mind. But the myth also represents an awakening to an inner wisdom that is passed along to others. Through his teaching and mentoring, as well as through the care he provided to others, Chiron modeled the value of self-awareness, the importance of connecting with those in suffering, and the freedom to choose how to live, which comes from accepting one's mortality. Such an acceptance increases the ability to make conscious choices, set meaningful goals, plan for the future in light of a transient and finite existence, and live life with a greater sense of clarity, awareness, and fullness. Paradoxically, this striving to lead a fuller life coexists with a striving to ensure immortality through one's children, achievements, and deeds and the transmission of knowledge, experience, caring, and wisdom to others.

The ultimate gift that dying and bereaved people offer us is an opportunity to awaken to the freedom to choose how to live life in light of the awareness that we are mortal. Thus, the rewards of caregiving are associated not just with the care we provide to others, but also with the realization that we are responsible for making choices that allow us to live a life that is both self-fulfilling and other-enhancing.

NOTE

1. According to Kobasa (1979), hardiness is a set of personality traits that characterize people who have a greater sense of (1) *control* (i.e., the feeling that they are able to influence events in their lives), (2) *commitment,* which they display by becoming involved in relationships, events and activities in which they find purpose and meaning, and (3) an ability to view difficulties as *challenges* and as incentives or opportunities for growth rather than as threats or disasters.

SECTION III

The Team in the Face of Death

8 Caregiving Organizations and Death

To embrace, to grow attached, to lose, to suffer and to transform before the experience of repeated deaths, consecutive bereavements, multiple losses—such is the challenge of an interdisciplinary team.

(De Montigny, 1993, p. 12)

My first encounter with a large organization was when I was hired as a psychologist at a public pediatric hospital. At that time, more than 25 years ago, dying children were isolated in a room at the far end of a ward, often on the top floor of the hospital. Nurses and physicians would enter the room only to ensure that there was nothing else they could offer patients and quickly left them to the care of their families. Professionals did not actively accompany the children and their parents through this difficult phase, since the responsibility was assumed by family members.

One of our patients was Anneta, a 4-year-old girl who was dying alone, as her teenage mother had left the hospital to return to her village when she learned of her terminal condition. Restless and anxious, Anneta seemed comforted only when I held her in my arms and talked or sang to her. What I distinctly remember to this day is not her actual death, but the response of care providers to her dying condition. During the last hours of her life, every so often the door would open slightly, and several care providers would peek into her room located at the end of the ward at the top floor of the building, curious to observe what was happening. I saw the faces of staff personnel and of interns I had never seen before. Despite the animation outside Anneta's room, no one came in. I quickly became aware that I was doing something out of the ordinary that went against the established order of operation in this setting.

In this hospital, dying was a family affair and death was carefully kept out of sight. In fact, when a patient died, his or her body was immediately transferred to the hospital's morgue, which family members were not allowed to visit. Instead, they were rushed away from the hospital. Those who lived in the city were expected to see their deceased child at church shortly before the burial, while those who lived in rural areas hold a wake at home the night before the funeral proceedings (Papadatou & Iossifides, 2004).

The hospital's morgue was always locked, and the only people who had access were the hospital employees who transferred the body, and the funeral home employees who dressed the deceased before transferring him or her to church. I once asked for the key to the morgue in order to say farewell to a beloved patient who had died suddenly during the night. It was refused to me, and I was sent to the hospital's administrator to obtain permission! Faced with my undeterred persistence, he finally gave in. My visit to the morgue was both a shocking and enlightening experience in terms of how the organization perceived and coped with death. The hospital's morgue was located in a corner of the hospital's yard, next to a small cabin in which small animals were kept for research purposes. The smell was unbearable, and the interior was cold and unfriendly. It was obvious to me that death was perceived as something remote, dirty, and ugly. Following my visit to the morgue, I wrote a letter to the hospital's board of directors, suggesting the need to renovate the site, transfer the cabin, and create a dignified space that would be open to bereaved families. My letter was totally ignored. So I wrote a second letter and paid several visits to the hospital administrator. Eventually, the morgue was painted and the cabin was removed, but the morgue remained off limits to parents and staff members. A few months later, I was surprised to find that the area around it had been turned into a dump where the hospital's construction garbage was thrown. It became obvious to me that I could not fight the system's established order alone. Death was perceived as a dirty affair, and the organization refused to integrate the dying, the deceased, and the bereaved into its structure and mode of functioning. I found myself being made a scapegoat and called "Ms. Death" and "Ms. Funeral" by members of the hospital personnel because I dared to challenge some of the established practices.

In response, I persisted in standing by children and families throughout illness and death and refused to be cloistered behind the closed doors of an office, expecting patients or families to be referred to me. Instead, I worked mostly on the wards, in hospital rooms, in the lounges of various units, and in the hospital's playroom, making my services known and available to others. Gradually, members of the hospital personnel—ranging from cleaning ladies to head nurses and department chairs—began to approach me to ask questions about patients or share personal problems and secretly confide their approval of my behavior. It was not long before I was invited to give a lecture to nurses and medical interns about seriously ill children and their families. Soon, I discovered that several colleagues were eager to share their experiences and concerns and consider alternative ways of approaching and communicating with patients and patients. At that time, a pediatric oncology unit was being developed, and along with the leading oncologist, who was open minded and good hearted, I collaborated closely to organize the psychosocial services that would be provided to young patients and their families throughout their illnesses.

Today, the situation has changed significantly. New units for children with acute, chronic, and life-threatening diseases have been created, while hospital leaders and interdisciplinary teams have established a new ethos of practice that allows for a significantly greater degree of integration of dying children into the organization's system.

SUFFERING IN THE WORKPLACE

Caregiving organizations have become increasingly complex. They provide specialized services and have to collaborate with each other. Those who work with the sick are expected to work with palliative care specialists, who, in turn, must coordinate with clinicians specializing in bereavement. No longer can organizations work as closed systems. This openness creates an ongoing turmoil but holds the potential for innovation, change, and evolution.

What is an organization? It is not a building or a facility, as is commonly assumed. An organization is a *multinuclear system of relations.* We are members of this complex system of relations. We do not work in isolation but belong to a team that usually interacts and collaborates with other teams within a larger context. Each organization has connections and collaborations with other professionals, teams, and organizations in the community. This entire system of relations operates according to a set of priorities and directives, which are often determined by the country's national health care policy. This policy reflects specific sociocultural values, beliefs, and attitudes about dying, death, and bereavement, which are not imposed or adopted as such; instead they are operationalized and transformed into concrete forms of action by each organization and affect the services that are offered.

In order to better understand how an organization addresses the needs of dying and bereaved people, we must first look into its history and psychology. According to Kaës (2003), each organization has its own history and characteristics that are independent of the characteristics of individual care providers. In other words, the psychology of a caregiving organization differs from the psychology of the individual care providers within it. Every organization transmits—in explicit or implicit ways—to providers a set of values, rules, and regulations; a specific code of communication; and a mode of functioning. It affects how professionals think, express their feelings, behave, and function when caring for ill, dying, and grieving individuals. This explains why some care providers display certain behaviors—for example, they may become abrupt, cynical, and distant—that are not apparent in their personal lives, in which they maintain warm, loving, and caring relationships. Not only does an organization affect its members, but it also is affected by their knowledge, expertise, personality, investments, achievements, dreams, and hopes, as evidenced in my personal experience with death in a large pediatric hospital.

According to the relationship-centered approach advocated in this book there is a shared space that extends beyond the person–professional relationship (see chapter 1) and incorporates the larger organization. This space belongs neither to the care provider nor to the organization but to their unique relationship (Kaës, 2003). By exploring this relationship, we can better understand how suffering is created, tolerated, mitigated, or transformed into caring acts and growth opportunities in organizations that belong to a specific community.

Thus, suffering stems from relationships that are developed at various levels:

1 *Relationships between the professional and the individual(s) who seeks care.* Forming and maintaining a partnership in the shadow of separation or death often evokes suffering for both partners.

This suffering is further aggravated when personal unresolved loss issues are triggered by the reality of death and are brought into the caregiving relationship by either care seekers or care providers.

2. *Relationships among team members (intra-team relationships).* Intra-team tensions, conflicts, communication problems, and collaboration difficulties absorb our energy as well as the team's energy and distract us from the people we serve.
3. *Relationships with other professionals, teams, or organizations (inter-team/inter-organization relationships).* Coordination difficulties with other professionals and teams are at the heart of a suffering that is commonly shared. Conflictual or mutually avoidant relationships may, for example, develop between a palliative care team and a cure-oriented team in the same organization. Each team functions as a closed system and avoids collaborations while members who enter the team stay forever and grow old together.
4. *Relationships with the larger community.* Suffering stems from the social discrimination we experience in our encounters with a society that stigmatizes our job, which is perceived as "dirty" or macabre, or idealizes our services to the dying and bereaved by contributing to our marginalization and alienation (see chapter 5).

These sources of suffering affect how we perceive and how we relate to self, to the people we serve, to our colleagues, to other teams or professionals, to administration officials, to the government and its health care policies, and to the community in which we live.

In conclusion, suffering is unavoidable in a multinuclear system of relations that are confronted with loss, death, and bereavement. When it is unacknowledged and suppressed, it tends to be expressed in subtle, indirect ways that become apparent through dysfunctional patterns of interaction and inappropriate solutions that perpetuate and aggravate suffering by allowing issues to remain unresolved. In other words, we do not suffer solely from the losses, disruptions, or conflicts we experience in our relationships with care seekers, our co-workers, superiors, and administrators; we also suffer from the way we cope with these challenges.

To better explain the context in which we offer services to dying and bereaved individuals, I wish to discuss the organization's ideals, primary tasks, and mode of functioning, since they affect the experience of suffering as well as the satisfaction and growth that we experience in this field of work.

THE ORGANIZATION'S MYTHS AND IDEALS

Every organization has a history that relates to its development and growth. This history is related to a myth that gives purpose and meaning to the organization's existence. The myth represents an ideal toward which all actions and efforts are oriented and enables the organization to define its mission and primary tasks and assign roles and responsibilities to individual care providers and teams. The myth is reflected in a story about the origin of an organization; its real or imagined leaders or heroes; their dreams, passions, and goals; and its overall mission. It consists of accounts about individuals who played a significant role in the organization's development and descriptions of significant events that took place with the passage of time. Every myth becomes imbued with symbolic meaning.

The organization's myth functions as a collective ideal and is internalized and adopted by care providers, whether they are aware of it or not. It unifies and guides their actions toward the accomplishment of commonly shared goals and offers a collective identity to those who work within the same setting. Moreover, it determines the organization's reason for being and provides members with a sense of belonging and orientation toward the achievement of one or more primary tasks.

Consider the myths that prevail in three different organizations. According to legend, a wealthy couple founded a large pediatric hospital in memory of their only son, who bled to death following a car accident. The couple donated their entire estate in order to create this pediatric medical center and made sure it was equipped with the most sophisticated technology, and staffed by renowned medical experts. The myth that prevailed in this organization was one of medical *expertise and omnipotence* over any life-threatening disease or critical health condition.

A different myth, one of *benevolence and sacrifice,* permeated a home care service for AIDS patients that was developed by a group of volunteers. They conducted a major fund-raising campaign and solicited the services of health care professionals, who agreed to design, develop, and supervise the program on a pro bono basis.

A myth of *excellence* prevailed in a bereavement center that was founded by a team of experienced mental health professionals who selected, trained, and supervised psychologists, psychiatrists, and social workers, who were subsequently hired to provide grief counseling and therapy to bereaved children, adults, and families.

We need to be aware that sometimes an organization or service has parallel myths, and that older myths may be replaced or embellished by new ones in order to explain the past, present events, and future organizational aspirations. Myths are reflected in narratives that describe the birth of an organization or service, the role of leaders, and its perceived achievements, glories, failures, losses, and traumas that shape the history and identity of the organization. They are transmitted from one generation of care providers to another through various channels, including narratives (e.g., informal discussions, speeches delivered on special occasions, information contained in leaflets), rituals (e.g., commemoration of founders, awards to leaders or members for outstanding achievements, celebrations of significant dates or events related to the history of the organization), and symbols (e.g., portraits, logos, religious and other representations that are integrated in the work environment).

It is not by coincidence that the myths of palliative and bereavement care organizations refer to the stories of death-related experiences encountered by their leaders, which served as the trigger for humanitarian actions and a profound social contribution.

For example, Cicely Saunders always referred to her brief but intense relationship with one of her patients, David Tasma, a dying Jewish émigré from Poland. She had shared with him her dream of founding a nurturing home where dying people like him could find peace and live meaningfully at the end of their lives. David Tasma left Cicely Saunders £500, along with a note that said: "I will be a window in your home" (Clark, 2002, p. 7). Today, when one visits St. Christopher's Hospice, one cannot help but observe a big window next to the entrance door, along with the inscription of Tasma's words to Saunders. He was St. Christopher's "founding patient" and Cicely Saunders' inspiration. His legacy remains at the core of the organization's myth. St. Christophers continues to serve as a window of hope to the international hospice movement and serves as a model of end-of-life care for thousands of hospices that have been developed across cultures and settings. Its philosophy of care is captured in the act of companioning people through terminal illness, reflected also in the name that was chosen for the hospice: St. Christopher is the patron saint of travelers and a symbol of Christian faith. The deeply religious Cicely Saunders developed a model of care into which she integrated her religious beliefs and ideas. The importance of spiritual care is reflected in the hospice's logo, the religious symbols that decorate the building, and the central space occupied by its chapel. Over the years, as multiculturalism has spread in the United Kingdom, St. Christopher's Hospice has progressively broadened its spiritual approach to incorporate faiths and rituals that are practiced by individuals of different cultural backgrounds.

Every organization perpetuates its myths. Quite often, a newly hired care provider who is not aware of the history and evolution of the organization may be caught in a mode of collective functioning that perpetuates one or more of the myths specific to the work setting. Enriquez (2003) cautions, however, that all myths must be maintained at some distance so that care providers can develop their own modes of thinking and functioning without having to blindly conform to a preestablished mode of operation. When a myth pervades the daily life of an entire organization, it risks stifling progress, creativity, and growth within the organization.

Unfortunately, nowadays, the increased need for specialized services for chronically ill, elderly, dying, and bereaved individuals has led business entrepreneurs whose motives are primarily economic to develop for-profit organizations that provide end-of-life and bereavement care. The underlying myths of such organizations are more product than people oriented. This negatively affects the nature and quality of services that are provided, as well as the experiences that both care seekers and care providers encounter in the face of death.

THE ORGANIZATION'S PRIMARY TASKS AND MODE OF FUNCTIONING

Every organization determines its primary tasks based on its history and myths. According to Rice (1963), the primary task of an organization is that which it must perform in order to survive. Sometimes an organization is responsible for parallel tasks that compete for primacy. For example, the task of caring for people who are sick, dying, or bereaved may coexist with the task of conducting research and/or the task of training medical, nursing, or psychology students. Other times, significant social developments force caregiving organizations to review their tasks and expand them. For example, the recent growth of the palliative care movement, along with the institution of the patients' bill of rights, has led several medical centers (whose primary task was the care of the sick through the use of expert knowledge and advanced technology) to define parallel tasks for the care of people who do not choose aggressive treatment or experimental protocols when a cure is not available. These parallel tasks have led to the development of new subspecialties in medicine and nursing and the establishment of palliative care units, home care programs, and bereavement services for families within existing organizations.

Problems occur when organizational tasks are unrealistic or tend to exhaust all available resources, leading to frustration and disappointment. For example, setting as a task the achievement of a 'perfect' death transforms the dying person and his or her trajectory into a personal or institutional success story. Similarly, striving for a 'perfect' bereavement through the open expression of feelings, management of unfinished business, and maintenance of an ongoing bond with the deceased may not always reflect the needs and desires of dying or bereaved individuals, to the dismay of health care providers.

Realistic tasks aim at ensuring an *appropriate* death or bereavement by taking into consideration the personal and cultural needs and preferences of individuals and families, who collaborate with a team of professionals to achieve goals that are meaningful to both. Marquis (1993) cautions organizations to avoid introducing primary tasks that make a success of all deaths and bereavements, something like a trophy in the art of dying and of mourning.

Instead, organizations should develop their own tasks and modes of functioning by assigning specific positions, roles, and functions to care providers, individuals, and families; by determining effective channels and modes of communication; and by establishing codes and rules that help temper suffering and enhance the potential of growth in the face of death. Each organization must structure and organize itself in order to cope with some major challenges that are associated with the humanization of the care of dying and bereaved people. What are these challenges?

- Integrating the dying, the death, and the bereaved into the organization
- Regulating suffering that is caused by death-related experiences
- Managing time by restoring a sense of continuity, which is irreversibly broken by death

Integration of the Dying, the Dead, and the Bereaved

An organization integrates the dying, the dead, and the bereaved into its reality when it defines tasks, goals, and a mode of functioning that acknowledge people's experiences and respond to their needs. In other words, it accepts the inevitability of death; validates the experiences of the dying by attending to their physical, psychosocial, and spiritual needs; and supports the bereaved through their grieving before and after the experience of loss. Moreover, a space is reserved for the dead, and rituals help to mark the end of life.

This integration is important for those who seek care, as well as for those who provide services. Instead of denying or hiding death, or giving up on each other, they address the reality of loss, which becomes shared.

Organizations that do not integrate the dying, the dead, and the bereaved into their goals, tasks, and operation disregard the needs and concerns of those whom they serve and condemn them to a social death. In other words, they organize their mode of functioning so as to isolate them and hide their experiences, as evidenced in the example of my early experiences in a large pediatric hospital.

Regulation of Suffering

Faced with death, organizations regulate the suffering that both care seekers and care providers experience and display. Such regulation is achieved through rules and norms that prescribe how individuals—but, most importantly, professionals—should think, feel, and behave in death situations. Psychodynamically oriented clinicians suggest that regulation is achieved through the development of a social defense system that protects part of the organization and its members from anxiety. This social defense system—which has been studied mostly by researchers from the Tavistock Institute (e.g., Menzies-Lyth, 1988, 1990; Rice, 1963)—becomes an aspect of each organization's reality with which old and new staff members must come to terms.

According to Menzies-Lyth (1988), who conducted a seminal study in the psychiatric department of a general hospital in England, every social defense system results from "the collusive interaction and agreement, often unconscious, between members of the organization" (p. 51). Once established and integrated into an organization's prevailing mode of functioning, it mitigates anxiety and facilitates the accomplishment of professionals' tasks. Behaviors such as the depersonalization of or detachment from patients and families, the ritualization of clinical performance, and splitting behaviors are common defensive mechanisms through which anxiety is tempered and suffering is regulated at an institutional level. Menzies-Lyth (1988) suggests that such behaviors reflect primitive types of immature defense mechanisms (such as denial, avoidance, splitting, and projection) commonly used by infants in their attempts to deal with severe anxiety.

Along similar lines, Kaës (2003) argues that every organization develops an unconscious pact or agreement with its members that aims to ensure order and continuity and protect care providers from anxiety, disorder, destruction, and suffering. This agreement forbids acts of violence, transgressions of rules, splits, and differences among care providers. Any event that threatens the organization's continuity, stability, established myths, and tasks by causing disorder, anxiety, or suffering is rejected, denied, or masked.

Time Management

Death abolishes time. In death there is no past, no present, no future. Organizations that provide services to the dying and the bereaved attempt to introduce an element of temporality in order to manage the rupture or void that death creates at a temporal level. How do they accomplish this? Usually by structuring their functioning according to time schedules to which professionals, individuals, and families have to abide. Schedules (e.g., for lab tests, medical rounds, appointments, patient visiting hours, number of counseling sessions) provide structure and minimize the unpredictable, the unknown, and the uncontrollable that the imminence or reality of death creates for the dying, the bereaved, and for the care providers. The latter choose interventions that aim at prolonging or restricting time's perceived duration. For example, through high-tech interventions they strive to prolong one's life time and instill hope for a possible future. Conversely, through palliative care services, they strive to pace time and help families to use it constructively in order to share meaningful interactions and prepare for death. In grief counseling and therapy they introduce an element of temporality by enabling the bereaved to visit the past, cope with the present, and contemplate the future.

In conclusion, the organization's mode of functioning determines how death experiences are perceived and managed, and how suffering is regulated. In an interesting early study, Miller and Gwynne (1972) studied organizations that delivered services to people with incurable, physically disabling illnesses. They identified two models of care by which organizations integrated dying patients into their reality and regulated the suffering of care providers: the medical or humanitarian model and the anti-medical or liberal model of care. While both models maintained an illusion of prolonging life, they had distinct ways of integrating people with incurable diseases into the organizations, and of managing staff members' anxiety.

The medical or humanitarian model developed a mode of operation that was based on the assumption that prolonging life was a good thing. Care providers collaborated with patients and families to preserve and prolong life in the face of death, which was not necessarily denied. What professionals did deny, however, was patients' anticipatory grief, depression, lack of fulfillment, and sense of futility. A good patient was anyone who passively and gratefully accepted being looked after, depended upon staff, and collaborated toward the achievement of medical goals—if not to prevent death, at least to prolong life in the face of death. Such an approach protected care providers from exposure to patient suffering.

The anti-medical or liberal model of care aimed at providing patients with opportunities to develop their potential. This model was built upon the assumption that quality of life is determined by the person's ability to remain active and involved in living. The patient with an incurable disease was perceived as normal, "just like everyone else," able to lead a full life. Care providers were responsible for offering opportunities for the development of abilities and consistently denied disabilities, and patients' complaints or suffering. A good patient was anyone who was independent, self-reliant, active, and happy, in spite of the possibility of impending death. Such patients were praised by staff members. Some patients responded well to such a model of care, since they wanted to fight deterioration, but those who wished to accept their declining condition and find relief at the end of life were highly distressed. Roberts (1994) points out that when a model is imposed and applied indiscriminately to all patients, based on the belief that it is the "right" way, it functions as a defense against the unbearable anxiety that care providers experience in the care of incurable individuals.

9 Team Functioning in Death Situations

Caregiving organizations expect care providers who provide services to dying and bereaved people to function as a team rather than as a group of clinicians who work individually and independently of each other by serving their own agendas. A team approach to care implies mutual collaborations among professionals who possess an awareness of how they affect and are being affected by their co-workers, and a deep understanding of the dynamics involved in teamwork.

To understand team functioning, we must begin by looking into ourselves. What is the personal baggage that each of us brings with when we join a team? It is the baggage of life experiences, which affect relationships not solely with the people we serve, but also with our co-workers, supervisors, and leaders. Within a team, we strive to ensure belonging. We adopt strategies that we used in our families of origin to gain parental attention, approval, love, and recognition, and to ensure a unique place alongside our siblings, in our transactions with authority figures and colleagues. If we learned early in life to form dependent or symbiotic attachments with our parents, we are likely to strive to establish similar bonds with our superiors or colleagues, to whom we cling whenever we are confronted with loss, separation, or death. If, on the other hand, we have learned to distrust others and have developed avoidant relationships in our families of origin, we are likely to maintain distant relations and rely solely upon ourselves. If we experienced secure attachments early in life, then we are likely to form relationships characterized by both individuation and interdependency. Basically, it is during childhood that we all learn how to cooperate with, to compete with, or to avoid others; thus, we tend to reproduce certain learned patterns of interactions in our relationships with peers and superiors at work. As a result, some of us thrive in collaborations and derive satisfaction from shared and collective efforts; others thrive on competition and derive satisfaction from having control, power, and authority; and still others like to work alone, independently of others.

While it is important to recognize what we bring to the team, it is equally important to acknowledge how we are affected by the team's history and mode of functioning, as well as by the larger culture of the organization.

To better understand the dynamics that come into play, let's imagine the team as a system with a two-sided membrane. (Figure 9.1). The internal part of the membrane comprises the internal world of the team, in other words its microcosmos; it is characterized by a structure that

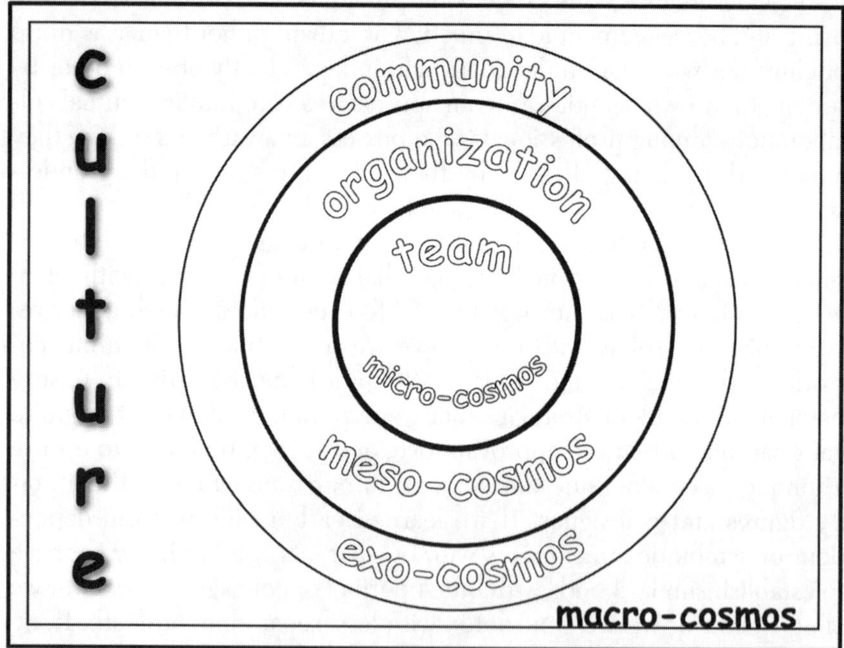

Figure 9.1 Team in context

assigns positions, roles, and functions to professionals and to people it serves; it defines specific goals and tasks to be achieved; and it operates according to a collective mode of functioning.

The external part of the membrane separates the team from—and concurrently unites it with—the intermediate world of the organization. In this mesocosmos are other professionals, teams, and administration officials with whom we are in direct or indirect communication. Through its external membrane, the team projects an image that is more or less congruent with its private reality. When the projected image is in dissonance with its private reality, then we feel confused, insecure, inauthentic, and dissatisfied with the care we provide. Such dissonance may invite criticism from the larger organization or resentment from care seekers, who sense a gap between what they experience when they enter our team and what is projected beyond its microcosmos.

Finally, the team's microcosmos and mesocosmos are embedded in the vast world of the community and are affected by the sociocultural beliefs, values, and practices of a given society with regard to dying, death, and bereavement.

Therefore, to fully understand the dynamics involved in caregiving, we need to look beyond our inner selves and explore the reality of our team through its interaction with the larger organization, the community, and the society we live in. These realities, although interrelated, are of a different order.

Before I discuss in further detail how teams are affected by death situations, I wish to raise a critical question: Can the people who seek our services be considered members of our team? According to the palliative care approach, individuals who seek our services and their family members are expected to participate actively in decisions and be responsible for shaping their trajectories at the end of life and through bereavement. It is assumed that they know best what is of value and significant to them. This family-centered approach places them at the center of the professional team and accords them a membership status (Egan, 1998). In my view, dying and bereaved individuals and their families can never become members of a team. There is an asymmetry in the relationship that is always present. Sick and grieving individuals inhabit the microcosmos of the team only temporarily. They do not share the team's experiences, history, and trajectory through time, nor do they adopt its mode of operation, rules, and values, even though they may conform to or be affected by them. The team does not have to reorganize itself in order to integrate them as members, even though it adapts its services and, sometimes, its practices to their individual needs. Moreover, the team's homeostasis is not threatened when a person dies or a bereaved individual leaves the team after having benefited from its services. It does so only in rare situations when a death is perceived as a nadir experience (see chapter 7) that causes a crisis or a major turmoil that threatens and alters the team's mode of functioning.

The relationship between a dying or bereaved person and the team is one of partnership; he or she is not a member of the team. Based on mutual trust and respect, partners strive toward the achievement of goals, which are defined according to each person's or family's values, needs, and preferences. Care providers learn from those who seek their services how best to assist and support them during this critical transitory period of their lives. The partnership places the person and family in the driver's seat and assigns the team the role of a companion who guides, orients, and shares with them the challenges of their journey. While the "driver" experiences the journey for the first time, the traveling companion, already familiar with the map and the territory of dying and bereavement, becomes reacquainted with the trajectory through the eyes and experiences of the driver. No journey is similar to any other.

Most often team membership is stable, with care providers working toward the achievement of mutually agreed-upon goals for which they are held accountable. Some teams, however, have a temporary structure and are made up of professionals who are brought together because of their particular skills in order to complete a project (Speck, 2006b). This chapter focuses on the psychology of teams that are stable; eight principles are offered to describe their functioning in the face of death (Box 9.1).

PRINCIPLE 1

Team functioning is affected by the organization's culture

Teams that belong to the same organization present more similarities than differences, since they are affected by the culture of their organization. This culture is determined by the myths, ideals, primary tasks, underlying beliefs, and values and priorities with regard to health, illness, dying, death, and bereavement. It reflects, among other things, how the dying and the bereaved are integrated into the system, how suffering is

Box 9.1

PRINCIPLES REGARDING TEAM FUNCTIONING IN DEATH SITUATIONS

Principle 1: Team functioning is affected by the organization's culture.

Principle 2: Team rules determine how professionals should care for dying and bereaved people and cope with suffering.

Principle 3: There are no functional or dysfunctional teams—only teams that use functional and dysfunctional patterns to cope with loss, death, and suffering.

Principle 4: The chronic use of dysfunctional patterns renders a team vulnerable to various types of disorganization.

Principle 5: Team crises are inevitable; they hold the potential for team disorganization as well as team growth.

Principle 6: All teams have the potential to function with competence.

Principle 7: Interprofessional collaboration is an unfolding process that is reflective of a team's development and growth.

Principle 8: Resilience is enhanced by the team's ability to effectively cope with suffering, and to creatively use its resources to foster change and growth.

regulated, and how time is managed. An organization's culture permeates its functioning, despite the fact that sometimes some teams adopt very divergent philosophies and practices of care.

Consider the following example. A large private health care center whose primary task was to relieve the suffering of the sick and the dying provided a wide range of services that addressed the individual needs of care seekers. Services included acute care and rehabilitation for patients with chronic diseases, as well as palliative care for terminally ill and bereaved people. Thus, hope was offered both to those who sought cure or life prolongation and to those who desired comfort and palliation at the end of life.

While the culture of the organization acknowledged and addressed issues related to dying and death, it nevertheless suppressed and systematically avoided facing the emotional suffering that such realities engendered in patients, families, and care providers. Suffering was perceived as unacceptable, ugly, and messy—an upsetting affair that should remain private and out of public sight. A culture of death awareness and of shuttered suffering permeated the functioning of both acute and palliative care teams. What happened in these teams, which had distinct goals yet maintained similar approaches to suffering?

In the critical care team, professionals openly and honestly discussed with families the patients' critical conditions and the possibility of death. An emphasis was placed on the undertaking of extreme measures and sophisticated interventions to save lives, control physical suffering, and postpone death. Patients were kept sedated, and transfers of patients to other units were rushed in order to regulate emotional suffering. Visiting hours for relatives were restricted to 30 minutes twice a day. During these visits, family members entered the unit one by one and stood at the bedside of the patient, since there were no chairs in the room. No waiting room was available to them, and no psychosocial or spiritual support was offered to patients and their families unless they displayed overt grief behaviors that disturbed the team's functioning or threatened the organization. When death occurred, families were informed by phone and invited to address their questions to the physician who was on call.

The palliative care unit appeared lively. Staff members were friendly but busy and often unavailable for long and in-depth conversations. It was with a sense of urgency that every patient or family member was attended to. Professionals found refuge from this commotion in a small room, where a sign on the door read: "Do not disturb." The team's psychologist and social worker provided support only to "difficult" patients and families who were referred to them by staff members, while the chaplain was involved only upon the families' requests. Rooms were luxurious, soundproof, and private. Doors were usually kept shut. A small sofa was located across from the escalators, placing visitors who sat there close to the exit of the unit.

While issues related to dying and death were openly addressed by staff, family members, and patients, emotions were kept at bay and hidden behind closed doors or busy schedules. In fact, when a person died, family members were expected to grieve in his or her room and leave unnoticed, without saying goodbye. Any door that was open was deliberately shut by nurses when bereaved family members passed through the corridor or when a body was removed from the ward. Everyone seemed isolated in his or her suffering, while signs (e.g., "Do not disturb") and rituals reinforced this privacy.

This example illustrates how the culture of the organization affected the functioning of two teams that had very divergent approaches to end-of-life care (cure versus palliative care orientation) yet perpetuated similar values, beliefs, and priorities that were critical to the organization.

PRINCIPLE 2

Team rules determine how professionals should care for dying and bereaved people and cope with suffering

Menzies-Lyth (1988) and other researchers and organizational experts (Kahn, 2005; Obholzer & Roberts, 1994) have described the social defense system adopted by caregiving organizations to counteract staff anxiety. Most of these observational studies stem from a psychodynamic perspective that overemphasizes the passivity of care providers who resist threatening situations; resort to immature, archaic defense mechanisms; and are affected by institutional forces that are beyond their control or awareness. This view dismisses a team's ability to affect and even change its mode of functioning by becoming aware of the underlying dynamics.

I view teams as active and dynamic systems that use alternative patterns and solutions to help them (1) cope with the challenges they encounter in the daily care of the dying and the bereaved, (2) manage the suffering that serious illness and death arouse in care providers, and (3) ensure continuity of functioning in the face of death. Team members are therefore perceived as active agents who can shape individual and collective responses to loss and suffering, instead of resisting threats and reacting passively to uncontrollable intrapsychic or organizational forces. They choose which coping patterns to use to manage suffering and achieve goals. Their choices are often affected by certain *explicit or implicit rules* that influence a team's mode of functioning and determine team members' roles, responsibilities, and expected conduct in death situations. When care providers choose to abide by these rules, they are rewarded by being assigned a secure place in the team; when they challenge or transgress them, they risk being criticized, punished, or isolated as a result of the threat they pose to the team's functioning and established homeostasis.

Team rules become apparent in the feelings, thought patterns, and behaviors displayed by most team members. These rules aim—among other things—at regulating the fluctuation between the experience and avoidance of grieving that professionals often experience in the face of death (see proposition 5 in chapter 6).

Each team develops its own rules. Teams that recognize professionals' grief and suffering, establish rules that facilitate mutual sharing, participation in consultation and supervision sessions, activities that promote self-care, team bonding, and the use of rituals that enfranchise grief (e.g., commemoration of deceased patients, prayer). In such teams, rituals are also used to mark separations from colleagues who retire or change work settings, and to encourage the open expression and sharing of feelings.

In contrast, teams that establish rules that disenfranchise or repress grief and suffering adopt coping patterns that protect professionals from experiencing any sense of loss. During highly emotional moments, for example, team members share cynical or macabre jokes; interrupt each other when feelings are expressed; engage in scientific debates about diseases, lab tests, or psychological assessments; and divert attention from suffering. Other times, team rules impose a false optimism and incite care providers to fight to prolong life, even against all odds. Such rules leave no room for the acknowledgement and management of suffering in both care seekers and care providers who encounter death situations.

Rules that determine caregivers' responses to loss and suffering are always in accordance with the team's primary task, goals, and strivings. In our studies, such rules became apparent only after we had interviewed all the physicians and nurses who worked in the same unit (Papadatou, 2000, 2006). When I presented our findings to the members of each team, not only did they confirm the rules that we identified, but they offered additional examples to illustrate how they maintained certain coping patterns to ensure an established mode of team functioning in the face of death. Interestingly, some care providers acknowledged that the way they felt, thought, and behaved at work was quite distinct from the way they coped with loss and suffering in their personal lives. They were honest enough to admit that at some point in their careers, they decided to adjust their individual functioning to a collective mode of operation and conform to some unspoken rules in order to be like everybody else and ensure belonging in the team. Once rules became explicit and their function became clear, team members were faced with the option of maintaining or changing them.

For example, the primary task of the pediatric oncology team was curing children. When this proved impossible, the task became one of palliation. During the terminal phase, team members were encouraged to maintain close relationships with children and their parents and support them through the dying process. There was a widely held belief that quality of end-of-life care is ensured through intimate and caring bonds. As a result, it was expected that team members would be affected by the loss of a close relationship and would grieve over the death of patients. There was, however, an implicit team rule that the professionals' grief should be tempered and controlled and never become so intense that it would impair clinical judgment or lead to emotional breakdown. There was also a rule that care providers' suffering should never become visible to sick or dying children or to their parents but should remain private and within the confines of the unit. In addition, care providers were expected to support each other and participate in formal or informal team gatherings. Personal experiences were shared during staff meetings, and during support groups that were led by an external consultant twice a month. Care providers developed various ways to support each other, as evidenced in the following account of a nurse, who reported:

> We have a ritual in our unit; it's like a sacred rule. We gather the day following a child's death and listen to the stories of the nurses who were on duty. They have a need to share their experiences. But, also, the nurses who were off duty need to know: How did the child die? Was it a peaceful death? Did we do the best we could? Could we have done anything more or different? We cover for colleagues who are deeply affected or take some time off to look after themselves, and we always accompany the one (a team member) who wants to attend the funeral of a patient. By attending the funeral, we pay our respect to the deceased child and to the family and at the same time support each other through our grief.

Different rules prevailed in the pediatric intensive care unit. The team's primary task was to save the lives of critically ill children at any cost. Due to the uncertainty of patients' prognoses, close relationships with patients and families were discouraged, and discussions with parents were kept brief to avoid emotional involvement. A basic rule encouraged the adoption of a detached approach. This was accomplished in one or more of the following ways:

- By not allowing relatives to enter the ICU outside the very limited visiting hours
- By keeping patients sedated, even when there was no real need
- By breaking down the workload into well-defined tasks, so that each provider performed a few tasks for a large number of patients

- By allowing professionals to replace each other in the care they provided to each patient
- By facilitating frequent transfers to other units

Death was perceived as the team's failure to save the patient's life, and rules discouraged the open display of suffering or grief. The implicit message was: "Do not grieve, at least not openly.... Be strong and brave in the face of death." Care providers limited their discussions to scientific issues and helped each other repress their grief by sharing jokes, by minimizing emotions, and by reinforcing a detached approach.

These examples illustrate how each team develops its own private code, values, and rules that acknowledge, deny, or repress suffering; facilitate or discourage grieving; and promote more or less functional patterns in the face of loss. Rules serve two basic functions. First, they determine the nature of the relationships that team members expect to develop with care seekers and co-workers, and second, they serve as tempering valves that regulate suffering and the fluctuation between experiencing and avoiding responses to loss and grief. As a result, they facilitate or hinder the integration of death experiences into the team's history.

What happens when rules are transgressed? The following example illustrates the experience of a critical care unit.

Chaos prevailed in the unit following the death of a 25-year-old patient who had been hospitalized for over a month as the result of a major head injury caused by a car accident when she was returning from her honeymoon. What triggered the crisis was not the patient's death, which was expected and perceived as inevitable, but the response of a newly hired physician, who invited the woman's family into the unit and stood with the relatives who shared their last farewells with their loved one. Moved by the family's loss, this physician shed a few tears. This incident threw the entire team out of balance, which, according to its established mode of functioning, never involved family members in the terminal moments of a person's life and disallowed the public display of care providers' emotions. The young physician had transgressed rules that were used to keep suffering at a distance. Team members were, consequently, exposed to both the family's and their colleagues' suffering and felt completely helpless to do anything for either. The crisis was resolved by the director of the critical care unit, who reprimanded the young physician for being too vulnerable and for her inappropriate conduct. Feeling guilty and ashamed, this young physician filed a request for a transfer to another unit, which was accepted. Order was reestablished, rules were reinforced, and the team went on with its usual mode of functioning.

In this example it becomes evident how a team can isolate and alienate a team member who transgresses sacred rules. Instead of exploring how loss, grief, and suffering affect all care providers, the team chooses to scapegoat one of its members who is perceived as having a problem or as being unprofessional, incompetent, and unable to function effectively. In this way, team members disown their vulnerability in the face of loss, death, and suffering and avoid identifying with the disturbing responses of their "malfunctioning" colleague (Catherall, 1999).

Unfortunately, it is more common for teams to over-regulate grief and suffering than to accept such responses as normal in the face of death. Over-regulation usually relies on the mistaken belief that care providers should never experience or show that they are suffering, should always control signs of emotional distress, and should always protect individuals and families from viewing their own vulnerability by projecting a facade of expertise, confidence, and absolute control over death situations. Over-regulation depletes the team's resources and deprives team members of opportunities for mutual support.

Equally disruptive are rules that under-regulate professionals' grief and suffering and dictate the display of certain emotions (e.g., sadness, grief, even guilt), without which care providers risk being labeled indifferent, cold, and distant. In such teams, members compete to appear most affected by the death or grief of a particular person in order to gain the team leader's attention, ensure the family's approval and gratitude, or project an ideal image of "false" compassion. These care providers attend every single funeral, where they grieve openly out of fear of being seen as not caring enough.

Fit and Misfits Between Team and Individual Coping With Loss and Suffering

Whenever the care provider's approach to loss and suffering is in congruence with the team's rules and mode of operation, then he or she feels at ease working in the team. This congruence, however, does not necessarily ensure quality of care, since it may mean that both the individual and the entire team maintain an avoidant approach to loss and suffering. It simply indicates a lack of difference between individual and collective patterns in coping with loss and managing suffering. This enables the care provider to know exactly what the team expects of him or her and to adjust accordingly. In response, the team provides the practitioner with a special place that enhances his or her sense of belonging.

Whenever there is incongruence between individual and collective patterns, then dissonance is unavoidable. To understand this dissonance, it is helpful to explore the concept of "emotional labor" proposed by the sociologist Arlie Russell Hochschild, who studied the role of emotions in organizations and published her findings in the book *The Managed Heart: Commercialization of Feeling*. She used this term to refer to the "management of feeling to create a publicly observable facial and bodily display" (Hochschild, 1983, p. 7). In other words, she suggested that emotional labor involves the management or modification of personal emotions when the workplace demands that certain emotions be shown or not shown to patients and clients.

How does the workplace demand the expression of certain emotions? Through *display rules* that determine which emotions are appropriate and which are not. For example, most health care organizations' display rules suggest that care providers show compassion and unconditional understanding toward seriously ill and bereaved individuals and control or hide personal feelings of frustration, anger, guilt, disgust, sadness, and despair, which are often elicited by loss, trauma, and patient suffering. When care providers enhance, fake, suppress, or adjust their own emotions in response to specific display rules, they experience *emotional labor*. Hochschild (1983) argued that emotional labor is useful to the organization because it increases the client's satisfaction with the delivered services. However, she also noted that the process of adjusting one's emotions to display rules is highly distressing and achieved in two distinct ways:

1. Through *surface acting*, which requires the regulation or manipulation of observable emotional expressions. For example, care providers display a false optimism regarding the condition of people who are fatally ill, or friendliness and compassion toward bereaved individuals for whom they experience pity or feel aversion.
2. Through *deep acting*, which requires the conscious and radical modification of one's feelings in order to express the desired emotion. For example, some care providers learn to suppress their grief over the death of a person in response to the demands of their work setting, which expects them to be strong and unaffected by death and suffering.

Different definitions of emotional labor have been offered by other researchers and theorists. For example, Ashforth and Humphrey (1993) expanded the concept of emotional labor beyond the process of managing emotions to include the display of appropriate behaviors that lead to task effectiveness. Morris and Feldman (1996) studied specific emotions—such as fear, sadness, joy, compassion, disappointment, anxiety, and enthusiasm—in relation to the frequency, duration, and intensity of their occurrence, and in accordance with each organization's expectations. Grandley (2000) went a step further and described how personal characteristics (e.g., gender, emotional expressivity, emotional intelligence) and organizational characteristics (e.g., supervisor and co-worker support) affect emotional labor and its outcomes. Despite these research efforts, the long-term effects of emotional labor upon practitioners, care seekers, teams, and organizations remain unclear and warrant further study.

I believe that incongruence between individual and team coping patterns is not always detrimental. In some cases it is beneficial and enriching. For example, when the team's display rules acknowledge suffering and encourage mutual support among colleagues within a safe holding environment, then individual providers who regularly repress their grief can be helped to accept aspects of their suffering, verbalize it, and find alternative ways to cope with loss within a permissive team environment, as illustrated in the following example.

Nick, a social worker who systematically avoided any display of disheartening emotions, worked in a nursing home in which rules encouraged team sharing of personal experiences in the face of loss. Popular among residents and staff members, Nick was able to reverse feelings of anger or sadness with his outgoing, cheerful, and humorous approach. He knew every joke about death and was willing to share them with anyone who was willing to listen. However, every time a patient died, Nick disappeared, became unavailable, and missed the consultation sessions during which experiences were shared and worked through.

When Nick's favorite resident died, he fell sick; missed the memorial service that was attended by staff, residents, and family members; and, after his return to work, refused to talk about the deceased patient. Instead, he acted as if nothing had happened and went on cracking new jokes. Concerned by his behavior, the team's consultant invited him to attend the consultation sessions as an observer rather than as an active participant. As an observer, he was expected not to intervene with personal comments or jokes but to wait until the end of each session and offer some observations of the team's process of addressing difficult issues and rewarding experiences. This position allowed Nick to assume a new role; listen closely to others; and observe how they coped, expressed, managed their grief, and made sense of their experiences. He gradually grew to like his assigned role and made very astute observations and comments. At the same time the team discovered in Nick an insightful colleague who—behind his jovial facade—displayed great sensitivity and insight. By the end of the sixth session, Nick expressed a desire to actively participate in the group process by leaving behind his clowning and reacquainting himself with his fellow co-workers.

While rules that acknowledge suffering can be helpful to providers who tend to repress their grief or deny their vulnerability, in a converse way, rules that control emotional expression can be helpful to professionals who regularly become over-involved with patients and are overwhelmed by grief. These providers may gradually learn how to contain suffering, set boundaries in their relationships, and explore alternative ways of caring for themselves, as illustrated in the following example.

Barbara, a devoted nurse in a community home care program, was emotionally devastated whenever a patient was dying or died. She described in detail the privileged, intimate, and exceptional bond she had with each patient and demanded the ongoing and undivided attention and support of her colleagues, who began to resent her overwhelming grief. Her inability to set boundaries in her relationships with patients was also apparent in her relationships with her peers, whom she burdened with her uncontrollable suffering. During one staff meeting, the team decided to set aside a sharing hour once a week to discuss distressing and rewarding experiences while having pizza and dessert. This relaxed gathering became important to all team members, who listened to each other, supported one another, and had fun together. "Looking after ourselves" became an established practice and team rule. This new approach enabled members to set boundaries on Barbara's overwhelming, ongoing, and endless accounts, which were heard only during sharing hour. During that hour team members eventually confronted her about her need to monopolize everybody's attention, and she slowly learned how to listen and offer support to her colleagues, who had quieter and more subtle ways of expressing both their suffering and the satisfaction they derived from caregiving.

Incongruence between personal and collective coping patterns over team rules benefits not only the individual care provider, but sometimes the entire team. This usually occurs in situations where one or a few providers—often authority figures—challenge display rules that over-regulate or under-regulate suffering and invite members to review the team's mode of functioning. The following example illustrates this situation.

Following the insistent complaints of a bereaved relative concerning what she perceived as the staff's indifference to her needs and concerns, the director of an HIV/AIDS unit invited his team to review its practices regarding the support that was offered to grieving families. The review process brought to the surface an unacknowledged suffering over repeated loss encounters and gave team members the opportunity to express their resentment at not being supported by co-workers, leaders, and the administration. They felt that the organization expected them to act heroically in a tough and uneven battle against death and neglected their own needs. Behind a facade of indifference to bereaved families, they experienced a genuine concern for them but chose to hide it out of fear that they would appear unheroic or helpless. They were vigilant and careful not to come too close to HIV/AIDS patients and had fantasies of being totally engulfed by their complex needs. Regular discussions enabled care providers to challenge expectations and display rules, accept their own suffering, and develop activities to expand their resources. This was accomplished through team-building activities, training in bereavement care, supervised clinical practice, and the development of a close collaboration with a community bereavement center that offered counseling services to grieving families and individual consultation for professionals who asked for it. Changes in the team's mode of functioning—through the review of its goals, rules, and resources—took place over time and care providers benefited personally and collectively by actively participating in the process.

PRINCIPLE 3

There are no functional or dysfunctional teams—only teams that use functional and dysfunctional patterns to cope with loss, death, and suffering

There is no such thing as a functional or dysfunctional team. We should reconstruct our perceptions and avoid labeling teams dysfunctional or pathological and highly functional or healthy. There are only functional and dysfunctional patterns and solutions to problems that teams mobilize in order to cope with stress, loss, death, and suffering. This suggests that individuals and teams have the ability to reflect on, evaluate, consider, and choose from alternative patterns and solutions if given an appropriate context to reflect upon their experiences and work through relationships that suffer.

We can hypothesize that when dysfunctional patterns and solutions become established, the suffering of professionals who encounter death situations becomes prolonged. It is important, however, to note that all teams occasionally resort to less effective patterns and solutions, especially when they are faced with a threat or a crisis that destabilizes them. In other words, dysfunctional patterns are used from time to time, as part of a team's effort to cope with a new situation that is unknown, threatening, and anxiety provoking. This is different from situations in which dysfunctional patterns and solutions are built into the team's mode of operation and become established as the prevailing method of coping with loss, death, and suffering. Under those circumstances, they preclude alternative choices, approaches, and solutions and forbid differentiations among team members.

Conditions That Favor Functional Versus Dysfunctional Patterns

To understand the context within which patterns and solutions develop and are perpetuated, it is helpful to explore how a team first, delineates and adjusts boundaries; second, operates in dying, death, and bereavement situations; third, copes with care providers' suffering; and fourth, perceives and manages time.

Team Boundaries

Teams with clearly defined boundaries that are flexible and permeable are most likely to adopt functional patterns. Such boundaries enable interdisciplinary collaborations and promote open teamwork. In contrast, teams with rigid or diffused boundaries are more susceptible to developing dysfunctional patterns. Rigid boundaries force a team to function as a closed system in which transactions are tightly controlled. Similarly, diffused or blurred boundaries expose team members to intrusions and invasions from within or outside and cultivate chaotic transactions that render intra- and inter-team relationships a source of considerable suffering.

Team Process

When the team's goals are clear, specific, and realistic, and the roles and functions of team members specified, then care providers develop functional patterns that facilitate mutual collaboration and task achievement. Loss and trauma issues are processed, and team resources are effectively used to manage crises and challenging situations. In contrast, unclear or unrealistic goals and blurred roles and functions tend to diffuse responsibility among team members, who compartmentalize care and work independently of each other. The team's mode of functioning is never reviewed, and changes are systematically avoided or arbitrarily imposed without ever being elaborated on by members.

Suffering

Functional patterns are most likely to occur in teams that recognize and address care providers' suffering and provide an appropriate environment that enables them to openly express, contain, explore, and transform it. A supportive community is available to both those who seek care and those who provide services. In contrast, dysfunctional patterns are perpetuated in teams where professional vulnerability is dismissed and rules over-regulate or under-regulate suffering. The mismanagement of professionals' suffering leads to distant or enmeshed relationships with the dying and the bereaved.

Time

When a team paces time, it encourages care providers to elaborate on their work-related experiences, learn from the past, integrate knowledge into present practice, and strive toward future goals that aim at increasing the quality of care. Such an approach to time also helps dying and bereaved people use time to live lives worth living. In contrast, when the team strives to accelerate or immobilize its subjective perception of time in order to evade death and suffering, then experiences are lived only in the immediacy of the present and are not integrated into the team's daily experiences and history.

Here we examine some of the most common dysfunctional patterns and solutions adopted by teams in their encounters with death. Functional patterns are later described in reference to team resilience (p. 260–265).

Dysfunctional Coping Patterns and Solutions

These patterns are not unique to palliative or bereavement care teams but are recognizable in any team that offers services by means of a helping relationship. To better understand them, it is important to focus on the purpose they serve when they become established rather than only seek the causes that lead to their creation. What are some of the purposes served by dysfunctional patterns and solutions?

- *To avoid suffering triggered by loss and death and protect members from its disturbing effects.* When suffering is not acknowledged, accepted, and worked through, care providers try to push it out of consciousness and seek relief through patterns that allow them to distance themselves from the source of their distress. For example, a team may adopt a series of anti-grief patterns by becoming overactive or underactive and protecting its members from the anxiety and pain caused by a person's death or grief.
- *To hide or keep at a distance a traumatic experience that has never been processed by the team.* When a team has experienced a traumatic experience that remains unprocessed (e.g., a medical mistake, suicide, the illness of a leader), dysfunctional patterns enable the team to avoid situations that revive the trauma, which remains suppressed and ignored.
- *To avoid further loss and change.* Change requires energy, new investments, and reorganization of team functioning. By using dysfunctional patterns, the team avoids the loss of familiarity and the undertaking of changes that are perceived as too threatening, risking to uncover its fragile balance and lack of resources.
- *To validate the prevailing myths, tasks, rules, and codes according to which a team operates.* In other words, if the team's myth is one of omnipotence, then dysfunctional patterns serve to protect members from experiencing vulnerability while encouraging them to maintain a facade of power, control, and super-competence.

What seems paradoxical about dysfunctional patterns is that they are tolerated and maintained in spite of the suffering they foster. Care providers acknowledge they are unhappy and distressed, yet they do not seek patterns or solutions that would effectively change the way they operate as a team. Sometimes they adopt new patterns; however, on closer examination, it becomes evident that these reinforce rather than change the mode of functioning that is familiar to team members. Challenging or changing a team's homeostasis may prove more threatening than perpetuating dysfunctional patterns.

Although dysfunctional patterns vary, all reflect a certain degree of inertia in the team's development and growth. Box 9.2 describes some

Box 9.2

DYSFUNCTIONAL TEAM PATTERNS IN DEATH SITUATIONS

- Fragmentation of care
- Violent acts and behaviors
- Scapegoating
- Splitting and forming subgroups with rigid boundaries
- Inhibition or disqualification of reflection
- Systematic avoidance of change
- Overinvestment in and over-eroticization of relationships
- Collective somatization of suffering
- Idealization of care

of the most common dysfunctional patterns that teams use in their daily functioning and confrontation with death and suffering.

Fragmentation of Care

Fragmentation of care allows a team to divide an experience that is perceived as too threatening, into small manageable aspects in order to control its distressing effects. When we fragment care, we are protecting ourselves from being directly exposed to the depth of human suffering evoked in death situations and concurrently protect the people we serve from seeing the team's fragility and inability to contain suffering.

Palliative and bereavement care teams often fragment care by adopting models that—even though holistic in theory—tend to label the needs of people as medical, psychological, social, or spiritual. Thus, professionals with different expertise address only a minor aspect of an individual's or family's experience and work in parallel rather than in collaboration with each other. No context exists for the comprehensive integration of services that view the person and family as a system.

Furthermore, fragmentation diffuses responsibility. Too many care providers are responsible for too many individuals and families, and each focuses on a limited domain of care. Despite the availability of diverse services, these are offered in a standardized way that precludes the formation of personal bonds.

"All patients deserve the same kind of care" is often heard in teams that fragment care. It is assumed that dying and bereaved individuals are similar in their needs and concerns at the end of life or through bereavement, and care providers know—well in advance—what they require, and which team member must respond to their concerns and needs. Tasks become more important than relationships. It shouldn't matter to professionals who the recipient of care is, nor should it matter to individuals and families who attends to their needs. In fact, they are often told that "All professionals—within their area of expertise and degree of experience—are equally capable." Individuality is lost in sameness. Team members are interchangeable. Individuals and families evaluate, thank, or reject the team as a whole without personalizing their recognition or criticism. As a result, individual care providers are deprived of the opportunity to learn what has been helpful or unhelpful in the delivery of their services (Menzies-Lyth, 1988). Finally, little or no satisfaction is derived from caregiving as well as from teamwork in death situations.

Violent Acts and Behaviors

Death has a violent impact on human relationships, which are threatened, broken, and irreversibly ruptured. Moreover, death annuls efforts to save a person's life and evokes deep suffering in the bereaved. The caring relationship often becomes the target of death's violence and elicits a wide range of feelings, such as anger, anxiety, helplessness, and despair. Usually these feelings are channeled into constructive behaviors and caring acts or the pursuit of socially acceptable goals (e.g., heroic measures to save a person's life, the pursuit of the most comfortable death possible, companioning of the bereaved through suffering).

Other times, however, teams channel these feelings into destructive behaviors, which are expressed through violent, socially unacceptable acts, such as neglecting patients, dismissing their needs, omitting planned interventions, or tolerating unethical practices by colleagues. Thus, the team displays an overt or subtle collective violence against a reality that is perceived as too painful or threatening.

A violent act is a form of discourse with no voice. In other words, it is an intense experience that cannot be verbalized but, nevertheless, is communicated through actions. Team members act out their guilt, disappointment, or resentment at people for dying "on them" or for getting stuck in their grief; they neglect patients, make accusations directed at them, or draw them into team conflicts by placing them in positions in which they are forced to judge, to criticize other members of the team, or to side with one professional against another. Violence elicits further violence, and when people feel manipulated by care providers, they tend to manipulate them, thus creating further disorganization in the team's functioning. Other times, professionals direct violence at each other by engaging in chronic disputes, which can lead to lawsuits that drag coworkers into courtrooms.

I consider depersonalization and indifference extreme forms of team violence directed at individuals who threaten—by their dying, death, or bereavement—to arouse or unmask the suffering of care providers and annul the team's primary task and raison d'être. Both preclude the establishment of personal relationships. Through depersonalization, people are treated as if they possess no human qualities and are approached as a disease, a case, a room number, or a psychiatric disorder. Depersonalization elicits in dying and bereaved people anger, resentment, and hate that they sometimes display by depersonalizing care providers. They strip professionals of their individuality, forget their names or refer to them in an impersonal manner, and use their scientific knowledge or skills without ever connecting to them in a personal way.

While depersonalization deprives a person of human qualities, when one is indifferent, he or she treats others as if they do not exist. This is probably the most severe form of violence a team can ever direct at dying and bereaved people.

Scapegoating

Scapegoating is a term used to describe a process that took place in biblical times, when the ancient Hebrews would symbolically transfer their own sins to a goat and send it into exile in the desert, ridding the community of evil (Kahn, 2005). A similar practice was performed by the ancient Greeks, who made two convicts scapegoats, called *farmakoi.* These convicts became the protagonists of rituals that took place during spring festivities, when Greeks prayed to their gods for a good harvest. The *farmakoi* wandered from one town to another in order to absorb evil and free men and women from their sins and misdeeds, which could engender punishment from the gods and cause harm to the harvest and the well-being of citizens. Afterwards, these two men were chased beyond the cities' borders, thrown into the sea, or burned. The word *farmakoi* derives from the word *poison* (*farmaki*) and the word *medicine* (*farmako*). It reflects the functions of scapegoats, who absorb the "poison" and negativity of the community, while at the same time, through a cathartic process, serving as a remedy that cleanses others of evil.

Scapegoating occurs when a team—unable to contain and tolerate suffering—projects feelings and thoughts that are too threatening or distressing upon an individual or group. Care providers ally with each other against a real or imagined enemy. The role of the scapegoat can be assigned to a difficult and rebellious patient or client, to an ungrateful family, to an insensitive colleague, to an incompetent leader, to a rival team, or to a harsh and unjust board of administrators. Collective forms of violence are enacted against the scapegoated person (or the scapegoated group), against whom accusations are made, and who is rejected and marginalized.

For scapegoating to occur, the person or group must assume the role of the scapegoat and adopt the projected thoughts and feelings by acting difficult and rebellious, ungrateful, insensitive, and inadequate. Without always being aware of it, the scapegoat sacrifices him- or herself for the benefit of the team, which displaces its suffering, which consequently remains disenfranchised. Like the *farmakoi* in ancient Greece, scapegoats become the target and container of distressing thoughts and feelings, facilitate a collective catharsis, and help care providers remain united in the face of loss, separation, and suffering.

In a cardiology department, care providers resorted to scapegoating every time the team's illusion of omnipotence was threatened. There was a widespread sense of pride among team members, who often bragged, "We are the best team in the country," "We have the highest rate of patient survival," "We fight death and save lives." Families who doubted their reputation or asked for a second opinion and individual care providers who dared to question the established practice or interventions were immediately scapegoated. Professionals projected their personal doubts, fears, guilt, inadequacies, vulnerabilities, and limitations on these scapegoats, which allowed them to avoid confronting these feelings as a team.

Splitting and Forming Subgroups With Rigid Boundaries

Splitting is indicative of a team's failure to integrate conflicting experiences, which are common in the face of death. These may involve, for example, conflicting desires to form an intimate bond and to distance ourselves from the dying or bereaved individual; to prolong and to end the life of a person; to grieve and to remain stoic; and to rely upon colleagues while remaining self-sufficient. When these conflicting experiences are not acknowledged, tolerated, and integrated, care providers divide their feelings and thoughts into differentiated elements and project them upon others within or outside their team (Halton, 2000). Care providers act as if certain characteristics belong to a certain subgroup, while opposite characteristics belong to another subgroup. Members of one subgroup attribute positive qualities to themselves and project negative qualities onto members of the other subgroup. For example, care providers in a bereavement center who are unable to manage and integrate their desires to come close and to remain distant from grieving children develop splitting patterns to manage their anxiety. They form rigid subgroups that accuse each other of being too compassionate and unable to maintain appropriate boundaries or too cold and distant in their interactions with bereaved children and adolescents.

Splitting leads to the formation of subgroups. It is important, however, to note that it is not the formation of subgroups per se that is destructive to the team, but rather the impermeability of each group, which develops its own private code of values and communication rules that bar other team members from belonging to it. Subgroups develop into cliques with rigid boundaries and engage in ongoing fights between the good and the bad ones, the sensitive and the insensitive, the conservatives and the rebels, the responsible and the irresponsible, the compassionate and the detached, or those who support euthanasia and those who oppose it. Such splits become apparent in staff meetings, which are dominated by ongoing conflicts.

Kahn (2005) describes different types of splits that are common in caregiving organizations and negatively affect their functioning:

1. *Hierarchical splits* are marked by relatively impermeable boundaries between hierarchical groups (administrators are disconnected from care providers as well as from care seekers).
2. *Functional splits* undermine collaboration. They are marked by impermeable boundaries with regard to the functions of different teams (e.g., ICU team versus palliative care team versus home care team), or the functions of professionals with different disciplinary backgrounds (e.g., nurses and physicians versus psychologists and social workers).
3. *Internal team splits* are marked by the formation of subgroups with diametrically opposed positions on a key issue related to the team's primary task (e.g., those for and against euthanasia).
4. *Identity group splits* are marked by rigid boundaries between groups whose members share similar characteristics (e.g., gender, religion, ethnicity).
5. *Care provider–versus–care seeker splits* reflect a serious disruption of the team's primary task. Individuals who seek help are

perceived as the enemy or the intruder and are kept at a distance by care providers, who avoid developing relationships in order to evade suffering.

Overall, splitting patterns are indicative of a team's failure to collectively address its suffering and integrate the painful and conflicting experiences that are common in the care of people experiencing life-and-death situations.

Inhibition or Disqualification of Reflection

Another common dysfunctional pattern involves the systematic inhibition of or attack on a team's attempt to reflect and process distressing work experiences. How is this accomplished? By a colleague, for example, who monopolizes discussion with his or her personal anxieties, complaints, or experiences, leaving no time for others' accounts; by team members who systematically ridicule any emotional expression (e.g., "You are too immature and inexperienced"); by professionals who put an abrupt end to the sharing of personal experiences (e.g., "Let's not talk about sad things"); or by colleagues who systematically create confusion around expressed ideas, thoughts, and feelings.

With the tolerance of the entire team, personal accounts are interrupted, everybody talks at the same time, and new topics of discussion are introduced and immediately sidetracked by irrelevant comments, jokes, or distracting activities. Such patterns become dysfunctional when they are repeated over time and silently condoned by all the team members, who attempt to prevent reflection and elaboration of threatening, painful, or traumatic experience that elicit suffering. As a result, the team's ability to work through its experiences is compromised and care providers move from one difficult situation to another at an incredible speed, with no time to reflect on or integrate their lived experiences into a meaningful discourse. Action replaces the verbalization of experiences and becomes the enemy of thought and reflection.

Systematic Avoidance of Change

Death and trauma engender changes and new adaptations for care providers, who often have to concurrently attend to work tasks, as well as to their own suffering. When a team is regularly exposed to death, it often over-regulates grief and suffering by adopting patterns that systematically avoid any form of loss and change. Care providers cling to their familiar mode of functioning and rigidly abide by rules, even when these prove countereffective. Nursing and medical procedures become rigidly standardized, psychological assessments are performed in a ritualistic manner, and prescribed interventions are applied to all problems. New decisions and initiatives are downplayed, discarded, and sometimes aborted for being unrealistic or doomed to fail. Statements such as "This is the way we function in this team," "There is no need to try something else," and "It won't work" silence suggestions of any alternative approach, proposal, or solution to a given situation. New projects or ideas are resented and systematically sabotaged. Knowledge derived from evidence-based research is not used to enhance practice or incorporated into the team's mode of functioning. In crisis situations that demand an altered mode of team functioning, quick and prescribed solutions are applied. Any new and unknown situation is perceived as threatening, engendering losses, discomfort, and uncertain outcomes—despite any potential benefits it might offer. The systematic use of avoidant patterns immobilizes the team in its course of development.

Overinvestment in and Over-Eroticization of Relationships

Some teams develop patterns through which they attempt to annul the disruption that death creates in human bonds by over-investing in relationships with individuals, families, and peers. Therefore, in response to loss, they develop symbiotic relationships without maintaining appropriate boundaries. In such teams, care providers are devastated or feel rejected, betrayed, or abandoned when a person dies (e.g., "He died on me") or when a family gradually moves away from the team and on with its life (e.g., "They gave up on us").

Fused and enmeshed patterns of interaction are common even among team members. Holidays and family celebrations are *always* spent with co-workers, who "adopt" each other's spouses and children. There is an implicit expectation that care providers' primary emotional commitment is to their team, which functions as a big family and incorporates, protects, and nurtures anyone who is significant to its members' lives. Attempts at individuation are criticized, while professionals who maintain private lives totally independent of the team are subtly marginalized or made to feel guilty.

In some teams, fused and enmeshed patterns lead to an over-eroticization of relationships in the face of death. Care providers systematically flirt and fall in love with each other and sometimes with the people they serve. These behaviors are silently tolerated or condoned by the team. It is important to distinguish the natural tendency to invest in relationships and activities that offer a sense that one is alive, loved, and in love from the persistent involvement in relationships and erotic activities that serve to counteract the anxiety over loss, death, and suffering.

Skogstad (2000) offers the example of a cardiology department where nurses and physicians, under the strain of several deaths, developed a highly sexualized atmosphere and flirted with each other in an open and provocative way in the presence of patients. By exciting each other, they distanced themselves from death, decay, and suffering. Thus, they were reassured that they were alive, sexually active, and distinct from dying people and bereaved individuals, who were deprived of relationships with their loved ones.

Collective Somatization of Suffering

In teams that systematically disenfranchise grief and suffering, members often display somatic complaints and physical problems. This somatization sometimes takes the form of an epidemic, with all or most team members presenting identical symptoms. Behind this collective "contagion," care providers who identify with each other's pain share their suffering in silence. Physical symptoms replace words and reflective sharing.

This dysfunctional pattern was adopted by care providers in a dialysis care team that encountered a major crisis that was never addressed. Team members hid their distress and projected an image of super-competence and efficacy, worked extra hours, and remained focused on tasks that kept them busy. Within a week, the large majority of them felt sick, and patients were transferred to other dialysis units in the local community. A few months later, a similar somatization occurred again when the team was faced with the death of three patients within a short period of time. The team's leader experienced whiplash and had to wear a neck brace; soon after, two other care providers wore similar braces as a result of an identical muscular dysfunction! By the end of the week, the team's social worker had left a note on the office's bulletin board, in which she noted: "I'll be away for a few days. I can't *swallow* any more death experiences." This note triggered staff discussions about the symbolic meaning of the collective somatization that had replaced words, and team members were eventually able to verbalize and share their suffering. Soon after, patterns of collective somatization disappeared, and the team began to consider alternative ways of coping with loss and death issues.

Idealization of Care

Idealization of care allows team members to attribute qualities and powers to their team that it does not possess in order to avoid confronting limitations and vulnerabilities that are evoked by loss and death. Care providers thrive on an illusion of excellence that is never questioned or reviewed and preclude the consideration of alternative courses of action or the examination of team shortcomings. There is a tacit agreement among care providers to keep within the team's boundaries any person or situation that reinforces the illusion of excellence, and to reject or exclude any person or situation that threatens its idealized image.

Through patterns of idealization, interpersonal conflicts, unresolved loss and trauma experiences, and suffering are hidden or masked. The team presents itself as the best, capable of outstanding achievements, while staff relations appear free of conflict and harmonious yet undifferentiated. Team members become openly or subtly aggressive whenever a colleague adopts an alternative approach to care, when a family seeks a second or third opinion, or when another team or organization seeks recognition. The team's energy is expanded toward the maintenance of an ideal image that precludes adjustment to the ongoing demands of a changing reality.

In summary, dysfunctional patterns reflect fragile relationships among staff members and a team's difficulty separating the lived experience of a painful or threatening situation from a reflective process upon these experiences. The team remains stuck in its evolution because it resorts to dysfunctional patterns in order to avoid, distort, or minimize the suffering evoked by the care of seriously ill, dying, and bereaved people. Paradoxically, the perpetuation of dysfunctional patterns creates more suffering and renders the team vulnerable to various forms of disorganization. It only requires a trigger to cause a major crisis that reveals the underlying suffering and brings to the surface interpersonal conflicts, as well as unresolved losses and traumas in the team's life trajectory.

While psychodynamic therapists suggest that dysfunctional patterns represent the team's unconscious resistance against anxiety and change, systemic clinicians perceive dysfunctional patterns as indications of a system's prudence in the face of loss, suffering, and change, rather than a defense against it (Ausloos, 2003).

Teams need a safe space, time, and distance from their experiences in order to reflect on, evaluate, consider, try out, and experiment with alternative patterns and solutions that can help them cope more effectively with the challenges they encounter in the face of death.

PRINCIPLE 4

The chronic use of dysfunctional patterns renders a team vulnerable to various types of disorganization

Dysfunctional patterns have long-term effects that become evident in various forms of team disorganization. Imagine team organization on a continuum. At each end of this continuum there is an extreme form of disorganization that reflects the system's level of entropy—in other words, its tendency toward disorder, degradation, and death. These aspects of disorganization involve ongoing overactivity and over-agitation that leads to *team chaos*, and a sustained inertia that leads to *team* marasme *and immobility*.

We should not assume that all teams that use dysfunctional patterns end up in chaos or immobilization. Most oscillate between the two and experience periods of inertia that alternate with periods of overexcitation and overactivity. Problems occur when dysfunctional patterns become chronic and the team's entire functioning is built around chaos or immobilization. Under these conditions, the team creates a new order out of the disorder that is maintained by the perpetuation of dysfunctional patterns. An organized disorganization is established that aims to protect care providers from facing loss, death, and suffering.

I have found relevant to the understanding of team disorganization the work of Guy Ausloos, a Canadian family therapist who has observed and analyzed families that present major dysfunctions. In his book *La compétence des familles: Temps, chaos, processus,* Ausloos (2003) describes forms of extreme disorganization that become apparent in family transactions that are either too rigid or too chaotic. He suggests that families with rigid transactions perceive time as arrested ("temps arrêté"), while families with chaotic transactions experience time as eventful ("temps evenementiel"). Both types of families misuse information that could help them understand their disorganization, as a result of which they are unable to make necessary changes that could contribute to their growth. The past cannot be used as a learning experience that can enhance the family's functioning in the present, while the future remains unforeseeable. Unable to situate themselves in time, these families live in the present with no perspective on their future.

A parallel can be drawn with teams that systematically use dysfunctional patterns to cope with loss, death, and suffering. In such teams, the *misuse of information* and a *discontinuous relation to time* compromise team functioning and the potential for change, evolution, and growth. With regard to the first, pertinent information that is helpful to effective team functioning is not appropriately used to benefit the dying and bereaved, as well as care providers. With regard to the latter, team members fight against the passage of time in a desperate effort to stop or slow it down so as to prevent death and avoid being affected by it, or they strive to speed up time in order to evade the suffering that death evokes. How do they accomplish this? Either by systematically filling time with activities, tasks, interventions, events, and crisis episodes that lead to team chaos or by freezing time through the suspension of actions, decisions, and interventions, which leads the team to apathy, inertia, and immobilization.

Both forms of team disorganization compromise change, progress, and growth (Figure 9.2).

Team Chaos

Chaos prevails in teams where members maintain chaotic transactions. Care providers engage in situations that lead to ongoing overactivity and over-agitation as they move frantically from one stressful event or crisis episode to another. Such over-agitation is not a temporary response to increased job demands, but a permanent condition that results from the team's attempts to avoid anxiety-provoking relationships, threatening circumstances, suffering, and death. Care providers attend to individuals and families, to team problems or conflicts, to bureaucratic or administrative issues, and even to secondary tasks that absorb all their energy with an acute sense of urgency. They overinvest in work tasks and leave no space or time to invest in relationships with people.

In such teams, time is determined by a sequence of events and crisis episodes that are often created or perpetuated by the use of dysfunctional coping patterns. Time for such teams becomes "eventful time." Acting and reacting are ongoing and vital to the team's survival, since underneath this frantic over-agitation lies an unrecognized need to escape

Team Chaos	**Team Immobilization**
Mode of Operation	
Ongoing overactivity Ongoing overagitation Over-investment in tasks & crises Disinvestment of relations	**Underactivity - Inertia** Facade of order and control No or minimal investment in tasks Disinvestment of relations
Relations/Transactions	
Chaotic, **Impersonal**	**Rigid, formal** **Impersonal, distant**
Relations to time	
"Event-full" time determined by sequence of events/crises	**"Frozen" time** determined by suspension of actions/decisions
Focus on the present	**Focus on the present**
Overstimulation of information Failure to use it for learning or change	No circulation of information Failure to use it for learning or change
"Let's move on. We are running out of time..."	"Let's buy some time. Let's no rock the boat".

Figure 9.2 Extreme forms of team disorganization

from death, loss, and pain. The perception of time is distorted in ways that make only the immediacy of the present moment count. What precedes or follows an event or crisis episode is not integrated. There is an over-stimulation and overload of information that is not assimilated or used appropriately. Incoming information that could be relevant and useful to the team functioning remains fragmented, sporadic, and superficial. Experiences cannot be stored in memory, integrated, elaborated on, and storied in a coherent way. Questions such as "What really happened?" "Why did this event or crisis occur now?" "What precipitated it?" "How did it affect our relationships, our interventions, and the functioning of our team?" "What patterns or solutions proved effective or ineffective?" "What can be learned from this event or crisis episode?" remain unanswered.

A dictate prevails that suggests: "Let's move on! We are running out of time. We have no time for chats with individuals, families, or colleagues. Duty calls." There is a manic pace of work that is reinforced by task demands, ambitious goals, and rushed decisions, often in view of incomplete information. Personal conversations with dying patients and grieving relatives are perceived as chats, while the significance of emotional bonds is dismissed. The implicit message in such a team suggests: "It's too risky to slow down in order to develop personal relationships and reflect upon our experiences. Any form of elaboration may reveal the vulnerability and suffering that we experience and may prove our attempts to be stoic and strong in death situations futile."

The team's culture is one of action and reaction, with care providers avoiding processing their experiences through the persistent use of dysfunctional team patterns. Sometimes this over-agitation is maintained by the unduly frequent moves of personnel or by prolonged staff absenteeism. Sudden transfers or the unstructured integration of staff members, students, interns, and volunteers in a service, as well as frequent absences due to sickness, business trips, or other responsibilities, blur the boundaries of the team, which has to constantly redefine itself and adjust to an ongoing process of change. Faced with such turmoil, the team learns to avoid close relationships with individuals, families, and co-workers. This excessive over-agitation increases chaotic situations and transactions and paradoxically contributes to the maintenance of disorganization. Thus the team organizes its functioning around chaos and disorganization and creates a new order out of the non-order.

Team Immobilization

Immobilization occurs in teams with rigid transactions. It is preceded by an under-activity and generalized passivity indicative of team *marasme. Marasme* is a Greek word that means "fading away," "dying," "leading to death and decay." It is used to describe a progressive degenerative process that leads to team immobilization, which is maintained by dysfunctional patterns. Sometimes immobilization is hidden behind the pretence that everything is fine. Underneath this facade, care providers experience burnout and low morale and feel trapped in a job from which they derive little or no satisfaction. They are more absorbed by team conflicts than by their encounters with the people who seek their services. They do not invest in work tasks, and relationships with the dying and the bereaved become distant or strictly formal. Interventions are performed "by the book" in a ritualistic, mechanical manner to the point that professionals often forget that they are applied to people. In fact, dying and bereaved people are perceived as a burden and, as a result, are resented and often treated with aggression. When this happens, professionals experience guilt and compensate by overinvesting in work tasks and relationships. However, this erratic investment is short lived, because they quickly exhaust themselves (since they possess little or no energy) and resort to a new cycle of inertia and apathy that causes further resentment and despair. They often hide away in an office and spend long hours in staff meetings that are sterile, repetitive, and boring, reflective of the team's stagnation. Whenever a care provider acts differently, introduces innovative ideas, or develops intimate bonds with care seekers, he or she is immediately made a scapegoat or alienated.

Death-related experiences are lived in the immediacy of the present and quickly forgotten or suppressed. Names of individuals and families, their stories, and their clinical experiences are erased from memory. Information that could be useful to team functioning does not circulate among professionals. Everything remains unchanged. Time is frozen.

The past is perceived as irreversibly lost. It is forgotten or idealized. Idealization, however, renders it painful since the reminiscence about the good old days causes more despair than comfort. Statements such as "There is no point in looking back to the past. It hurts too much to remember our team's glory days" are quite common.

Concurrently, the future is perceived as a mere repetition of the present. There is a belief that nothing can change. "What's the point of trying something different? We will always continue to do the same things over and over again… forever." There is no innovation, no creation, no movement forward, since there is no anticipation, no hope, and no dreams.

Immobilization maintains the team's mode of operation and its dynamics. Everyone minds his or her own business or task, while crises are systematically avoided since they demand increased energy when resources are depleted. The message that prevails is: "Let's buy some time. Let's not rock the boat." However, it covertly suggests: "We barely manage to survive. Moving forward requires more energy than we possess and causes more anxiety than we can tolerate. Let's not stir up situations that will reveal our suffering." Care providers are merely interested in surviving in a job that provides them with a salary and economic security, but no satisfaction.

In summary, chaos and immobilization allow the team to remain unchanged and compromise its evolution and growth. In both situations, dysfunctional patterns are perpetuated over time and organized around a chaotic or immobilized mode of operation. There are no opportunities for reflection and elaboration on experiences, which would allow care providers to circulate information and use it constructively to learn from their experiences, address their suffering, and make appropriate changes in the team's functioning. Boundaries are either too rigid, in which case team members develop distant relationships that prevent the circulation of information, or too diffused and enmeshed, in which case team members lose sight of their roles and separate functions. The overall feeling is one of job dissatisfaction.

Organized in their disorganization, such teams become extremely vulnerable to chronic disputes, frequent resignations, and pervasive suffering among providers, who experience a sense of utter loneliness, often reflected in statements such as "No one cares. No one can really understand what we are going through." This sense of loneliness becomes a source of suffering that is even more painful than the actual confrontation with death.

Intervention in a Team's Disorganization

In extreme forms of team disorganization, the need for an appropriate intervention by an experienced consultant (who is external to the team and the organization) is imperative. Consultation can help the team review and deconstruct its "organized disorganization" and discover or use its resources in the pursuit of a new equilibrium. This is accomplished when the team with a chaotic mode of operation is helped to learn how to slow down and pace time in order to use the available information and move out of chaos. Conversely, the team that becomes apathetic can learn how to mobilize time and facilitate the flow of information in order to move out of inertia. The latter can be achieved through the introduction of a change or a crisis at a team level that offers possibilities for the exchange of experiences among team members (Ausloos, 2003).

Any intervention should aim at introducing an element of temporality by inviting care providers to construct stories of their experiences and of their collective trajectory through time. Narration can help them discover a thread that links the past with the present and future and permits the integration of lived experiences into a historical context.

PRINCIPLE 5

Crises are inevitable; they hold the potential for team disorganization as well as team growth

A team's confrontation with death may be experienced as a challenge, a crisis, or a distressing or neutral event. This depends upon a number of variables. Some are developmental and intrinsically related to the team's prior death experiences and current mode of functioning in the face of loss; other variables are situational, associated with concurrent stressors experienced by the team (e.g., bereavement overload, cutting of funds, staff changes); and still other variables are appraisal and value related. When reality does not conform to the team's values, beliefs, expectations, and experience, death is likely to be perceived as a threatening and highly distressing event. A death that is highly distressing to one team may not be to another.

For example, in our studies, members of a critical care team perceived as most distressing, the slow death of patients who were hospitalized for an unusually long time and with whom care providers had developed an emotional bond; in contrast, members of the oncology team perceived as most distressing sudden and unexpected deaths that deprived them of the opportunity to save a life or to develop a meaningful relationship with the person who died (Papadatou et al., 2002). Different types of encounters with death challenged each team's values and practices, causing discontinuities in their familiar modes of functioning.

Sometimes a death experience can trigger a team crisis. In an attempt to understand the dynamics involved, I offer some of my views on team crisis in Box 9.3 and discuss various forms we encounter in our work with dying and bereaved people.

Pinel (1996) distinguishes between two types of crises: the mutative crisis and the explosive crisis. The difference between the two is not related to the nature of the event that triggers the crisis but to the way the event is perceived and managed by the team or organization.

Mutative Crises

A mutative crisis usually occurs during transitional periods, when a team reviews and restructures its goals, values, and mode of functioning. The

Box 9.3

BASIC ASSUMPTIONS ABOUT TEAM CRISES

- Crises are unavoidable in every team.
- A crisis temporarily throws the team's established dynamics and mode of operation out of balance and confronts care providers with chaos, disorder, destruction, and a sense of meaninglessness. However, crisis also offers opportunities for change through the discovery of a new order, of alternative views of reality, and of new coping patterns and solutions.
- Death-related experiences can trigger a crisis when they are perceived as too threatening to the team's myth, primary tasks, or mode of functioning; its goals, values, and expectations as to what is appropriate in dying and bereavement.
- Dysfunctional team patterns may cause, precipitate, or aggravate a crisis, while functional team patterns tame the temporary chaos that a crisis creates by using its potential for innovation and change.
- Not every crisis is necessarily detrimental to the team, nor should all crises be controlled or avoided at all costs. A crisis introduces new information. When this information is used constructively, it can lead to new adaptations or changes.
- Adaptations ameliorate aspects of team functioning, while changes restructure the team and its mode of functioning and bring new order and balance following a crisis.

crisis may be triggered by an external, painful, or traumatic event, or the accumulation of several minor or major stressful events. The outcomes of the crisis largely depend upon how care providers perceive the crisis, how they cope with the challenges evoked by an unknown or highly distressing situation, and how they move from a familiar to an unfamiliar reality.

Consider the following example. The suicide of an individual who was grieving the death of a family member created a mutative crisis in a hospice team and forced professionals to take the time to review the nature of the services they provided to grieving families, the effectiveness of their interdisciplinary collaboration, and the collective patterns they used to cope with death, bereavement, and suffering. The suicide occurred during a period when team members were voicing frustrations and concerns about the quality of care that was being provided to grieving families, and engaging in long debates about alternative forms of action. The suicide reinforced a reflective process that was underway and accelerated the implementation of changes to the team's mode of functioning and interdisciplinary collaboration.

Explosive Crises

An explosive crisis occurs suddenly and without warning and creates a major rupture in the team's structure or mode of functioning. Consider the previous example of the bereaved person's suicide. The same event could be experienced as an explosive crisis in a team that interprets the suicide as a fatal failure to serve the needs of bereaved families, and a severe blow to the team's reputation and goals of excellence.

An explosive crisis sometimes reflects the team's inability to cope with mutative crises that are managed through dysfunctional patterns that preclude the review of team goals and modes of functioning. As a result, team members resort to destructive and violent acts and use scapegoating or splitting patterns to manage the suffering that a traumatic event elicits.

Not every explosive crisis leads to team chaos and disorganization. In Hong Kong, the SARS epidemic some years ago caused the death of 67 people, 6 of whom were health care professionals. This created an explosive crisis among care providers, who were suddenly forced to work in an unfamiliar way that caused a discontinuity to their existing goals and mode of operation. Every patient and co-worker was perceived as a potential enemy. Death was a threat both to the layperson and to the professional. Palliative care became particularly taxing for health care professionals, who were required to wear gowns, masks, and gloves and, through an impersonal and alien demeanor, attempted to maintain personal and human relationships with terminally ill patients and grieving families. Bereavement services were in high demand. The SARS epidemic quickly overtaxed care providers, depleted their resources, and confronted them with their own suffering and increased levels of burnout. They worked under highly stressful conditions and under the constant threat of death. Anxiety, grief, and suffering could not be dismissed or neglected.

Out of this explosive crisis sprang a nonprofit organization founded by a group of health care professionals in Hong Kong. This nongovernmental organization—with the financial support of the government—developed a center called Oasis, which currently provides professionals with a safe space in which they can receive professional counseling, engage in relaxation or meditation activities, listen to music, watch movies, interact with colleagues at their leisure and attend to their needs. The center was created as a response to an explosive crisis, and as a proactive attempt to cope with the distress and suffering that affect care providers in their daily work as well as in extraordinary situations caused by a disaster or pandemic.

Multiple Team Crises

Sometimes, a crisis provokes a series of parallel crises in a team that has consistently used dysfunctional patterns to cope with challenges and difficulties. In fact, a triggering event brings to the surface prior unresolved issues or traumas that have been suppressed for a long time and creates secondary losses that the team is unable to manage.

Consider the following example. In an adult oncology unit in which there was high staff and administrative turnover, an overdose was administered to a patient, whose condition deteriorated suddenly and became critical. The medical director called a staff meeting and requested a detailed account of events from the young nurse who had administered the overdose. The nurse, unaware that she had administered an overdose, accused the head nurse of not having drawn her attention to the new labels and dosages that the pharmaceutical company had issued for the drug in question. Instantly there was chaos in the unit, with all staff members shouting at each other and making accusations. In the midst of the turmoil, the head nurse, who felt hurt and unjustly accused, announced her resignation from the team. This drew attention to her, and the team engaged in a long debate in an attempt to convince her to reconsider. Discussion moved from the medical error to another crisis caused by the potential loss of one of its leaders. The situation was further escalated when the social worker, who had remained quiet through the staff conflict, left the room, declaring that his time was better spent at the bedsides of patients than among his troublesome co-workers, and slamming the door behind him. His dismissive attitude triggered a new crisis that redirected discussions toward long-term conflicts among team members that had gone unaddressed. Chaos was met by further chaos, as team members moved with an incredible speed from one crisis to another to avoid coping with the guilt, pain, and suffering that the medical error had created. Eventually, the young nurse was scapegoated and was expelled from the team. This critical incident was experienced as a collective trauma that was never again addressed. It deprived the team of an opportunity to use pertinent information in a productive manner, address conflicts, learn from experience, and move forward in its growth.

A mutative or explosive crisis sometimes elicits prior unresolved conflicts or trauma issues. When the team spends its energy on denying or dismissing them, opportunities for change and growth decrease.

Other times, a crisis can be aggravated by the impact it has upon certain individual care providers. Diet (1996) analyzes the destructive behavior of some highly vulnerable care providers with personal histories of unresolved loss that they display only when the team undergoes a crisis. He argues that their destructive behavior is not apparent at other times, but only during a crisis episode that reactivates their personal experiences of trauma. Threatened by suffering or emotional breakdown, these care providers exercise a power of destruction against any collective effort to work through the crisis. They sabotage every form of elaboration of events, reject or cast doubts on proposed interventions and changes, and deny the anxiety and suffering that the crisis evokes in them. They forestall the circulation of information (e.g., "Let's forget what happened and move on") and seek allies among other care providers who are also ambivalent and threatened by the crisis. Together, they cultivate splits and create confusion, miscommunications, and discontinuities that affect the entire team. For example, by developing exclusive relationships with some colleagues (e.g., "I can say this only to you") they secretly attack any team member who represents the team's ideals or is capable of containing the chaos and facilitating a process of learning and change.

Diet (1996) suggests that these extremely vulnerable care providers cope with their personal suffering by creating more suffering and destruction in the team. However, it would be mistaken to assume that they are responsible for the team's crisis. Their difficulties are further aggravated when the team is unable to provide a holding environment for its members and opportunities to work through the chaos that the crisis creates. In such an environment, dysfunctional dynamics are perpetuated among co-workers whose personal histories of loss resonate with the team's loss history.

The Risks and Benefits of Team Crisis

As has already been suggested, every crisis holds the potential for change and innovation. Sometimes the only hope for change is for a mutative crisis to turn into an explosive one in order to mobilize the team's creativity and resources and provoke reorganizations. Other times, an explosive crisis is better managed if it is turned into a series of mutative crises, over which care providers have a greater sense of control and efficacy.

Not every crisis is detrimental to a team. Although distressing, a crisis always holds the potential for positive changes and growth. Changes, however, are not always welcomed by the team. Why? Because, as Menzies-Lyth (1988) suggests, "Change is inevitably to some extent an excursion into the unknown. It implies a commitment to future events that are not entirely predictable and to their consequences, and inevitably provokes doubt and anxiety" (p. 62).

This explains why it is difficult for a team to change its established patterns of coping with death, loss, and suffering, despite the fact that team members accurately perceive the need for a change. Changes cause increased anxiety and elicit fear of chaos and destruction. A team must be able to contain its anxiety and fears in order for change to occur.

Rouchy and Desroche (2004) distinguish *changes* from *adaptations*, which occur as a result of a crisis or planned intervention. According to them, changes require a thorough review of the team's goals, values, structure, and mode of operation. No change is possible without the adoption of new perceptions, beliefs, and values, all of which are translated into new forms of action. Adaptations, in contrast, integrate new behaviors and practices into a preexisting system of values and beliefs. Even though adaptations can ameliorate a team's functioning through the implementation of bright ideas and initiatives, they nevertheless allow the system to remain unchanged by reinforcing its myth, primary tasks, and established mode of functioning.

Team growth occurs mostly through changes that demand a process of working through challenging experiences and team crises. According to Levy (1973; cited in Rouchy & Desroche, 2004), this process is often slow, anxiety provoking, and difficult and involves an element of risk. However, it enables a team to reframe its experiences in new ways, so as to acquire new meanings. Traditional practices, values, and team rules are challenged or disconfirmed, and established patterns of interaction invalidated. A lack of order is almost inevitable before new meanings, values, and patterns are discovered and adopted.

Ausloos (2003) suggests that change occurs as a result of a system's ability to *tame* the chaos that a crisis creates, instead of striving to control it. He argues that we tame chaos when we develop a genuine interest in the accidental, the different, the unexplainable, the lack of order, and when we are able to stand in the dark, not understanding or making sense of a situation, yet trusting that the team will expand its way of thinking, will explore that which it cannot fully understand, and will learn from experience. We tame the chaos that a crisis creates by seeking to use new information and learn from novel or unfamiliar experiences, as well as by using the team's potential for creativity, innovation, and change. Changes that derive from such a process are reflected in the team's functional patterns, as well as in care providers' positive representations of themselves, their teams, and the people they serve.

PRINCIPLE 6

All teams have the potential to function with competence

No matter how disorganized a team may be, it always has the potential to develop functional patterns and operate with competence, as long as certain conditions are fostered. What are these conditions? Little do we actually know. The existing literature on teams describes a number of characteristics that make teams effective or high functioning.[1] Teams that do not present certain positive attributes tend to be pathologized, while proposed interventions aim at managing team problems and dysfunctions. My intent is not to outline these fixed characteristics, since their presence or absence does not determine, in my view, team functioning. What determines team competence are certain conditions that facilitate caregiving and care receiving in an environment that is supportive of both those who seek care and those who provide it. Three basic conditions exist that enhance the team's ability to function with competence in death situations: *commitment* to clearly defined tasks and to each other, a *holding environment* for care seekers and care providers, and *open teamwork* through interdisciplinary collaborations (Figure 9.3).

When the triangle is equilateral (i.e., all sides are of equal length), then care is likely to be satisfactory for both care seekers and care providers. Professionals are committed to shared goals and to each other, work in a holding environment that enables them to process their experiences and cope with distress and suffering, and are open to meaningful collaborations with other teams and professionals. Recognizing which of these three conditions is underdeveloped can help a team plan appropriate actions and interventions.

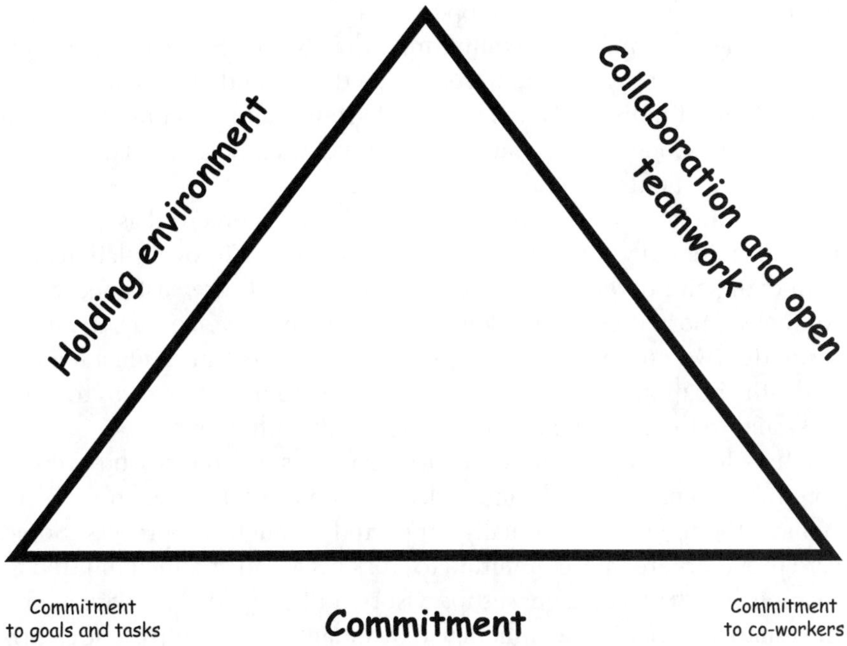

Figure 9.3 Conditions that promote team competence in death situations

Condition 1: Commitment

According to Ketchum and Trist (1992), who conducted extensive research on organizations, "commitment to work is central to people's lives" (p. 14). However, such commitment "is conditional on the work experience" (p. 15). The authors define "work experience" as the way work is organized. Through their qualitative studies, they distinguish between good and bad work experiences. A care provider is most likely to commit him- or herself when certain psychosocial factors (variety and challenge, continuous learning, autonomy, recognition, support, the sense that one is making a meaningful contribution, desirable future) and socioeconomic factors (adequate pay, job security, benefits, safety) are present. In fact, a good work experience lies at the core of what these researchers describe as 'quality of work life'.

Caring for dying and bereaved individuals is often so distressing that to remain committed in this field of work, we must attach meaning to both what we are doing and how we achieve our goals. While team goals orient our actions, in reality supportive and collaborative relations help us to achieve them. Thus, commitment has two components: (1) commitment to clear, realistic, and well-defined goals and tasks that promote the welfare of individuals, families, and groups, and (2) commitment to each other through collaborative and mutually supportive relationships. These components are closely interrelated.

The more committed we are to tasks that are perceived as meaningful and potentially rewarding, the more we invest in our relationships with dying and bereaved people. Such investments are sustained when we feel supported by our work environment. In a reverse way, the more supported we are by co-workers, supervisors, or organizational leaders in death situations, the more likely we are to commit ourselves to work tasks and to the development of caring bonds with others.

In a few words, committed care providers are those who are devoted to meaningful goals and tasks, rely upon each other in order to achieve them, and are mutually supported through the process. Some care providers are only committed to work tasks and are uncommitted to relationships with colleagues, supervisors, and team leaders, with whom they share competitive, conflictual, or avoidant relationships. With a primary concern on doing the job right and projecting an image of self-efficacy, they fail to develop a genuine interest in others and work with team spirit. Their services are ego centered or theory driven, rather than relationship centered.

Commitment to Goals and Tasks That Promote the Welfare of Individuals and Families

Commitment to goals and tasks is facilitated when they are *clearly defined,* thus orienting care providers to their individual and collective pursuits; *realistic,* with defined criteria to determine effectiveness; *meaningful* to all members of a team; and *open to review* from time to time.

These goals take into account the welfare of both the individual and the network of significant others to which he or she belongs.

Goals and tasks should be operationalized into concrete forms of action and must not remain mere descriptions of good intentions. In addition, specific criteria should determine whether goals and tasks have been achieved. If, for example, the goal of a bereavement team is to support bereaved children by extending psychological services to significant people in their lives, then interventions that include them should be developed (e.g., parents' groups, peer support programs, seminars for educators). In assessing whether the team's goals were effectively achieved, evaluation should focus upon the well-being of bereaved children, as well as upon their sense of belonging among significant others (e.g., family, school, community). Moreover, assessment should further extend to the well-being of the family, school, or community, which may have benefited from available services.

Clear goals and tasks also help to define and delineate the roles and responsibilities of care providers who work in close collaboration. When these are vague and unclear, professionals assume roles that do not belong to them and offer services that are off task. A psychologist, for example, assumes the role of an overprotective parent toward bereaved children, or a nurse adopts the nurturing role of a spouse toward a seriously ill patient, or an entire team functions as a family, with leaders acting as parents, team members as children, patients as "adopted" children, and relatives as rivals and outcasts. These off-task roles contribute to dysfunctional patterns that foster splitting, scapegoating, or the idealization of team members or leaders.

One of the main problems in palliative and bereavement care is that teams often strive to achieve unrealistic goals with tasks aimed at a perfect death or a perfect bereavement (Marquis, 1993). This is often reflected in their striving to achieve a death that is totally free of physical and emotional suffering, with the person dying in acceptance and harmony with him- or herself and others, and the relatives having settled all their unfinished business. Bereavement teams may also strive to achieve a perfect bereavement, which is determined by the person's open expression of feelings, accomplishment of grief tasks, and attribution of a positive meaning to loss.

Unrealistic goals exhaust care providers. Clinical practice shows that sometimes people do not have a good death, and many believe that there is no good way to die. Moreover, not every bereaved person wishes to openly express grief, maintain a continuing bond with the deceased, or even find positive meaning in a devastating loss. Some bereaved people find purpose and pleasure in delving into suffering, and others are relieved by the death of a significant person (e.g., an abusive spouse, a mentally ill relative) and happy to develop a new life on their own.

Realistic goals and tasks acknowledge the limitations of what care providers and teams can offer. We cannot always avoid death or prolong life, nor can we promise relief from grief. The only thing we can commit ourselves to is a caring relationship in which we are present, available, and able to introduce continuity in the midst of loss, separation, and suffering. Such a relationship can be developed when the work context enhances interconnectedness at a team level.

Commitment to Co-Workers

Commitment to co-workers requires an involvement in relationships with our colleagues. Acknowledging the suffering that we, the care providers, often experience in death situations is not always enough. In committed relationships, there is a willingness to do something about distress and suffering. This may be accomplished in various ways: by providing information or feedback to a peer, by being present at the side of a grieving co-worker, by responding in a humane way to a distressed colleague, by offering and receiving emotional support, and so forth. Committed care providers show care and concern. They do not offer each other counseling or therapy but refer others or ask for help whenever such needs arise. Mutual support is compromised whenever team members are too absorbed in themselves, engulfed in their own suffering, or overconfident about their ability to manage difficulties on their own.

Sometimes we mistakenly believe that being committed to each other requires a high degree of emotional bonding and intimacy with co-workers. Even though this is common in palliative and bereavement care teams, it is not always the case. Some teams prefer to maintain a high degree of bonding that is limited solely to the pursuit and achievement of specific goals. They collaborate, respect each other's knowledge and skills, and are mutually supportive in the performance of well-defined tasks.

Commitment to each other involves a sense not only of shared responsibility for the welfare of others, but also of solidarity among co-workers. Solidarity, according to Tessier (1993), constitutes "the most important coping mechanism when [one is] facing death and the intense distress that necessarily goes with it" (p. 1). In fact, solidarity—referred to in the literature as social support—is the ingredient that sustains care providers in this field of work.

We must broaden our perspective on solidarity and recognize its multiple aspects. Through our studies, we identified four aspects of support that we seek and expect to receive from colleagues:

1 *Informational support* involves the exchange of information about the people we serve, and about the team's mode of operation; it comprises mutual feedback about and evaluation of

individual or team performance with opportunities to expand one's knowledge and skills.

2. *Instrumental support* involves helping each other with practical issues (e.g., sharing of workload), and the coordination of efforts toward the achievement of specific tasks. Shared goals, role clarity, and trust in each other's knowledge and skills enhance this form of support.
3. *Emotional support* involves opportunities for sharing personal feelings and thoughts in a safe environment in which one feels heard, understood, valued, and appreciated. Sometimes the mere presence of another colleague during stressful moments is all that one needs.
4. *Support in meaning construction* involves opportunities to reflect on and work through work-related experiences and invest individual and collective efforts with meaning. Care providers help each other understand their responses, correct distortions, and reframe a situation in ways that make sense to them (Papadatou, Papazoglou, Petraki, & Bellali, 1999).

Each team values and encourages different aspects of support at different times. For mutual support to be effective, it must be timely and responsive to the specific needs and preferences of care providers, which vary from one team to another, and at different times or under different circumstances. Usually emotional support takes precedence when a traumatic experience affects the entire team (e.g., the illness or death of a colleague, or a beloved patient), while informational and practical support becomes a necessity when tasks require the coordination of services (e.g., family and community support following multiple deaths). Whether mutual support is provided often depends on a team's goals, rules, and mode of functioning, which determine which aspects of support are desirable and acceptable (Papadatou et al., 1999).

In an intensive care unit, for example, team members valued informational and instrumental support, which helped them perform their tasks and save people's lives. They were very efficient in exchanging information, teaching skills to younger colleagues, and coordinating complex interventions. Team rules demanded that they keep their emotions under control so as to avoid any interference with their clinical judgment. Their need for emotional support was totally ignored, and several professionals complained about the lack of care and concern among co-workers. They hardly ever shared their experiences as a team, while several raised ethical and existential concerns that others avoided bringing up out of fear of rocking the boat. To cope with the lack of emotional and meaning-making support in the unit, some practitioners invited colleagues into their family lives by offering them the roles of best man, maid of honor, and godparent, while a few got married to each other. Thus, they integrated opportunities for emotional support into their personal lives, which the rules of the work environment discouraged.

In contrast, in an oncology team that reinforced close relationships with patients and families, care providers effectively supported each other at an emotional and meaning-making level, to the detriment of informational and practical support. While they bragged about solidarity in the face of death, they also complained about role blurring, and unsatisfactory coordination of interventions due to the limited exchange of pertinent information on clinical issues.

In summary, truly committed care providers are those who devote themselves to meaningful goals and tasks and rely upon each other's support in order to achieve them. They do not devote themselves to abstract ideals, unrealistic goals, or charismatic leaders. They strive to meet the needs of dying and bereaved individuals through caring relationships, which are simultaneously supportive to them. They operate according to the assumption that "to be cared for is essential for the capacity to be caring" (Gaylin, 1976, p. 63).

It is not by chance that some research findings suggest that the perceived lack of support among care providers is one of the primary factors—if not the most significant—contributing to professional burnout and suffering and affecting the decisions of professionals who work with the dying and the bereaved to leave this field of work (Papadatou et al., 2001; Vachon, 1987, 1997).

Condition 2: Holding Environment

The concept of the holding environment was first mentioned by Winnicott (1960/1990) in a paper entitled "The Theory of the Parent-Infant Relationship," where he described the nature of effective caregiving between parents and infants. He argued that a holding environment is provided by a "good enough mother," who physically holds the child, expresses love, and creates reliable and safe boundaries for her infant that protect him or her from any external disruption, threat, or danger. Such behaviors function as a continuation of the protection that her womb previously provided to the unborn child. Yet a holding environment offers more than protection. It offers a sense of order, predictability, and continuity that enables the infant to move from the safety of the parental relationship into the external world, which is unknown to him or her. In this holding space the infant feels valued and secure. From this space the mother progressively introduces the outer reality to her child in small doses and helps him or her learn how to cope with what Winnicott referred to as the "difficulties of life." Elements of the external world are brought into the safety of the parental relationship and are gradually assimilated into the child's evolving personality. The holding environment provides both a safe space and a sense of continuity between the inner and outer realities. It also provides continuity between the failures and achievements that every child experiences as he or she gradually develops his or her identity and adjusts to the social environment.

Each of us carries within ourselves the experience of a holding environment from childhood that we re-create in adulthood. Our holding environment is comprised of family and friends, co-workers, the social institutions, the legal system, and the government policies of our country, all of which provide what we perceive as conditions of safety, order, predictability, and continuity, which are critical in times of trouble and uncertainty. In this holding environment, we safely experience and work through life's difficulties. When faced with work challenges, we expect our team to provide these same conditions, which can help us cope with the ambiguity, uncertainty, adversity, and losses that the care of dying and bereaved individuals engender (Papadatou, 2006).

When our team offers a holding environment, we allow ourselves to feel safely overwhelmed by loss encounters. We acknowledge and accept our suffering as natural and lean temporarily upon others who understand, validate our experience, and encourage us to trust our insight, knowledge, and abilities to manage work challenges. Being securely attached and held by others also enables us to become self-reliant, as suggested by Kahn (2002).

Consider how the following challenges were met adequately when a holding environment was in place in three different units.

A young nurse who had never been confronted with death was terrified of the prospect that during her night shift one of her favorite patients might die. She talked about it with a senior nurse, who listened attentively and volunteered to share the shift. The head nurse accompanied the young nurse, who assisted the dying individual and his family in their last moments together. By offering feedback and guidance, she was available and supportive when the young professional needed someone with whom to share her feelings.

Team members avoided entering the room of a terminally ill patient who devalued and verbally assaulted them. The team ceased providing appropriate care, which aggravated the patient's fury against members of the hospice personnel, who then neglected his needs even more. Team members repeatedly discussed the issue at staff meetings, proposed alternative approaches that consistently failed, and eventually sought consultation. The consultant helped them to understand the underlying feelings of helplessness, inadequacy, and despair that both the patient and team members experienced in the face of impending death, and to acknowledge the dysfunctional patterns through which a cycle of violence was established between the team and the patient.

Members of a neurology team whose beloved leader suddenly died from a heart attack experienced intense grief. The administration decided to assign an external leader to the team in order to avoid emotional turmoil and reestablish order. This decision was met with strong opposition by staff members, who resented both the immediate replacement of their leader and the disenfranchisement of their grief. Instead, they proposed an alternative plan. Two senior team members offered to act as temporary co-leaders, and a number of rituals and activities would be organized by the team in commemoration of the deceased leader. Some rituals were aimed only at team members, and other rituals were addressed to the entire organization (including patients treated at the unit), and a conference in the deceased's memory was planned for the scientific community of specialists in neurological disorders. Administrators accepted the team's proposal, and a follow-up meeting was scheduled to evaluate its outcomes.

In each of these examples, care providers experienced an upsetting situation that triggered intense feelings of anxiety, anger, despair, or grief that temporarily threw the team or organization out of balance. However, in each situation there was a key person (a colleague, a consultant) or a group (a team, a board of administrators) who created a safe environment and assumed a holding function, enabling team members to express their feelings and concerns instead of disguising or avoiding them, and to seek alternative forms of action in order to cope with the death or loss experience. This holding environment did not disempower care providers by overprotecting them, imposing decisions, and excusing their shortcomings in the delivery of care. Instead, it provided a refuge to which they could retreat and where they could deposit their anxiety, anger, grief, or insecurities, which were heard and acknowledged. It also helped them move forward and assume new responsibilities or become involved in activities that enhanced both their sense of control and their sense of continuity in the delivery of care. While therapy per se was not offered, a supportive and secure space was provided that had therapeutic value for team members who experienced distress. In this milieu, relationships were characterized by "mature dependence," which, according to Kahn (2005), is marked by a healthy collective respect for autonomy and relatedness. Moreover, professionals who assumed a holding function did not give up their roles as colleague, leader, consultant, or manager in order to become a therapist or surrogate parent for helpless children. They maintained the roles of mature adults who created a partnership with care providers in distress, whom they perceived as competent to think and act for themselves. They offered appropriate and timely support, which enabled staff members to face a distressing experience rather than to avoid it. Care providers were held accountable and responsible for their actions and were helped to use available resources.

The senior nurse, for example, took the time to listen to the younger nurse, who felt anxious about her first confrontation with death. By sharing the night shift, she did not attempt to replace her but provided feedback, valued her role, and accompanied her, offering various forms of support (informational, emotional, practical, and meaning-making support) that helped her make sense of her first encounter with death.

In the case of the abusive patient, the consultant did not offer interpretations and solutions but helped team members explore and understand how they reinforced the patient's fury by becoming abusive. They were encouraged to reframe reality and adopt alternative approaches that took into consideration both the patient's cry for help and support and their own need for respect and recognition.

Finally, the crisis caused by the sudden death of the unit's leader was managed efficiently because the team created a holding environment in which the needs of both patients and care providers were appropriately met. Moreover, clear boundaries protected team members from external disruptions or imposed decisions and ensured continuity in the face of death.

Kahn (2001, 2005) describes three types of holding behaviors that enable care providers to move toward rather than away from difficulties and anxiety-provoking situations. Care providers who display holding behaviors may engage in (1) *containment* by making themselves available to attend to, listen to, and contain part of another person's experience; (2) *empathic acknowledgment* by exploring the other person's experience in ways that make him or her feel understood and valued; and (3) an *enabling perspective* by helping the other person make sense of his or her experiences and move toward task achievement. What basic functions does a holding environment fulfill?

1. *It contains experiences.* In other words, it holds experiences that are painful or threatening without dismissing, repressing, masking, distorting or dividing them into smaller parts. Care providers—particularly those with insecure attachments—cannot emotionally survive in a work setting where loss is so profound without the containing function of a team. Others with secure attachments and an advanced level of individuation discover this containing function in themselves and effectively manage loss experiences and suffering.
2. *It facilitates the elaboration of experiences.* Elaboration requires a process of working through difficulties. It is enhanced by the circulation of information among team members, who use it constructively to learn and eventually change and grow as individuals, and as a team. Such elaboration involves an ongoing evaluation of the caregiving process and its impact on those who receive and those who provide care.
3. *It tempers or transforms suffering in creative ways.* A holding environment provides opportunities to recognize and transform suffering in different ways, such as by reframing painful events, constructing meaningful narratives in the face of loss and adversity, planning activities and rituals that enfranchise grief, and using resources creatively to build team resilience.
4. *It promotes interconnectedness and interdependence among team members.* Care providers are concerned not only about the well-being of the people they serve, but also about the well-being of their team. Mutual respect and shared responsibility are at the core of effective collaborations.

Teams vary in their abilities to create holding environments and in their desire to be held and hold others. Moreover, team rules and values can enhance or hinder the development of a nurturing environment.

Even though establishing a holding environment seems desirable, it nevertheless involves a risk: the team's confrontation with fear, anxiety, despair, powerlessness, and other aspects of personal and collective suffering. Along with this risk comes a responsibility to review dysfunctional patterns of working and relating to one another. Some teams are not able or willing to engage in such a process, which may cause turmoil in an already fragile homeostasis. Kearney (2000) suggests that for a team to function as a container, it has to build its containing functions, a process that involves deliberate and conscious effort. He argues that the "containment of the containers" is facilitated through clinical supervision and the services of an external facilitator who can help a team develop awareness of the patterns it uses to cope with work challenges and death situations.

In essence, a holding team environment serves as an antidote to suffering. Since we cannot relieve all the suffering we experience in the face of loss, we can at least recognize, share, and learn how to temper and transform it, so as to avoid its power to negatively affect the quality of our services.

Condition 3: Open Teamwork

Open teamwork requires the development of external relations and collaborations with other professionals, teams, organizations, or services within the larger organization or community in order to respond to the needs of dying and bereaved individuals and care providers. Such openness is possible only if team members shift perceptions from themselves to the world of their team, the larger context of their organization, and the vast community, and vice versa. This inward-outward look is necessary for the team's network building within the organization, the community, and the larger social environment (Payne, 2000).

Open teamwork is facilitated when the team provides a secure base for its members, who go out into the community and collaborate with different individuals and groups, which are subsequently drawn into the team. This going out–drawing in process is critically important in the care of seriously ill, dying, and elderly people, whose needs shift from hospital care to home care and to hospice services, as well as for bereaved families, whose needs require coordination among members of the palliative care team, the school community, the work agency, and mental health centers.

Open teamwork necessitates permeable team boundaries. Whenever boundaries are rigid, information does not circulate beyond the team's microcosmos. Care providers cultivate an illusion of collective omnipotence and team sufficiency and isolate themselves as well as those whom they serve in a secluded world that places itself at the margins of society. This, in fact, constitutes one of the risks of modern palliative and bereavement care teams, which often function as closed systems. By providing individuals, families, and care providers with a cocoon-like environment, they reinforce the social marginalization of the dying and the bereaved, stigmatize or discriminate against care providers, and protect society from exposure to death experiences, which are hidden from public view.

Open teamwork necessitates meaningful collaborations that prevent such marginalization, discrimination, and alienation. Collaborations that integrate different approaches and services for the benefit of the dying and the bereaved are meaningful. Care providers with different forms of expertise do not simply coexist or juxtapose their services. Instead, they strive toward developing an integrated explanatory framework in which biological, psychological, social, pastoral, and other services are linked in ways that foster a deeper understanding of the complex reality that dying and bereaved people experience in the sociocultural contexts in which they live. Such integration is at the core of a humanized and personalized approach and relies upon coordinated efforts among various professionals and teams that respond to people's needs in the most appropriate ways.

Service integration is a characteristic of teams that function with competence. As open systems, they communicate effectively and confront rather than avoid challenges, while their members, who respect and trust each other, invest time and energy in ensuring a collaboration that is meaningful both to the people they serve and to their team.

The following example shows some of the challenges of open teamwork, and how these were managed in a small community. Three teams were responsible for the care of terminally ill individuals and bereaved families: (1) an oncology team that was cure oriented, (2) a palliative care team that provided home care services to families who chose palliation at the end of life, and (3) a mental health care team that offered bereavement support through a local nongovernmental agency. Although the goals of these teams were complementary, their approaches became a source of constant conflict and compromised continuity and quality of care. Members of these teams blamed each other for incompetence, superficial interventions, and impersonal care. The situation was aggravated by the teams' leaders, who were trapped in an ongoing battle. They devalued each other, criticized their approaches as too symptom oriented or too emotion oriented, avoided exchanging information about patients and families, and spoke negatively of individual staff members. Care seekers were caught in this conflict and took sides by supporting one team against the other. The absence of administrative intervention enhanced splitting rather than the integration of services.

The situation was so desperate that a popular journalist whose spouse had recently died conducted a thorough investigation on end-of-life care, interviewed families and published an article in the local Sunday newspaper on the problems that families encounter. The article suggested that—in addition to the suffering caused by the dying process and death of a loved person—families experience stress as a result of the lack of communication between teams and conflicts between professionals, all of whom were perceived as highly competent and qualified in their areas of expertise. The journalist raised the issue of professional burnout and posed a number of questions about the non-integration of services that are critical to dying and bereaved people. Readers responded with personal stories that brought to light several issues caused by the lack of teamwork with regard to the care of seriously ill, dying, and bereaved people. The journalist mailed these stories to the managers of these three organizations, who decided to meet and take action.

During this meeting, they agreed to use the services of a consultant, who invited them to address the challenges of open teamwork. Through this process they came to realize that their organizations were trapped in a conflict that had originated several years before, when two leading oncologists fought over conflicting ideologies and approaches to the care of people with cancer. That conflict resulted in the development of separate units, and the foundation of different scientific societies whose members were in constant competition with each other. The split was projected onto patients and families, who created two nonprofit cancer associations in the same community! Everyone had to pick a side.

Eventually, the managers of these organizations invited all the care providers who belonged to these three teams to engage in a fruitful dialogue that was later extended to include families and representatives of local cancer associations. In a safe environment, organizational myths and primary tasks were discussed, and conflicts addressed, and the circulation of information allowed for new opportunities for networking and collaboration.

Open teamwork facilitates new initiatives and developments, but it also enables professionals to value their work, to realize what society gains from their services, and to derive satisfaction from the care they provide.

PRINCIPLE 7

Interprofessional collaboration is an unfolding process that is reflective of a team's development and growth

When a team adopts an approach that medicalizes dying or pathologizes bereavement, it focuses exclusively on symptoms and disorders that require treatment or management. Specificity becomes the focus of care among professionals who share a common view, approach, and language of communication. In contrast, a holistic focus demands close collaboration between professionals with different educational backgrounds, knowledge, and skills, who must communicate in the languages of different disciplines and coordinate their services. This is not an easy task. It can become even more complex when too many experts become involved and/or function under the assumption that everybody can do everything (Clark, 1999). To avoid the negative side effects of the plurality of services, teams are challenged to develop creative and discrete ways to meet the multiple needs of the people they serve.

Collaboration among care providers with diverse areas of expertise may take different forms. Collaborating teams have been described as multidisciplinary, interdisciplinary, and transdisciplinary (Payne, 2000; Reese & Sontag, 2001; Rowe, 1996; Schofield & Amodeo, 1999; Speck, 2006b). What are the differences?

In *multidisciplinary teams,* which are usually hierarchically organized, care providers work independently and are unaffected by each other's disciplines. They do not feel compelled to adapt their roles, knowledge, skills, and responsibilities to fit with the roles, knowledge, skills, and responsibilities of professionals of a different discipline. Leadership is usually held by the highest-ranking care provider, and interactions among team members are limited. Traditionally, information is communicated via the medical or psychological file of the dying or bereaved person or via staff meetings, during which each team member reports his or her assessment or intervention, which is added to rather than integrated into the patient's care plan.

Interdisciplinary teams, in contrast, are organized around common problems that are addressed by care providers with different forms of expertise, who share information and the responsibility for care. Team members work interdependently and in close collaboration with each other in order to develop a plan of care and achieve shared goals. There is a higher degree of interconnectedness among team members, who value the identity of the team over their personal identities. They believe that care providers can achieve as a team much more than the sum total of the contributions of the individual members. Ongoing interaction and communication among team members are vital to task achievement, while leadership, responsibility, and accountability are shared.

Finally, in *transdisciplinary teams,* care providers train one another and broaden their knowledge and skills, which are subsequently used in clinical practice, without duplicating services or creating role confusion. This form of collaboration allows practitioners to learn from each other, expand their skills, and acknowledge the limits of their abilities. Hall and Weaver (2001) suggest that transdisciplinary collaboration is an advanced stage of team development, while Connor, Egan, Kwilosz, Larson, and Reese (2002) believe that it is a component of high-functioning teams.

It is my belief that we can learn more about team collaboration if we adopt a developmental perspective. Teams evolve and go through stages of development that allow for increasing degrees of openness and reflexivity over experiences, and deeper understandings of the human experience in the face of loss, trauma and death. Parallel to team development, team collaboration can evolve in distinct stages (Morasz, 1999). These stages are depicted in Figure 9.4.

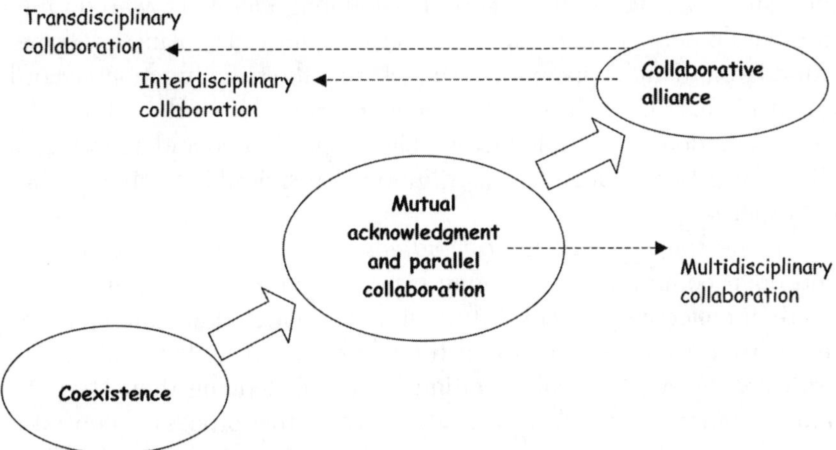

Figure 9.4 Developmental stages in team collaboration

During the *stage of coexistence,* each discipline delimits its boundaries and mode of functioning with regard to the care of an individual or family, whose needs are fragmented and compartmentalized. Care is divided, and representatives from each discipline assume the responsibility of a limited aspect of care, under specific conditions. Transactions among professionals are rigid, and communication limited. Collaboration usually takes the form of referrals. Individuals or families are referred to an "expert" when professionals who belong to a different discipline exhaust their knowledge, skills, and resources, or when they wish to protect their team from unsolvable problems and suffering. For example, when physicians and nurses have nothing else to offer a terminally ill patient who is depressed, they ask the team's psychologist or social worker to intervene as a last resort. Similarly, when a team is at a loss because a family is aggressive toward or abusive of care providers, then a psychiatrist is called in to manage the family and spare the team from its own distress or suffering.

Interventions are further fragmented when psychologists, psychiatrists, or social workers do not return to the primary team to share information that could be useful to physicians and nurses who made the initial referral, out of fear of giving up their power and control over the people they serve.

At the *stage of mutual acknowledgement and parallel collaboration,* care providers recognize each other's knowledge and skills and collaborate in parallel and complementary ways. They use each other mostly as consultants in their disciplinary pursuits. Transactions are more open, but communication remains superficial among members, who do their jobs but do not necessarily integrate services into an explanatory framework. Even though appearances suggest that the team functions according to a biopsychosocial-spiritual model of care, this model is limited to the recognition of multiple factors that are juxtaposed and addressed in clinical practice through the distribution of responsibility among different experts.

At the *stage of collaborative alliance,* focus is placed on effective and open communication among experts who plan, offer, and evaluate their collective services. Information circulates, and team members learn from each other, broaden their horizons of understanding, and critically review their collaboration by acknowledging their strengths and limitations in the face of death. A reflective process is central to their collaboration. This process is not limited solely to the identification of the content of care (e.g., management of specific problems, challenges, or needs) but expands to the understanding of the process by which services are offered and integrated into a comprehensive model of care. Mutuality, interconnectedness, and the fostering of a sense of community and belonging are key aspects of such an alliance. In fact, through them, care providers are able to confront death and mortality, accept their vulnerability in death situations, and temper their suffering.

A collaborative alliance makes transdisciplinary work possible. This is particularly important at the end of life, when the family does not wish to become involved with several care providers yet wants to maintain a few relationships with professionals who are significant to the dying and the bereaved. A team that works at a transdiciplinary level allows some aspects of a care provider's primary function to be undertaken by members of other occupational groups without being threatened. For example, with the appropriate guidance of the psychologist, a nurse who spends many hours at the bedside of a dying patient may be helped to assess his clinical depression and provide appropriate support or intervene at a family level to facilitate communication and decisions among family members. Similarly, an informed social worker can respond to the dying person's questions about his or her prognosis and explore the family's expectations regarding his or her declining condition.

For a collaborative alliance to develop, care providers must spend time working together, rather than isolating themselves in offices that separate one discipline from the other. The time that is shared allows for the exchange of different points of view and understandings, enhances the acquisition of new knowledge, clears up confusion, and reinforces team building. Gradually a common language is established that does not involve the use of jargon, which tends to exclude some team members from participation in discussions. The responsibility of care is assumed by a community of professionals rather than by individual care providers. This mode of functioning replaces the traditional hierarchy that often prevails in multidisciplinary teams, where one leader gives orders and directions or assigns responsibilities to be performed by team members.

Teams that adopt a truly interdisciplinary or transdisciplinary approach function as open systems that use information to integrate services into a framework of care that is meaningful to individuals and families as well as to care providers. Team members derive satisfaction not only from the provision of services but also from their collaboration with one another. They form a team identity that supersedes individual identities, of which they are proud.

PRINCIPLE 8

Resilience is enhanced by the team's ability to cope effectively with suffering, and to creatively use its resources to foster change and growth

Resilience is not a trait, as is often assumed, but the result of an ongoing process. To better understand it, we must look beyond a team's ability to "bounce back" from adversity by returning to an original position or equilibrium. Resilience develops when the team is exposed to highly distressing events and losses and involves a forward movement toward coping with reality through the use of functional patterns and solutions. This doesn't mean that a team may not experience transient perturbations in its normal functioning, but that it manages to benefit from these experiences and create opportunities for team learning and growth. Instead of avoiding discussing and reflecting on its losses, traumas, or crises, it develops an enlarged view of reality that enables team members to perceive, feel, think, and behave in new, even divergent, ways, and to address key questions, such as "Is the care we provide worthwhile?" "How can we best achieve our goals?" "How do we cope with the short- and long-term effects of caregiving in death situations?" "What is the nature of the suffering we experience?" "What are the rewards?" and "How can these be enhanced or lead to personal and team growth?"

A team that fosters resilience is not invulnerable or omnipotent. It recognizes both its strengths and limitations, reflects upon experiences, works through adversities, learns from mistakes, and transforms suffering into opportunities for change and growth. This metamorphosis enables members to move beyond loss and death and value the preciousness of life, accept mortality, and appreciate the process of caregiving. It is achieved when the team mobilizes functional patterns and solutions, and uses creatively its resources to enlarge its view of reality in ways that foster change and growth.

Functional Patterns and Solutions

In contrast to dysfunctional team patterns that reflect a certain degree of inertia in a team's development, functional patterns (Box 9.4) are indicative of team resilience and increase the likelihood of team growth.

Box 9.4

FUNCTIONAL TEAM PATTERNS IN DEATH SITUATIONS

- Personalization of care
- Integration of services through interdisciplinary collaboration
- Working through loss and death experiences
- Acknowledgment of both the universality and uniqueness of care providers' responses to loss and death
- Instillation of hope
- Solidarity through caring acts and behaviors
- Use of play patterns and humor
- Development and use of rituals
- Risk taking and change

To better understand functional patterns, it is helpful to explore the purposes they serve, which involve helping team members:

- To accept, temper, and/or transform suffering by minimizing its disturbing effects
- To cultivate connectedness, collaboration, and mutual support among co-workers who are repeatedly exposed to loss and death situations
- To promote innovation and change that foster team growth
- To ensure quality of care for dying and bereaved people

The functional patterns and solutions described below can be grouped into two major categories: (1) patterns that promote team cohesion, interdependence, belonging, and mutual support; and (2) patterns that enhance differentiation, individuation, risk taking, and openness to new experiences, to meaningful collaborations, and to change. Both categories of patterns are necessary to foster team resilience.

Personalization of Care

Team members look beyond the diseased body, the bereavement process, or the theoretical model they adopt in their interventions and engage in caring acts and behaviors that promote relationships with dying and bereaved people, whose needs and concerns are identified and addressed. Caring for a person who has a name, a unique personality, and a life story demands a relationship-centered approach. This does not mean that the identification of specific tasks and reliance upon a theoretical framework are not important, but these are not superimposed or rigidly applied so as to dismiss the uniqueness of the people we serve. The humanization of care demands the establishment of partnerships or bonds, through which suffering is contained, mitigated, and transformed.

Integration of Services Through Interdisciplinary Collaboration

Sharing the responsibility of care does not involve the division of tasks into manageable parts, but rather the integration of services into a comprehensive context of care that is meaningful for care seekers and care providers. Interconnectedness and interdisciplinary collaboration permit the assessment of problems and challenges from different perspectives, and the development of interventions that require coordinated efforts. Collaboration becomes more important than the egos of individual providers or the identity of disciplinary groups. A team that brings together professionals who work interdependently, share the responsibility for care, and support each other tempers the suffering caused by loss and death and increases opportunities for collective rewards and enrichment.

Working Through Loss and Death Experiences

The ability to reflect on and work through experiences presupposes a work environment where team members feel safe enough to share personal views, opinions, and feelings, no matter how confusing, painful, or threatening these may be. Sharing often has a cathartic effect, especially under stressful situations. However, it is not sufficient in and of itself. When there is no holding, sharing can prove destructive to providers who feel threatened by the intensity of emotions or unduly exposed without being supported. Sharing is beneficial only when it occurs in an environment in which personal experiences can be discussed and opportunities are offered to explore and work through them.

What does *working through* involve? It involves a process that allows care providers to take some distance from their lived experiences in order to understand, interpret, and/or reframe them; attribute meaning to them; integrate them into a narrative that makes sense; and finally develop a plan of action that addresses the challenges created by circumstances. Therefore, patterns that cultivate open emotional sharing along with cognitive reflection and reframing of experiences enable care providers to make informed decisions about how to cope in a given situation, and to concurrently support each other. This is particularly critical when the team is faced with traumatic events that affect everyone involved. Functional coping patterns are used to work through the trauma and learn from this process.

Acknowledgment of Both the Universality and Uniqueness of Care Providers' Responses to Loss and Death

Collective patterns that recognize the impact of death upon care providers and challenge irrational and obstructive beliefs about their responses to loss, trauma, and death (e.g., "You get used to death," "One must be strong," "Grief is a sign of weakness or incompetence") are critical to effective team functioning. There is a collective acknowledgement that some aspects of professionals' suffering are universal and unavoidable in death situations. Grief responses are normalized and perceived as indications of one's capacity to be human, empathic, and compassionate. Existential and spiritual issues are addressed and viewed as integral to growth and maturity.

While certain team patterns acknowledge some common and universal responses to loss and death, other patterns accept the individuality of each care provider and his or her unique responses to death. In this way, team members increase their tolerance of alternative responses without judging, criticizing, or inhibiting them. Instead, they provide opportunities to explore, learn from, become enriched, and integrate them into the team's history and development.

Instillation of Hope

Hope introduces a sense of temporal perspective that is important both to care providers and to the dying and the bereaved. Team members avoid giving false hope and never promise anything they cannot provide in death situations. They instill hope by being fully present to people and families who want to be accompanied through dying and bereavement. They also instill hope by being available to each other and by developing secure bonds that allow team members to move forward, change, and grow.

Solidarity Through Caring Acts and Behaviors

Mutual support is critical to the establishment of a safe and holding work environment in which providers feel held, supported, and validated in what they are doing. Marquis (1993) suggests that those who work for several years in palliative and bereavement care without burning out are those who belong to one or more support networks that are present on an ongoing basis, rather than during times of distress. These care providers acknowledge their needs, they are not afraid to seek care, and they benefit from available support. Being emotionally held by colleagues and loved ones makes one better able to hold others in return.

Use of Play Patterns and Humor

Play is critical to effective team functioning as well as to team growth. According to Gosling (1979) openness to change is related to the degree to which a team permits playfulness among its members. Play involves creativity, which in turn allows team members to consider alternative views and approaches to new situations.

Constrained team patterns restrict playfulness, since the team is guided by a strict agenda that leaves no room for the exchange of new ideas, creativity, or risk taking. Under-constrained team patterns involve an ongoing playfulness that minimizes or devalues problems. Team members compete for attention, recognition, power, and control and engage in transactions characterized by games. In contrast, moderately constrained team patterns invite the exchange of different views, opinions, ideas, and approaches. Through trial and error—which is associated with the capacity of play—these are implemented, evaluated, and integrated into the team's mode of operation.

Humor, like play, involves an alternative view of and approach to reality. It evokes laughter and the release of energy and is highly therapeutic under distress, especially if providers do not laugh at but laugh with a situation, a person, or themselves. Play patterns transform an experience that is potentially frustrating, painful, or dramatic into an experience that can also elicit laughter and a hopeful perspective on reality. Teams that engage in playful and creative activities and use humor in their daily functioning are more likely to take risks and facilitate a process of innovation and change in the face of loss and adversity.

Development and Use of Rituals

The integration of rituals into the team's functioning helps care providers recognize their losses and enfranchise their grief in death situations. Through formal rituals, they commemorate people who were significant in their lives (e.g., by lighting candles, praying together, sending cards to bereaved families) and cope with suffering (e.g., through staff support groups, rest, and recreation activities). Formal or informal ritual activities help them affirm their bonds with each other and enhance connectedness and a sense of belonging to a team that is able to contain suffering and provide opportunities for change and growth.

Risk Taking and Change

Risk taking involves the freedom to engage in innovative actions and alternative solutions and express different or opposing ideas without the fear of being rejected or criticized. Team members are not threatened by diversity and conflict but have faith in their ability to constructively manage differences of opinions or different approaches, which are openly shared and respectfully heard without being dismissed. Responsibility is shared by care providers, who seek creative ways to achieve identified goals and derive satisfaction from belonging to a team that changes and evolves.

Regular Review and Validation of Services

Another effective pattern involves the regular review and assessment of the team's competence and the quality of delivered services. Team members reflect critically upon their work and contributions. Moreover, they participate in assessing intra-team collaboration, as well as collaborations with other individuals, teams, and community organizations or services. Emphasis is placed on the positive aspects of team functioning, while shortcomings are not neglected. Appropriate action is taken to optimize care for the dying and the bereaved but also to provide support to care providers. Through regular assessment, the team learns from experience and improves. Its contribution to society is recognized and validated, and care providers remain committed to a job from which they derive significant satisfaction.

Availability and Creative Use of Resources

Functional teams patterns are critical to effective team functioning; however, they are not enough. Teams must have also easy access to material and to human resources through adequate staffing and effective collaborations with other teams or organizations. While the availability of resources is important, it is their appropriate and creative use that determines the quality of care.

It is in times of major economic strains that restrict funding for the care of dying and the bereaved people that we need to be most creative in how we use the resources that are available to us. Moreover, we, the care providers, must act as a resource to the community by sensitizing and educating laypeople on the value of actively supporting and accompanying their friends, families, and fellow humans at the end of life and through bereavement. In this way, dying and bereavement need not become the exclusive responsibility of "experts," but a reality that is shared by society.

Box 9.5

TEAM FUNCTIONING IN DEATH SITUATIONS

Answering these questions can help you clarify whether your team meets the three basic conditions that enhance effective team functioning in death situations: (1) a commitment to clearly defined tasks and to each other, (2) the presence of a holding environment for care seekers and care providers, and (3) open teamwork through interdisciplinary collaborations. Moreover, it allows you to explore the collective patterns that your team mobilizes in coping with loss, death, and suffering, and encourages you to consider the value of your work.

- How does your team function in the face of loss and death?
- What helps your team function effectively in such situations?
- What obstacles does your team encounter in the process of caring for dying and bereaved individuals?
- What is the degree of commitment to work goals and tasks among team members?
- How committed are care providers to each other?
- In what ways does your team show care and concern (holding behaviors) for its members?
- Which types of mutual support (e.g., informational, emotional, practical, meaning-making support) are promoted, and which need further enhancement?
- How is the suffering of team members processed in your team? Which are the collective patterns used to mitigate and/or transform suffering? How functional or dysfunctional are these team patterns?
- Which factors enhance, and which hinder, inter-team collaboration?
- How does your team promote collaborations with other professionals, teams, and organizations for the care of dying and/or bereaved individuals?
- How is appreciation for services communicated?
- What contribution does your team make to your community?
- What would enable your team to function with competence and offer better care?
- Imagine your team 10 years from now. Is your view a desirable one? In what ways can you influence the future through your present actions and behaviors?

In summary, team resilience has nothing to do with invulnerability or resistance to adversity. It involves a process in which a team transforms suffering—through the use of functional patterns and available resources—into a tolerable experience that contributes to adjustment or into an enriching experience that fosters growth. The team's ability to transform suffering becomes its trophy (Cyrulnik, 1999). It expands its view of reality and helps care providers develop a consciousness of the preciousness of life and of the value of human relations.

NOTE

1. A detailed analysis of these characteristics is offered by Malcom Payne (2000), who conducted an extensive review in his book *Teamwork in Multiprofessional Care,* and by Connor and his colleagues (2002), who focused on the characteristics of teams that provide care to people at the end of life.

10 The Good-Enough Team

Teams that are regularly confronted by death situations learn with time and experience not to strive for perfection, but toward becoming good enough in the face of death.

Good-enough teams, as shown in Figure 10.1, are more likely than others to display growth and evolution. Their boundaries are clear, flexible, and permeable, allowing members and other professionals to move in and out of the team and use valuable information that fosters collaboration and interdisciplinary teamwork. Transactions are characterized by liveliness, authenticity, and genuineness toward both people who are served and co-workers. Team members are committed to goals that are realistic, meaningful to them, and appropriately adjusted to the needs of individuals and families.

Such teams invest in both relationships and work tasks. Partnerships are formed with the dying and the bereaved in the pursuit of the accomplishment of well-defined tasks. Partnerships are also developed among co-workers, who trust each other and have great respect for autonomy and interdependence (Kahn, 2005). Care providers develop a holding environment in which they can openly express themselves without the fear of being criticized, attacked, or ridiculed and work through team conflicts and tensions. They also use functional patterns and make creative use of available resources in their coping with loss, death, and suffering.

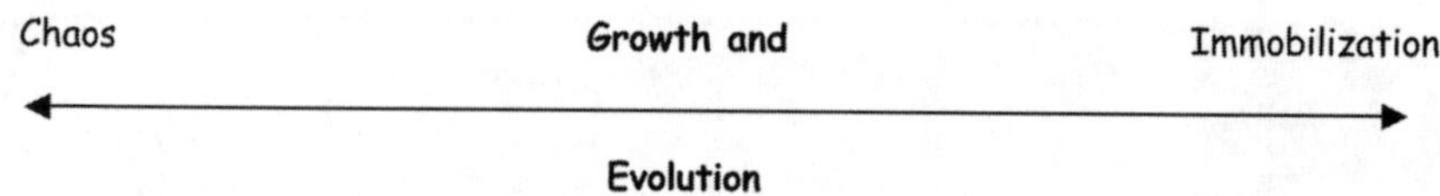

Mode of operation
Openness to experience
Commitment to goals, tasks, and relationships
Establishment of holding environment
Promotion of collaboration and interconnectedness among team members

Relations and Transactions
Openness to relationships
Autonomy and interdependence
Aliveness, authenticity, and empathy

Relation to time
Paced time
Elaboration of experiences
Use of pertinent information for learning and change
Integration of experiences into past-present-future

Figure 10.1 The good-enough team

Time is paced in order to allow care providers to relate to each other, to share experiences, and to reflect and elaborate on and integrate them into a past-present-future continuum reflected in narratives that are coherent and meaningful to them. Time is used to explore opportunities for perceiving and doing things differently. The team's message to its members suggests: "Let's take the time to reflect and process our experiences. Let's use *pertinent information* in ways that promote new opportunities, alternative approaches, and a process of learning and evolving."

Pertinent information is any information that is relevant to care providers because it increases their understanding of how they operate as a group in the face of death, how they manage suffering through more or less functional patterns, how they use or misuse their resources, and what rewards they derive from the caregiving process. Through the use of pertinent information, teams develop collective narratives that allow for the integration of both positive and negative experiences into their history.

TEAM NARRATIVES OF TRAUMAS AND ACHIEVEMENTS

Good-enough teams acknowledge their strengths as well as their limitations because they are open to experience. This is evidenced in the stories they create about major achievements and successes, as well as about major losses and traumas they have experienced in their encounters with death. These stories are shared representations of events that have a lasting impact upon the team, its development, and its history; they affect how team members construe meanings and cope with loss, trauma, and success in their daily encounters. What really happened in a given situation is less important than what is remembered, how the event is perceived, how it is narrated, and which meanings are attached to it by care providers. Focusing on the narration of major achievements and traumas illuminates a team's immobilization, resilience, and growth.

Narratives of achievements and successes represent events with which team members associate positive feelings of pride, satisfaction, contentment, and security. These stories are about extraordinary interventions or innovative approaches that had a positive impact on the care that was provided to dying or bereaved individuals, or about specific individuals (care seekers or care providers) who affected the team through their behavior, contribution, or social action.

Success or achievement narratives affirm the myths, primary tasks, and values of a team. They contain shared meanings about the team's positive qualities and elicit a sense of pride, satisfaction, purpose, and hope. They enhance team bonding and collective esteem. In times of distress, success narratives are often restoried to activate hope and cultivate the expectation that crises can be overcome.

Narratives of losses and traumas recount selected events that have caused a major disruption in the team's structure or functioning, triggering intense grief, shame, guilt, humiliation, resentment, rage, feelings of helplessness, and other powerful emotions. Usually they are built around an acute or traumatic event that occurred with no warning and affected the entire team and its functioning. For example, the medical error that caused the death of a patient, the undignified dying process of a colleague, the hospitalization of severely wounded children following a local disaster, the suicide of a bereaved client, and the cutoff of funds for bereavement services are events that are perceived as traumatic and affect both a team and the organization to which it belongs.

Occasionally, collective traumas result from the cumulative effect of highly distressing situations, such as the constant verbal harassment of care providers by families or superiors; prolonged exposure to deaths or disaster situations; and ongoing conflicts, splits, or lawsuits among team members.

As part of a research project that involved individual interviews with members of a dialysis unit, I asked care providers to describe the most distressing or traumatic experience they had experienced in their work lives (in other words, a nadir experience). All of them referred to a medical error that had happened eight years before as a result of miscommunication among team members. Interestingly, all interviewees used identical expressions to describe the incident, which was perceived as "thunder and lightning that struck [the team] in the midst of clear blue skies," leaving team members stunned and paralyzed. In addition, they all referred to the subsequent decision of the medical director to retire prematurely, which "shook the ground" under their feet, as he was charismatic, highly competent, and respected by all.

Affected by forces that unexpectedly confronted them (thunder and lightning) and deprived them of a secure base (unsafe ground), team members felt lost, helpless, and guilty both for the medical error and for the director's early retirement. Their organization dealt with the medical error through sanctions that quickly "shoved the issue under the carpet." The team experienced a mute suffering that affected relationships among co-workers, who progressively became estranged from each other.

Unprocessed traumas have a lasting negative impact and can remain unaddressed for decades, becoming dormant in the team's collective memory. They become reactivated when a crisis or distressing event triggers similar feelings, images, and representations. Under those conditions, the current crisis or stressful event is contaminated by the old trauma. These unexplored traumas are reflected in various forms of narrative disruptions that teams develop, which include:

1 *Absence of narrative.* Such an absence is the result of a conspiracy of silence. Care providers avoid making any reference or allusion to the loss or trauma event. There is an unspoken agreement to remain silent in order to avoid the underlying feelings of

guilt, shame, rage, deception, and utter powerlessness. Nobody speaks about the experience or about the feelings associated with it. The team functions undeterred, as if the event caused a minor disturbance.

2 *Disorganized narrative.* Various versions of the story are exchanged within the team, and these are enhanced by rumors and/or conflicting information. No one ever openly addresses the latter so that it will not have to withstand validation. Information is patchy, untested, and conflicting. Thus, the traumatic experience remains fragmented.

3 *Dominant narrative of a petrified memory.* This narrative is an enforced account that marginalizes alternative personal stories. It is well organized, and the plot appears far too cohesive (Neimeyer, 2006; White & Epston, 1990). Everybody in the team talks openly about it. Yet in spite of the detail in which it is told, and the clarity and vivacity with which it is described, it is recited in an identical way by all team members. Words, expressions, metaphors, and interpretations of events are exactly the same. Such narration excludes any form of elaboration, alternative interpretations, or even minor modifications. Team members reinforce each other's narratives in order to maintain the collective memory. Petrified, the memory of the event or of a specific image to which traumatic feelings are attached, remains unchanged over time. Correale (1996) refers to this phenomenon as the "memory's hypertrophy" ("hypertrophie de la mémoire"). The team avoids circulating pertinent information (regarding facts, thoughts, or feelings) that would enable members to process their loss or trauma. This rigidity enhances an illusion of control and prevents any elaboration that is perceived as too perturbing or threatening.

Overall, team narratives reflect the degree to which traumatic events are processed. Attention should be directed at teams that use solely a biomedical discourse or a psychological jargon to construct a narrative that is imposed upon all members. Similarly, caution should be taken with teams in which members who are reluctant to use an emotion-focused discourse are uncomfortable with the exclusive use of "feeling" language, while rational talk may be too constricting for other members who perceive it as cold and sterile.

It is important to remember that unprocessed collective traumas are transmitted from one generation of workers to the next and may affect the entire life of an organization. Occasionally, they lock or immobilize teams in a situation that prevents learning, growth, and forward movement and compromise a collective sense of resilience.

How does a good-enough team cope with loss and trauma? Even though elaboration of experiences temporarily increases anxiety and discomfort, the disturbing effects of trauma are minimized in the long run. Care providers cease spending their energy hiding, disguising, or ignoring the event and direct it toward circulating information, learning from their experience, developing resources, and building a sense of confidence. Eventually, they create a story that organizes their experience, in which order replaces pain and chaos. Such a story comprises descriptions of events or situations that temporarily threaten the team's functioning or identity, accounts of its impact, details of the reparative actions and solutions that were used to manage the loss or trauma, and lessons derived from the team's experience. Therefore, a collective story that is meaningful and coherent to team members consists of a plot about the traumatic event (what happened), the team's response (how the team's functioning was affected and what patterns were mobilized to cope with the trauma), and the lessons learned (which changes or adaptations occurred at a team level).

The important thing is not to create a collective narrative that is rigidly accepted by all care providers, but to establish an openness to formulating collective meanings and tolerating different discourses and stories of a shared event. A good-enough team allows alternative discourses to occur, as well as nondiscursive forms of expression. Thus, besides conversation and sharing, narratives are co-created through actions, rituals, and symbolic or creative activities that serve as bridges and salvage narrative continuity (e.g., a collage constructed by the team, an exhibition of the artwork of team members). The ability of a team to process traumatic experiences and integrate them into its life trajectory and story is far greater and more creative than the ability of any individual member.

In summary, quality of care does not solely require good-enough care providers who possess knowledge and skills and are committed to the people they serve and to each other. Quality care also requires good-enough teams that create the necessary space for members to experience, reflect on, understand, and process their losses, traumas, and achievements; to transform suffering through mutually supportive relationships; and to draw meaning and satisfaction from the caregiving process. Good-enough teams cultivate in care providers a sense that they belong to a compassionate group that can bear and transform suffering in creative ways, draw upon its strengths and resources, learn from mistakes, and evolve through meaningful collaborations that expand beyond the microcosmos of the team. In this process, the roles of leaders, supervisors, and consultants are vital.

LEADERS IN GOOD-ENOUGH TEAMS

We often assume that a leader (whether a manager, director, or head of a department, unit, service, or team) must possess certain traits or characteristics in order to be effective in his or her leadership role and functions. As Payne (2000) argues, it is hard to identify who has and who does not have these traits. A leader who is effective in one team may be less effective in another team. Moreover, different teams have different needs at different times in their development, so different traits and leadership styles are appropriate under different circumstances. Payne proposes a *situational and contingency view of leadership* and suggests that effective leadership depends upon the leader's ability to recognize and respond to the needs of a situation while taking into account the organization's or team's dynamics and developmental process. This invites for the use of diverse leadership styles that are appropriate to each work context at a given time.

This view of leadership is particularly relevant in teams and organizations that offer palliative and bereavement care services to populations with very diverse needs (e.g., children, adolescents, adults, elderly, family and community members who are affected by death). In spite of the diversity in leadership styles, underlying values must be consistent and promote mutual respect, freedom of choice, interconnectedness, and collaboration.

For any leadership style to be effective, it is necessary for leaders first to acknowledge how they are personally affected by loss and bereavement, and second to understand how dying and death affect their team. They must also be aware that, as a result of their key position, responses to loss and death are often projected upon them by care seekers and care providers, who scapegoat or idealize them. Effective leadership—regardless of style—requires solid knowledge and skills in group dynamics in order for a leader to avoid enacting various projections or becoming locked into dysfunctional team patterns of interaction.

Dutton, Frost, Worline, Liliius, and Kanov (2002), in an article entitled "Leading in Times of Trauma," suggest that organizational leaders have a critical role in facilitating the development of a compassionate environment for care providers who experience or witness loss and trauma. At one level (referred to as the "context of meaning"), they are responsible for creating an environment in which team members freely express and discuss their feelings, make sense of events and experiences, seek or offer support, and maintain an optimistic and hopeful view of caregiving. At another level (referred to as the "context of action"), leaders are responsible for creating an environment in which alternative ways of coping with suffering and promoting change and growth are considered.

In order to achieve both of these functions, leaders must be competent so that they are able to:

- Facilitate the development of a team's holding environment
- Assess, promote, and reinforce functional team patterns
- Activate a process of change when necessary
- Promote the coordination of action among professionals with different areas of expertise
- Facilitate intra-team communication and narrative construction
- Facilitate communication between the team and other teams, organizations, the community, and the world at large

Establishing a holding environment is not and can never become the sole responsibility of a leader. The leader must communicate the idea that such an environment is a shared responsibility to be assumed by all team members, who must display compassion through simple caring actions and thoughtful responses to their colleagues (Vickers, 2005). Nevertheless, a leader facilitates the development of a holding environment by acting as a positive role model and by engaging in holding behaviors and caring acts directed toward dying and bereaved people, as well as toward team members. Being cared for and held by leaders enables care providers to do the same with the people they serve.

In times of crisis, leaders may act temporarily as parental figures who provide professionals with the "roots" of a secure base and the "wings" to explore an unknown or threatening situation (Kahn, 1995, 2002). They are available when needed and withdraw when team members are able to rely on their own resources. In so doing, they avoid dependent relationships and they bring out in the open and into awareness the dynamics of clinging and symbiotic relations that practitioners sometimes develop in the face of adversity, loss, or death.

Leaders are responsible for helping care providers use or develop new knowledge, skills, and resources in the pursuit of desired goals. By providing information and feedback about the team's mode of functioning, they encourage team members to learn from mistakes and achievements and become enriched by their experiences.

Finally, leaders are responsible for facilitating open communication and maintaining clear and unambiguous boundaries that are neither too rigid nor too blurred. We should not forget that a leader inhabits the two-sided boundary (see Figure 9.1) that both separates the team from the larger organization and community and unites them. His or her role is therefore pivotal in facilitating the flow of information and the coordination of services within and beyond the team's boundaries.

In the microcosmos of the team, the leader must ensure the presence of *role boundaries* by helping members define their role and responsibilities in relation to team goals and tasks; *time boundaries* by determining the duration of work shifts, the beginning and ending of staff meetings, the timing for support or consultation, and the punctuality of appointments with care seekers; and *spatial boundaries* by ensuring that team members have a private space to withdraw to and a space to work together, collaborate, and connect (Kahn, 1995).

In the team's mesocosmos (intermediate world) and macrocosmos (external world), the leader is responsible for enhancing communication and cultivating relationships with peer leaders, administrators, and other community services and organizations in order to facilitate teamwork. A leader represents the team to the outer world and concurrently protects the team from external interferences or intrusions. He or she creates bridges that allow information to circulate and be used effectively. Pertinent information is introduced into the team from the outside (as input) and communicated by the team to others (as output) to achieve desired goals and ensure collaborations. This is critical in end-of-life care, when the needs of dying patients and grieving families increase and become urgent and demand the effective coordination of hospital, home, and community-based services, as dying individuals are often transferred from one unit to another or to a hospice or home care program, and back to the hospital. Psychosocial services can benefit bereaved children, adults, and elderly people; school communities; and community networks that are affected by death.

When boundaries are too permeable, and the leader is ineffective at protecting the team from external threats or intrusions, care providers feel exposed and resist or sabotage collaborations with other teams or professionals. Conversely, when boundaries are too rigid and the leader overprotects the team or controls any incoming information, then care providers become isolated and deny dying and bereaved people the opportunity to become integrated in a community that is sensitive to their needs, which are met through appropriate services and caring acts.

Speck (2006c) suggests that "in our present age, leadership has come to be associated more with inspiration, vision and the ability to relate to others, than with commands and orders" (p. 65). This observation is particularly significant in the context of palliative and bereavement work, where leadership is usually shared even though one person is designated the team's leader. It is common practice for a team member to take the initiative to decide on a plan of care in light of the rapid changes that a person or family experiences or to make decisions on the spot, which are then reported back to the team for discussion and evaluation. Such a form of shared or "distributive" leadership can be effective only if care providers show trust, respect, and confidence in each other's competence and skills; learn from each other; and focus on team building on a daily basis with the help of a competent leader.

SUPERVISORS AND CONSULTANTS

For a good-enough team, clinical supervision is not an option but a necessity. Through supervision, team members seek to acquire new knowledge, develop skills, and evaluate the effectiveness of their services. The primary task of a supervisor is to help team members provide quality care by focusing on (1) the services they provide and the relationships they develop with dying and bereaved people, (2) their collaboration with each other and other professionals or teams, and (3) the impact of caregiving upon themselves and the team. Clinical cases are discussed; personal, interpersonal, and interprofessional dynamics are examined; and alternative courses of action are planned. Through this process, team members are guided and supported. In fact, the palliative care approach underscores the necessity of ongoing support for care providers who are affected by death, loss, and suffering (International Work Group on Death, Dying, and Bereavement, 1979, 1993a, 1993b, 2002, 2006). Support is offered not only by leaders and supervisors but also by consultants.

Consultants are professionals external to the team and the organization who are invited to provide guidance and support through various interventions: support groups, Balint groups, stress debriefing sessions, consultation services, and discussion groups. Such interventions are distinct from staff meetings, which aim at organizing the team's work, supervising, and managing clinical cases. Consultants address specific issues of concern to care providers and concurrently collaborate with them to prevent burnout, develop functional patterns of coping with distress, promote the well-being of workers, and enhance team building.

When a team formulates a request for guidance or support, it is important to analyze its content as well as the process by which care providers decided to ask for consultation. Individual expectations vary and are sometimes conflicting or opposed. The analysis of a request can help a consultant understand what are the needs of care providers and what expectations they have for his or her involvement with their team (Morasz, 1999).

Most often, consultants are invited to offer expert advice and guidance during a crisis episode, to fix problems, or to assume the care of burned-out health care professionals who request straightforward and quick solutions to ease their suffering. To avoid assuming the role of saviors, consultants must possess knowledge and experience in group processes, organizational dynamics, and crisis intervention management.

Other times, a team formulates a request for regular support and expects the consultant to facilitate communication among members and help with change. Such a request may prove more beneficial, since team members build into their work a time, a space, and opportunities to explore their experiences and process how they affect and are being affected by them.

Not infrequently, team dynamics mirror the dynamics experienced by families in the face of loss and separation. As a result, care providers may develop highly dependent, conflictual, or avoidant relationships with each other or with their leader, supervisor, or consultant. The consultant's role is to help them understand these dynamics without imposing specific interpretations or solutions; he or she invites them to think through experiences and develop new insights. Thus, a consultant helps them learn (1) how to exercise reflective practice in order to broaden their perception of reality, (2) how to develop problem-solving skills in order to experiment with alternative solutions to challenges, and (3) how to effectively cope with suffering and make creative use of their resources. Through this process, team members develop competence and, concurrently, learn how to care for themselves and co-workers in the face of human suffering, loss, and death.

Methods of Supervision and Consultation

Supervisors and consultants adopt different approaches in their work with teams and use various methods of intervention depending on their theoretical background. One common approach focuses on the analysis of team functioning. Its goals, dynamics, functions, rules, and practices in death situations are discussed, reviewed, affirmed, disconfirmed, or changed. Team conflicts and tensions are exposed, addressed, and processed. The team is perceived and analyzed as a system, while emphasis is placed upon strengthening relationships among care providers, and upon developing team resources and a holding environment.

Another common approach focuses on the analysis of specific cases or events, along with their impact upon team members. Emphasis is placed upon understanding and managing specific work situations through the exploration of individual or team responses, skills, and competencies. Team members are helped to identify what facilitates and hinders possible options for actions and are invited to consider alternative coping patterns and solutions to problems elicited by a case or event. Priority is placed on doing a good job, and constructive feedback facilitates the achievement of specific tasks.

Even though these approaches have different foci, in reality they overlap and complement each other. When a team works on a case or a crisis, it inevitably addresses issues related to team functioning, and vice versa. It is my firm belief that supervision and consultation are most effective when they introduce opportunities for team members to review their responses to life-and-death issues that occur at work but extend to and affect their personal lives.

No supervision or consultation is helpful when it imposes a specific model of intervention upon a team, whose experiences are made to fit the model. There is no intervention that is effective for all teams. Different interventions are appropriate at different times and in different situations, and for different teams, the needs of which vary. Some teams benefit most from relating experiences to how care providers are being personally affected by their encounters with dying and bereaved people. Others who feel uncomfortable talking about themselves welcome interventions that focus on team relations and team functioning or prefer discussing a specific concern that preoccupies the entire group (e.g., a crisis episode, impending change, a traumatic death). Supervisors and consultants must be flexible and highly skilled in group psychology in order to work with care providers to meet their needs and enhance team growth.

TOWARD A COMMUNITY OF SUPPORT

Unfortunately, many leaders, supervisors, and consultants are trained to identify pathology and often forget to emphasize the effective patterns that a team uses to cope with loss, adversity, and suffering. Moreover, they tend to locate pathology in individual care providers who display behavioral or emotional problems instead of adopting a systemic perspective that focuses on relationships. As has already been suggested, there are no functional or dysfunctional care providers, nor are there functional or dysfunctional teams. Care providers and teams mobilize functional and dysfunctional patterns to cope with loss and suffering, which can be understood only in relation to the organizational and sociocultural contexts in which they occur.

Leaders, supervisors, and consultants are responsible for recognizing dysfunctional patterns; identifying—with the help of team members—the purpose they serve; and activating conditions for change. They are concurrently responsible for pointing out functional patterns and solutions and validating the team's effective use of resources. The latter is particularly relevant, especially in teams that have learned to focus solely on problems and dysfunctions.

Payne (2000) suggests that when one is conducting a team assessment, it is always helpful to consider the internal *strengths* and *weaknesses* of a team, as well as the external *opportunities* and *threats* that may impinge on its work (this process is referred to as a SWOT analysis). Such an approach emphasizes the importance of developing interventions that do not simply manage problems and difficulties but build resilience among professionals.

Those who act as leaders, supervisors, and consultants must also recognize their need for support in times of trouble and turmoil. Without opportunities to receive feedback and to be supported, they may feel utterly alone, become overwhelmed by responsibility, or be vulnerable to burnout. Everybody expects them to be as strong as a rock, in total control during crisis situations, and available on an ongoing basis. It is important that they do not fall into the trap of fostering such expectations in the people around them, and that they invest in the development of a holding environment where they can receive feedback, supervision, and support.

In closing this chapter, I would like return to a personal experience that I shared in chapter 4. Our nonprofit group was invited by the Greek Ministry of Education to organize a psychosocial intervention in nine school communities after seven adolescents were killed when the school bus carrying them to the Paralympics was overturned by a truck. My role was to design and coordinate an intervention in a rural area of 8,000 habitants, 400 kilometers away from Athens. I collaborated closely with 17 professionals who were actively involved in the program and formed four subgroups: (1) an experienced team of grief counselors and therapists, (2) a local team of psychologists who were assigned to the schools and provided services twice a week, (3) a research team that conducted psychological assessments of students at 2 and 18 months after the accident and evaluated the effectiveness of the intervention, and (4) a filming team that responded to the students' desire to record their story in commemoration of their deceased friends.

I traveled regularly to the area over three years. I led groups for educators and offered various seminars to sensitize them to issues related to trauma, loss, and resilience; held supervision sessions with local psychologists; and collaborated closely with local officials. At the end of each meeting, my colleagues and I gathered at a local taverna and treated ourselves to a delicious meal. The owner of the tavern, Mr. Ilias, served us many unique dishes, which we enjoyed over long hours of talk. Thus we established a ritual of sharing our personal experiences and food while Mr. Ilias looked after us, making sure that we were fed and content, and that our discussions were uninterrupted. I have often thought that this informal ritual served several functions: a need to fill with food the loss and emptiness caused by the deaths we encountered in our interactions with the traumatized youngsters and adults, a need to strengthen the bond among us, and a need to create a collective narrative of a work that acquired personal meaning for all of us.

At the end of each school year, our team instituted a more formal ritual by spending a weekend by the sea. We invited an external consultant, who facilitated a review process of our yearly intervention by addressing the frustrations and achievements that we had experienced, by exploring the benefits and shortcomings of our team collaboration, and by drawing our attention to the insights and lessons we had learned.

Coordinating this community project was a highly challenging and enriching experience for me. Not only was it rewarding to participate in the growth of an entire community, but I was impressed by the incredible transformation of the psychologists who made up the local team. Throughout the entire project, they remained open to the experience, and eager to be trained and supervised and to work through their losses, failures, and successes. Sometimes anxiety, grief, frustration, ambivalence, and anger permeated their accounts in supervision, while at other times joy, hope, humor, love, and affection prevailed. I was able to contain their suffering because I was also well supported by two senior colleagues who stood faithfully at my side when I needed to share my own agonies, dilemmas, and joys. Moreover, the recording of my experience in a diary and my active participation in the creation of a documentary about this intervention helped me temper my own pain and capitalize upon the rewards of caregiving through an innovative and creative project.

One of the major challenges I encountered in my role as a leader was an overwhelming sense of responsibility and aloneness during the early stages of the project, when critical decisions had to be made instantly, powerful projections had to be managed on the spot, and irrational demands to relieve the community of its excruciating suffering had to be addressed with sensitivity and compassion. Through this process, I learned that when we assume the role of a leader, supervisor, or consultant in death situations we need to fulfill two critical functions: First, we must act as a container of increased anxiety, of violent and depressive forces, of ambivalent feelings toward help and advice that is simultaneously sought, resented, and rejected, and second, we must serve as facilitators of movement in coping with trauma and grief, of change, and of growth. Through the process it is important to be supported in our leadership, supervisory, or consultative role, since prior experience does not make us immune to suffering. Finally, I believe that our ability to lead, to supervise, or to offer consultation is enhanced when we also maintain a dual role of *educators* who socialize practitioners into genuinely caring for others and for self, and of *learners* who benefit from new knowledge and skills that we integrate into our practice.

11 The Challenges of Educating Health Care Professionals

Despite the dramatic growth of knowledge in palliative and bereavement care over the past decades, education remains a major challenge in this field. Surveys of practitioners who provide services to terminally ill patients in different countries indicate a lack of formal courses in adult palliative care, but even more so in pediatric palliative care (Barclay, Wyatt, Shore, Finlay, Grande, & Todd, 2003; Dickinson & Field, 2002; Downe-Wamboldt & Tamlyn, 1997; Hilden et al., 2001; Oneschuk, Hanson, & Bruera, 2000; Sullivan, Lakoma, & Block, 2003).

Wass (2004) asserts that less than a fifth of American students in health professions are offered a full course on death throughout their studies. Most graduates attend one or a few lectures on issues related to terminal and bereavement care, as a result of which they are totally unprepared to care for the terminally ill and bereaved. They learn to provide services by trial and error or by observing senior colleagues (Hilden et al., 2001). Moreover, they lack role models and mentors who can offer helpful feedback and support them in their encounters with death (Sullivan, Lakoma, Billings, Peters, Block, & PCEP Core Faculty, 2003). Without appropriate education, guidance, and supervision, young practitioners tend to distance themselves from stressful situations and experience difficulties in their communications with individuals and families, who are dissatisfied by the services they receive.

The preparation of psychologists, counselors, and social workers on issues related to end-of-life and bereavement care is even more problematic. Basic textbooks provide little information about end-of-life and bereavement care that is usually limited to specific populations (e.g., those with AIDS, the elderly) and death topics (e.g., assessment for suicide) (Kramer, Pacoureck, & Hovland-Scafe, 2003). These mental health professionals often rely on workshops and seminars to learn how to accompany the seriously ill, suicidal individuals, and bereaved families.

There is no doubt that death education is sporadic and fragmented, and rarely related to issues of modern life, such as natural disasters, fear of terrorism, death by acts of violence, and death and multiculturalism (Chassay, 2006; McDermott & Demmer, 2008). Moreover, the word *death* is increasingly being taken out of educational programs and replaced by words such as *dying* and *terminal care;* expressions such as *life-threatening conditions, palliative care,* and *end-of-life care;* and abbreviations such as *EOL* and *EPEC.* According to Wass (2004), the use of these words and phrases do not make education and training more appealing or less threatening.

Since 1995, researchers who highlighted the shortcomings of palliative and bereavement care have made a strong case for the improvement of clinical practice through appropriate education (e.g., Fins et al., 1999; SUPPORT Investigators, 1995). In response, medical and nursing associations have developed educational curricula. Unfortunately, most of these curricula are tightly structured and packaged in kits that illustrate a step-by-step teaching procedure, offer detailed instructions for educators and learners, and provide slides and teaching materials. As a result, educators are deprived of the opportunity to be original, creative, and personal in their teaching. These curricula, however, are useful to educators who feel unprepared to teach several key components of palliative and bereavement care and are more concerned with the *content* being taught than with the *context* in which learning occurs or the *process* by which knowledge and skills are best acquired.

Unfortunately, education in palliative and bereavement care continues to be perceived as a "banking process" through which educators with expertise deposit knowledge in learners, who are expected to passively receive it and apply it in clinical practice. Such a philosophy of teaching compromises the preparation of novice practitioners.

In this final chapter, I outline five challenges that educators must address in order to ensure adequate education and training (Box 11.1). It is my firm belief that education is at the root of effective care. It is,

Box 11.1

CHALLENGES IN PALLIATIVE AND BEREAVEMENT CARE EDUCATION

1 Develop a philosophy of teaching that promotes relational learning and reflective practice
2 Develop curricula that include goals, learning objectives, and methods of teaching that focus on relationships with the dying, the bereaved, and co-workers
3 Integrate current knowledge into educational programs and supervised clinical applications
4 Evaluate training outcomes, as well as the context and process by which learning occurs
5 Integrate formal and informal learning activities into the work context

therefore, imperative to review *what* we teach our students, *how* we educate them to accompany dying and bereaved individuals and families, and *how* we prepare them to cope with life-and-death issues in their professional and personal lives.[1]

CHALLENGE 1

Develop a Philosophy of Teaching That Promotes Relational Learning and Reflective Practice

MacLeod (2004) argues that teaching should not be a technical business of well-managed information processing but should become an active process in which both the educator and the trainee are fully engaged and learn. In fact, the role of the educator is to arrange for conditions in which students understand what is being taught, reflect upon its content, and explore possibilities for implementing the acquired knowledge. "Teaching is more difficult than learning, because what teaching calls for is this: *to let learn,*" wrote Heidegger, who is cited in an interesting analysis on palliative care education by MacLeod. Indeed, the competent educator develops a genuine rather than a know-it-all authoritative relation with learners and creates conditions that encourage them to discover knowledge, attribute personal meanings to the acquired information, and experiment with alternative ways of using it in clinical practice.

Over the past decades we have witnessed a minor shift in education from a knowledge-centered approach to a learner-centered approach

(Attig, 1992; Coppola & Strohmetz, 2002; Corr, 2002; Morgan, 1987; Papadatou, 1997). Rather than using passive learning methods, students and trainees are exposed to less directive teaching approaches. They are helped to become actively involved in determining goals and practice-based learning objectives according to their needs and interests, identifying resources to achieve learning objectives, and defining criteria to evaluate whether objectives were achieved (Davies & Sharp, 2001).

Most recently, a new approach is being proposed by Browning and Solomon (2006) that focuses on relational learning. They suggest that learning is not a matter of knowledge and skill acquisition, but a complex interdependent process of social participation to which learners belong. Thus learning should stem from formal and informal educational experiences, all of which are firmly situated in relationships among students, instructors, individuals, families, and practitioners. The focus is placed on the context in which teaching and learning occur. Educators are responsible for creating a safe and trusting holding environment for trainees in which experiential learning, cognitive understanding, and emotional processing occur. In such an environment, different perspectives among learners, educators, dying and bereaved individuals are explored. Opportunities for reflection are encouraged, and new learning is incorporated into an acquired body of knowledge that affects skill acquisition. Furthermore, personal losses are recognized, grief is enfranchised, and creative ways to cope with and transform the learner's suffering are explored (Jellinek, Todres, Catlin, Cassem, & Salzman, 1993; Papadatou, 1997; Shanfield, 1981).

Relational learning is greatly facilitated when educators bring all of themselves into the educational process, involve trainees in the formation of the course's content, and act as role models by developing caring and supportive relations with them and effective collaborations with co-instructors.

CHALLENGE 2

Develop Curricula That Include Goals, Learning Objectives, and Methods of Teaching That Focus on Relationships With the Dying, the Bereaved, and Co-Workers

The recent shift from a strictly medical to a holistic model of care in health is reflected in educational curricula for physicians, nurses, health psychologists, and social workers. An increasing amount of information is provided with regard to the assessment of a person's physical, psychosocial, and spiritual needs and concerns in death situations. However, what is often neglected is the relational context within which such knowledge and skills are acquired and implemented. Students and trainees do not learn how to reflect on what they bring into their relationships with the people they serve and are not taught to process how they affect and are being affected by the caregiving process. Moreover, they totally ignore how team relationships and collective patterns of coping with death affect the quality of services that are provided to dying and bereaved people.

A relationship-centered model of care challenges existing educational curricula and supports revision of their goals, learning objectives, and methods of teaching. Learning should expand beyond the mere study of symptom management, pain control, assessment of the psychosocial and spiritual needs of the dying, and the grief responses and tasks to be achieved by the bereaved. Instead it should focus on understanding relationships, since it is through them that quality of care is ensured. Therefore, learning objectives must include an in-depth understanding of the psychic space or intersubjective field in which care providers and care seekers meet, plan, offer, and receive care (see chapter 1). The core of any educational activity must become the relationships among individuals, families, care providers, and organizations.

For example, teaching how to use interviewing and active listening skills or how to break bad news becomes meaningful if it is connected to real encounters with sick, dying, and bereaved people who provide trainees with feedback about their practice. Their lived experiences can become a valuable source of information and learning (Solomon & Browning, 2005) when educators integrate them into the educational process and allow their voices to be heard (e.g., through books they have published, filmed interviews, or the sharing of their personal stories in class). Finally, the use of reflective activities such as journal writing, role-playing, and vignette exercises can serve as teaching tools in the development of students' relational capacities and self-awareness with regard to loss, death, grief, and caregiving. In that respect, reflective learning can help reduce the gap between theory and practice.

Olthuis and Dekkers (2003) suggest that education should aim at three interrelated learning objectives: (1) the acquisition of theoretical knowledge, (2) the development of clinical skills, and (3) the establishment of a moral attitude that is reflected in the trainees' capacity to remain committed to the caregiving process and respond in a humane manner. Other educators suggest two additional learning objectives: (4) the capacity for self-awareness and reflective practice, and (5) the ability to engage in inter- or transdisciplinary work (Browning & Solomon, 2006; Burns & Bulman, 2001; Jasper, 2003; Kember, et al., 2001; Papadatou, 1997; Papadatou, Corr, Frager, & Bouri, 2003; Rosenbaum, Lobas, & Ferguson, 2005).

Training in teamwork should not be limited to a description of the professionals who make up a palliative or bereavement care team, and what their roles and functions are. It should rather provide opportunities for interaction and collaboration among students from different disciplines (nurses, physicians, psychologists, pharmacists, etc.) who seek to learn together and from each other.

However, learning must also occur through reflective practice that occurs at both the personal and group levels. Reflective practice is a concept that was developed in the 1980s and is widely used in the training of students and novice health care practitioners, particularly nurses. It involves consciously thinking about one's clinical experiences and developing new understandings that lead to new actions. Conscious action after a careful examination and evaluation of one's beliefs, feelings, and actions transforms the experience that is lived, and affects future action on the basis of what has been learned. Thus, reflective learning not only is a matter of using analytical skills to reflect upon something that has already happened but helps to plan and anticipate future action (Jasper, 2003).

CHALLENGE 3

Integrate Current Knowledge Into Educational Programs and Supervised Clinical Applications

Another major challenge is the integration of the accumulated knowledge on death, dying, and bereavement into educational programs offered in medicine, nursing, and allied disciplines. The care of dying people should not be limited to discussions of Elisabeth Kübler-Ross's five stages of grief theory, to euthanasia issues, or to Freud's concepts of eros and thanatos. Educators must be aware of current theoretical and research developments as well as of innovative programs and initiatives in the field. They must demonstrate how the available knowledge relates to clinical practice, and offer opportunities for trainees to get out of the classroom and enter clinical settings in order to spend time with dying patients and bereaved families and to subsequently record, reflect, and discuss their experiences (Block & Billings, 2005; MacLeod, Parkin, Pullon, & Robertson, 2003; Sartain, Clarke, & Heyman, 2000; Wilson & Ayers, 2004; Wilson, Egan, & Friend, 2003).

I would like to offer an example of a learning activity that we use in the training programs on pediatric palliative care that we offer to pediatricians, nurses, psychologists, and social workers. Early in the training, each trainee is introduced to the family of a seriously ill, dying, or deceased child. The family (initially approached by members of the child's caregiving team) is invited to act as teachers who help the trainee develop into a competent practitioner by sharing of their experience over the duration of the training (10 months). Trainees are required to keep a diary of their encounters with the family and record their personal feelings, thoughts, and insights. While they are offered the option of individual supervision, all of them participate in four general sessions in which they share the experiences, insights, and difficulties they encounter as they learn from and accompany families through dying or bereavement. The themes of these general sessions, during which common concerns are discussed and explored (e.g., personal boundaries, communication or collaboration issues, parental or child suffering), include (a) encounters with the child and family, (b) companioning the family through illness or bereavement, (c) acquaintance with the patient's caregiving team, (d) lessons learned.

At the last session, each participant presents a report of his or her experience of accompanying the seriously ill child and/or the bereaved family. The focus is placed on how knowledge that was acquired during the training has been used to understand the child's or family's experience, as well as the trainee's attitudes and responses to dying, death, and bereavement. This activity is completed when each trainee reports back to the child's health care team the lessons learned from the family that he or she accompanied.

CHALLENGE 4

Evaluate Training Outcomes as Well as the Context and Process by Which Learning Occurs

Training programs and curricula are rarely evaluated, and the impact of the training upon learners remains largely unknown. Assessment tools have appeared in the literature in the past few years and are currently being used to illuminate the strengths and weaknesses of diverse programs (Meekin, Klein, Fins, & Fleischman, 2000; Rawlinson & Finlay, 2002; Sullivan, Lakoma, Billings, et al., 2003; Wood, Meekin, Fins, & Fleischman, 2002). It is important that evaluation does not limit itself to the assessment of educational *outcomes* (e.g., What did participants learn? To what degree were the identified goals achieved?). Evaluation should also include the *process* by which learning was facilitated and achieved (e.g., How appropriate were the contents and methods of teaching? How was learning facilitated or compromised?). Finally, evaluation should focus on the *context or environment* in which learning occurred (Was the environment imbued with safety, trust, and respect? Did trainees feel safe to reflect on and discuss how the educational process affected their personal and professional development? Did they feel free to discuss discrepancies between what was taught and practiced?). While reflective practice is increasingly accepted as an important method of teaching and learning in health care professions, there is a lack of empirical evidence showing that it enhances the quality of care and benefits care seekers and care providers (Davies & Sharp, 2001).

To evaluate educational initiatives, we must always address some key questions: *who* assesses *what* and *when?* Are trainees and educators responsible for the evaluation, or should seriously ill and bereaved individuals be invited to evaluate the services that were provided to them by practitioners who completed a training? What are the short-term and long-term effects of training and education upon the learners and their practice? How do acquired knowledge, skills, and reflection bridge the gap between theory and practice and affect individual professionals and teams?

I have found it useful to assess the knowledge, skills, and attitudes of trainees prior to, immediately after, and six months following the completion of a training program, and to further compare participants' responses to those of a control group of non-trainees who work in the same context but do not attend the training. This approach has helped determine the impact of learning in day-to-day practice and to further identify which aspects of the educational program are effective, which require improvement, and how the learning objectives have met the trainees' educational needs.

Ongoing and careful evaluation of any educational activity is vital if our goal is to teach palliative and bereavement care practitioners to apply their knowledge and skills to a diverse range of situations and settings and cultivate ethical and caring relationships with individuals, families, colleagues, and themselves in death situations.

CHALLENGE 5

Integrate Formal and Informal Learning Activities Into the Work Context

It has been suggested numerous times that what practitioners actually do in their day-to-day work is quite different from what they are taught in the classroom and in workshops. This discrepancy has a profound effect upon inexperienced care providers, who progressively become disillusioned, experience moral distress, and feel guilty and ashamed of being less than perfect and vulnerable in the face of death. They gradually unlearn the knowledge and skills that they have acquired through formal training and become affected by the hidden curriculum that prevails in health care practice (Browning & Solomon, 2006; Hafferty & Franks, 1994; Wear, 1998).

Haidet and Stein (2006) suggest that the hidden curriculum in the medical culture is built upon value-based assumptions, such as the belief that doctors must be perfect, uncertainty and complexity should be avoided, the outcome is more important than the process, and hierarchy prevails. In psychology and social work, the hidden curriculum expects practitioners to help people change, provide solutions to problems, eradicate suffering, and display detached concern to protect self from burnout.

What is often described as the hidden curriculum reflects the goals, values, and rules that govern the operation of a given discipline, team, or organization. Unlearning what one has been taught in order to learn the values, goals, and rules that prevail in a particular work setting often results in the erosion of professionalism and deprives practitioners of the satisfaction of being compassionate, caring, and empathic with people in death situations. This obstacle is overcome when training and education are linked to clinical practice instead of remaining isolated activities that occur solely in academic settings. Such a link exposes the hidden curricula of educational and clinical institutions and invites reparative action.

End-of-life and bereavement care require a wide repertoire of knowledge and skills, and an ethic about life and death that cannot be taught by any single educational program. Existential issues related to the meaning of life and death are best addressed when learning occurs in clinical settings that offer opportunities for formal and informal teaching. Sahler, Frager, Levetown, Cohn, and Lipson (2000) stressed the importance of taking advantage of the numerous teachable moments available when one is actually caring for a dying person and supporting a bereaved individual. These can serve as valuable opportunities to address pertinent issues and teach skills or expand knowledge. Planned or spontaneous discussions among novice and more experienced professionals can be beneficial to both. Modeling alternative ways of managing the challenges of communication, of physical and emotional care, of ethical and existential concerns, and of personal distress is highly instructive. Furthermore, discussing the challenges of interprofessional collaboration can be a valuable experience for both learners and practitioners.

In a longitudinal study, Vazirani, Slavin, and Feldman (2000) found that not only do pediatric house officers begin their training feeling uncomfortable with death-and-dying issues, but it takes four years before they experience a change in their attitudes and begin to feel comfortable coping with issues related to pediatric palliative care. These researchers suggest that even though training programs may inform and familiarize participants with end-of-life issues, it is supervised clinical practice and professional experience that contribute to their preparedness and comfort.

Thus, educational programs should not remain independent of supervised clinical practice. Instead, they should encourage hospitals, hospices, home care services, nursing homes, and bereavement centers to integrate various formal and informal learning activities on how to provide adequate care to the dying; how to counsel the bereaved; how to reduce miscommunication, misunderstanding, and disorganization at a team level; and, most importantly, how to acknowledge, cope with, and transform personal suffering.

Through education on death and dying, students and trainees address issues that are related to the core of humanity. When we, as educators, provide them with a holding environment in which they can confront death and reflect upon their life trajectories, we contribute to their growth as individuals, to their competence as professionals who are able to empathize with and assist dying and bereaved people, and to their ability to enrich others' and their own lives.

NOTE

1. For example, the American Medical Association developed the "Education for Physicians on End-of-Life Care" (www.epec.net), and the American Association of Colleges of Nursing designed the "End-of-Life Nursing Education Curriculum" (www.aacn.nche.edu/elnect/curriculum.htm). The National Hospice and Palliative Care Association developed the "Training Curriculum in Pediatric Palliative Care" (www.nhpco.org/i4a/pages/index.cfm?pageid=3409), and the Initiative for Pediatric Palliative Care (www.ippcweb.org/curriculum.asp) was sponsored by the Education Development Center.

Epilogue

At the genesis of the cosmos, only gods existed, according to Greek mythology. The time came when they decided to create living beings, which they molded with earth, water, and fire. After giving them various shapes and sizes, the gods ordered two immortal titans, Prometheus and his brother Epimetheus, to give each creature a special trait, positive quality, or talent. Epimetheus gave small creatures the capacity for speed, wings to fly, or the ability to hide underground and endowed big creatures with the power to protect themselves from threats. He decorated some beings with a thick fur or a hard skin to withstand cold weather and gave others the necessary resources to survive in high temperatures. Although generous and creative, Epimetheus was both thoughtless and reckless. He used all the available traits, talents, powers and qualities and was left with none with which to endow on man. So when Prometheus inspected his brother's work, he found man naked, defenseless, and vulnerable. He decided to bestow upon man a power—unshared by any other living creature—that would bring man near to the perfection of the immortal gods. He thought about giving man the gift of fire. But fire was in the possession of the gods, who were unwilling to share it with humans. So Prometheus stole the fire from the gods and gave it to them. They accepted the treasured gift and immediately used it to cook, to create various tools, and to develop artistic and cultural pursuits.

Zeus was furious with Prometheus for stealing the fire, and with humans for accepting the gift. He decided to punish both. He chained Prometheus with unbreakable shackles to a huge rock on the Caucasus Mountain in Central Asia. Each morning an eagle ate his liver, and in the evening the liver would grow back again. Prometheus was therefore tormented for 30,000 years before Hercules killed the eagle and freed him from his chains.

To punish humans, Zeus sent Pandora to them. She was a woman created by Olympian gods, who had given her the gifts of beauty, charm, artistic and musical talents, cleverness, foolishness, cunning, and curiosity. In fact, her name means "she to whom all gifts were given" (*pan* = all, *dora* = gifts). However, she is also referred as Pandotira, "the one who gives everything," and as Anisidora, "the one who brings gifts from below" (Kakridis, 1986).

When Pandora was offered as a gift to humans by the gods, she carried along a large jar (*pithos,* in Greek) as a gift and was ordered never to open it. Being clever and distrusting of Zeus, Prometheus refused the gift and warned Epimetheus to do the same. But his brother, who was less thoughtful and impulsive, was seduced and fell in love with Pandora, whom he wedded. They lived happily until one day Pandora, curious to see the jar's contents, opened it. All the misfortunes and evils that affected humankind were released from the jar. Alarmed, she managed to shut the jar, leaving one thing at the bottom: hope (*elpis,* in Greek).

This myth suggests that human existence can be filled with adversities and suffering, but that with hope, an exceptional capacity that only humans possess, we pave our way through the difficulties of life. Hope infuses us with energy to move forward and change our world and provides us with wisdom to alter our view of a reality that we cannot change.

The myth of Pandora and Prometheus is a myth of hope and transformation. Prometheus gives hope to all humans—in the form of fire—providing them with opportunities to survive and use their knowledge to work, develop skills, and transform their lives for the better. Pandora, on the other hand, keeps hope within as a shield against the evils of life, and as a valued source of rebirth, renewal, and transformation from pain, adversity, and suffering.

In life, we need both: hope to anticipate, contemplate, and plan the future and move forward, as well as hope to learn from the past and live differently in the present. When we are confronted with the finality of death, hope abounds. We hope for a good death, to realize a dream or goal, to join our loved ones in an afterlife, or we hope that our life had purpose, meaning, or value to ourselves and to others. Hope enables us to accept, temper, or transform suffering and invest life and death with meaning.

Those of us who accompany people through dying and bereavement come to realize, sooner or later, that we cannot provide effective care, unless it is hope-*full.* Hopeful care is made available when we embrace and accept suffering as inevitable to human existence, and transform it through the development of caring and meaningful relationships.

Through this process we always risk being affected and changed as people, as professionals, or as a team. In this risk, however, lies the hope that we can humanize care and make it rewarding to dying and bereaved people, as well as to ourselves and to our colleagues.

This book was written with such a hope. Writing it was like a pregnancy for me, filled with joys, pains, and frustrations, along with the sheer anticipation of bringing to life aspects of my experience of accompanying dying and bereaved children and adults through death. May this book open up new avenues for reflection; opportunities for debate; and an increased awareness of what we, the professionals, bring into our relationships with the people we serve, and what we receive in return that enriches our personal and professional lives.

Appendix: Brief Description of Bowlby's Theory on Attachment

Bowlby argued that humans are all born with a fundamental need for safety and security that is achieved through emotional bonds that develop with nurturing caretakers. This need is present from the cradle to the grave and becomes apparent across the life span, particularly when one is vulnerable, distressed, sick, or threatened with loss. By observing the infant-mother relationship, Bowlby studied the patterns of interaction through which an infant and a parent (or primary caretaker) get to know each other and form an attachment bond. Even though he believed that this attachment bond is the "property" of both the child and the parent, his studies focused mostly on the child's care-seeking behaviors, and less on the parent's caregiving behaviors.

He stipulated that both sets of behaviors are biologically rooted and ready to develop when certain conditions are present. "Human infants, like infants in other species, are preprogrammed to develop in a socially cooperative way," he argued. "Whether they do so or not, turns in high degree on how they are treated" by their caretakers (Bowlby, 1988, p. 9).

In Bowlby's theory, care-seeking and caregiving behaviors are complementary and interdependent. What is their function? The main function of a child's care-seeking behaviors—generally referred to as attachment behaviors—is to seek and maintain physical and emotional proximity to the parent in order to achieve a sense of security. They fall into two categories: (1) those aiming to bring the caretaker to the child (signaling behaviors, e.g., crying, smiling, babbling, or calling) and (2) those aiming to bring the child to caretaker (approaching behaviors, e.g., following, seeking, and clinging).

According to Bowlby, attachment behaviors belong to a system that has its own form of internal organization. This system is activated and becomes most apparent when the parent-child bond is threatened or disrupted by temporary separation. The infant or child cries, protests, seeks the absent parent, and clings to him or her upon his or her return in an attempt to restore proximity and prevent lasting loss.

The child's attachment behaviors activate in the parent or caretaker a system of caregiving behaviors whose function is to ensure proximity and provide the child with a sense of safety that, subsequently, allows him or her to explore the world. Caregiving behaviors vary from one caretaker to another and affect the parent-child interaction in different ways. For example, an ordinary sensitive mother is attuned to the infant's desire for proximity and support, discovers what suits him or her best, and behaves accordingly. By responding to the child's needs, she enlists his or her cooperation. Feeling secure and relaxed, the child is then able to move away from the mother in order to explore the environment, knowing that he or she can retreat to an available and secure base in case of trouble. Other mothers rebuff the child for wishing to be near them or to sit on their lap, or for seeking cuddles and caresses, as a result of which the child—who becomes preoccupied with the mother's unavailability—responds with more clinging and crying. Depressed mothers who have a long history of deprivation are unable to respond to the child's attachment behaviors, and as a result he or she learns to rely upon him- or herself.

The interplay between care-seeking and caregiving behaviors accounts for the differences evidenced among children, some of whom develop secure attachment patterns, and others of whom insecure attachment patterns that affect their relationships with others later in life (Ainsworth, Blehar, Waters, & Wall, 1978; Main & Goldwyn, 1984).

Secure attachments are characteristic of children who are more open and cooperative with others who, in return, are consistently sensitive and responsive to their attachment needs. These children explore with greater confidence their environment. In contrast, insecure attachments are characteristic of children who view the world as dangerous, hostile, or indifferent and are intolerant of or anxious about separation. They develop insecure attachments that fall into one of the following categories:

- *Anxious/ambivalent attachments.* This type of attachment is characteristic of children who are in constant fear of losing their caretakers, who are sometimes unavailable and unresponsive, and at other times intrusive and overprotective by discouraging the child's need to explore the world.

- *Avoidant attachments.* This type of attachment is characteristic of children who perceive others as insensitive to their own needs and therefore learn to compulsively rely upon themselves in novel situations.
- *Disorganized/disoriented attachments.* This type of attachment is characteristic of children who have little trust in themselves, behave in an inconsistent and unpredictable way to separations from and reunions with caretakers, and oscillate between approaching and avoiding others, whom they mistrust.

We must keep in mind that children form attachment bonds with both parents as well as with other caretakers (e.g., grandparent, older siblings, nannies), who display different caregiving patterns in response to their attachment needs. As a result, they have different experiences. Their attachment histories may be simple, uncomplicated, and relatively consistent from infancy to adulthood (regardless of whether they are characterized by secure or insecure attachments), or they may be filled with loss events and changes (e.g., death, divorce, parental depression) that range from attachment security to attachment insecurity (Rholes & Simpson, 2004b). Each life story is unique and affected by the combination of multiple factors that determine a person's attachment orientation or attachment style in life.

To understand the role of attachment, it is helpful to explore what Bowlby referred to as an individual's *internal working model,* which is developed from early life experiences and comprises a set of assumptions about oneself, others, and the world. These assumptions are purely subjective; however, they are held to be true by the person. They provide blueprints for what should be expected, and what is likely to occur in different kinds of interactions in which one seeks safety and security (care-seeking patterns) or attends to the needs of others in times of trouble (caregiving patterns). In other words, a person's internal working model orchestrates behavior, cognition, and affect and provides direction about what to expect, how to behave, and how to explain interpersonal events and relations. Bowlby used the term *working* to suggest that even though an internal model is relatively stable over time, it is not fixed but remains open to revision and change, especially in situations of major life events, traumatic experiences, or attachment bonds that lead to new insights and corrections and modifications of assumptions about oneself, others, and the world. Thus, childhood attachment styles are not written in stone, and as a result, a person with an insecure attachment style in childhood may be able to develop a secure attachment style in adulthood if his or her life experiences and choices provide opportunities for the development of bonds with people who display a secure attachment style. Therefore, while early attachment experiences often explain attachment orientations with one's spouse, children, peers, and other adults in adulthood, they do not always predict these orientations. A number of longitudinal studies are currently illuminating how attachment bonds develop between individuals, how they change from early childhood to adulthood, and which processes generate changes (Grossmann, Grossmann, & Waters, 2005; Rholes & Simpson, 2004a). The field is open to a rich debate that will hopefully help us better understand attachment in caregiving situations, and particularly in relationships that develop between those who seek care and those who provide it in the face of death.

References

Abend, S. M. (1982). Serious illness in the analyst: Countertransference considerations. *Journal of the American Psychoanalytic Association, 30,* 365–379.

Adler, A. (1935). The fundamental views of Individual Psychology. *International Journal of Individual Psychology, 1,* 5–8.

Adler, A. (1937). Mass psychology. *International Journal of Individual Psychology, 3,* 111–120.

Adler, A. (1958a). *The practice and theory of Individual Psychology.* Paterson, NJ: Littlefield, Adams.

Adler, A. (1958b). *What life should mean to you.* New York: Putman & Sons. (Originally published 1932)

Adler, A. (1964). *Social interest: A challenge to mankind.* New York: Putman & Sons. (Originally published 1933)

Adler, A. (1971). *The practice and theory of Individual Psychology.* London: Routledge. (Originally published in 1923)

Aiken, L., Clarke, S., Sloane, D., Sochalski, J., & Silber, J. (2002). Hospital nurse staffing and patient mortality, nurse burnout, and job dissatisfaction. *Journal of American Medical Association, 288,* 1987–1995.

Ainsworth, M. D. S., Blehar, M. C., Waters, W., & Wall, S. (1978). *Patterns of attachment: A psychological study of the Strange Situation.* Hillsdale, NJ: Erlbaum.

Albery, N., Elliot, G., & Elliot, J. (Eds.). (1993). *The natural death handbook.* London: Virgin.

Alexander, J., Kolodziejski, K., Sanville, J., & Shaw, R. (1989). On final terminations: Consultation with a dying therapist. *Clinical Social Work Journal, 4,* 307–321.

Ansbacher, H. L., & Ansbacher, R. R. (Eds.). (1956). *The Individual Psychology of Alfred Adler.* New York: Harper & Row.

Ariès, P. (1974). *Western attitudes towards death: From the Middle Ages to the present.* London: Marion Boyars.

Ariès, P. (1981). *The hour of death.* London: Allen Lane.

Ashforth, B. E., & Humphrey, R. H. (1993). Emotional labor in service roles: The influence of identity. *Academy of Management Review, 18*(1), 88–115.

Attig, T. (1992). Person-centered death education. *Death Studies, 16,* 357–370.

Attig, T. (1996). *How we grieve: Relearning the world.* New York: Oxford University Press.

Ausloos, G. (2003). *La compétence des familles: Temps, chaos, processes.* Ramonville Saint-Agne: Editions Erès.

Baile, W. F., Buckman, R., Lenzi, R., Glober, G., Beale, E. A., & Kudelka, A. P. (2000). SPIKES—a six-step protocol for delivering bad news: Application to the patient with cancer. *The Oncologist, 5,* 302–311.

Balint, E. (1969). The possibilities of patient-centered medicine. *Journal of the Royal College of General Practitioners, 17,* 269–276.

Barclay, S., Wyatt, P., Shore, S., Finlay, I., Grande, G., & Todd, C. (2003). Caring for the dying: How well prepared are general practitioners? A questionnaire study in Wales. *Palliative Medicine, 17*(1), 27–39.

Barnard, D. (1995). The promise of intimacy and fear of our own undoing. *Journal of Palliative Care, 11*(4), 22–26.

Bauby, J-D. (1997). *The diving-bell and the batterfly* (J. Leggatt, Trans.). London: Fourth Estate.

Beach, M. C., Inui, T., & Relationship-Centered Care Research Network. (2006). Relationship-centered care: A constructive reframing. *Journal of General Internal Medicine, 21,* 53–58.

Behnke, M., Reiss, J., Neimeyer, G., & Bandstra, E. S. (1987). Grief responses of pediatric house officers to a patient's death. *Death Studies, 11*(3), 169–176.

Bené, B., & Foxall, M. J. (1991). Death anxiety and job stress in hospice and medical-surgical nurses. *Hospice Journal, 7,* 25–41.

Benoliel, J. Q. (1974). Anticipatory grief in physicians and nurses. In B. Schoenberg (Ed.), *Anticipatory grief* (pp. 218–228). New York: Brunner-Mazel.

Bion, W. (1961). *Experiences in groups.* New York: Basic Books.

Block, S. D., & Billings, J. A. (2005). Learning from the dying. *New England Journal of Medicine, 353*(13), 1313–1315.

Bonnano, G. A. (2004). Loss, trauma, and human resilience: Have we underestimated the human capacity to thrive after extremely aversive events? *American Psychologist, 59,* 20–28.

Bonnano, G. A., Wortman, C. B., Lehmna, D. R., Tweed. R. G., Hating, M., Sonnega, J., et al. (2002). Resilience to loss and chronic grief: A prospective study from preloss to 18-months postloss. *Journal of Personality and Social Psychology, 83*(5), 1150–1164.

Bowlby, J. (1973). *Separation: Anxiety and anger.* London: Hogarth Press.

Bowlby, J. (1980). *Loss: Sadness and depression.* London: Hogarth Press.

Bowlby, J. (1982). *Attachment* (2nd ed., Vol. 1). New York: Basic Books. (Originally published 1969)

Bowlby, J. (1988). *Parent-child attachment and healthy human development.* London: Routledge.

Bowlby, J. (2005). *The making and breaking of affectional bonds* (2nd ed.). London: Routledge.

Bram, P. J., & Katz., L. F. (1989). Study of burnout in nurses working in hospice and hospital oncology settings. *Oncology Nursing Forum, 16,* 555–560.

Britt, T. W., Adler, A. B., & Bartone, P. T. (2001). Deriving benefits from stressful events: The role of engagement in meaningful work and hardiness. *Journal of Occupational Health Psychology, 6*(1), 53–63.

Browning, D. M., & Solomon, M. Z. (2006). Relational learning in pediatric palliative care: Transformative education and the culture of medicine. *Child and Adolescent Psychiatric Clinics of North America, 15,* 795–815.

Brunelli, T. (2005). A concept analysis: The grieving process of nurses. *Nursing Forum, 40,* 123–128.

Burns, S., & Bulman, C. (Eds.). (2001). *Reflective practice in nursing: The growth of the professional practitioner* (2nd ed.). London: Blackwell Science.

Burton, A. (1962). Death as countertransference. *Psychoanalytic Review, 49,* 3–20.

Calhoun, L. G., & Tedeschi, R. G. (1998). Posttraumatic growth: Future directions. In R. G. Tedeschi, C. L. Park & L. G. Calhoun, (Eds.), *Posttraumatic growth: Positive changes in the aftermath of crisis* (pp. 215–238). Mahwah, N. J.: Lawrence Erlbaum Associates Publishers.

Catherall, D. R. (1999). Coping with secondary traumatic stress: Importance of the therapist's professional group. In B. H. Stamm (Ed.), *Secondary traumatic stress: Self-care issues of clinicians, researchers, and educators* (2nd ed., pp. 80–92). Baltimore, MD: Sidran Press.

Chalifour, J. (1998). L'infirmière face à ses deuils. *Soins, 623,* 39–42.

Chassay, S. (2006). Death in the afternoon. *International Journal of Psychoanalysis, 87,* 203–217.

Chiriboga, D. A., Jenkins, G., & Bailey, J. (1983). Stress and coping among hospice nurses: Test of an analytic model. *Nursing Research, 32,* 294–299.

Chochinov, H. M., & Breitbart, W. (Eds.). (2000). *Handbook of psychiatry in palliative medicine.* New York: Oxford University Press.

Clark, D. (1999). "Total pain," disciplinary power and the body in the work of Cicely Saunders, 1958–1967. *Social Science and Medicine, 49,* 727–736.

Clark, D. (2002). *Cicely Saunders—founder of the hospice movement. Selected letters, 1959–1999.* Oxford: Oxford University Press.

Clarke, P. J. (1981). Exploration of counter-transference toward the dying. *American Journal of Orthopsychiatry, 51*(1), 71–77.

Clarke-Steffen, L. (1998). The meaning of peak and nadir experiences of pediatric oncology nurses: Secondary analysis. *Journal of Pediatric Oncology Nursing, 15*(1), 25–33.

Connor, S. R., Egan, K. A., Kwilosz, D. A., Larson, D. G., & Reese, D. J. (2002). Interdisciplinary approaches to assisting with end-of-life care and decision making. *American Behavioral Scientist, 46*(3), 340–356.

Contro, N., Larson, J., Scofield, S., Sourkes, B., & Cohen, H. (2002). Family perspectives on the quality of pediatric palliative care. *Archives of Pediatric and Adolescent Medicine, 156*(1), 226–231.

Contro, N., Larson, J., Scofield, S., Sourkes, B., & Cohen, H. (2004). Hospital staff and family perspectives regarding quality of pediatric palliative care. *Pediatrics, 1114,* 1248–1252.

Cook, A. S., & Oltjenbrun, K. A. (1998). *Dying and grieving: Lifespan and family perspective* (2nd ed.). Fort Worth, TX: Hacourt Broca.

Coppola, K. M., & Strohmetz, D. B. (2002). How is death and dying addressed in introductory psychology textbooks? *Death Studies, 26*(8), 689–699.

Corr, C. A. (2002). Teaching a college course on children and death for 22 years: A supplemental report. *Death Studies, 26*(7), 596–606.

Correale, A. (1996). L'hypertrophie de la mémoire comme forme de pathologie institutionnelle. In R. Kaës, J. P. Pinel, O. Kernberg, A. Correale, E. Diet, & B. Duez (Eds.), *Souffrance et psychopathologie des liens institutionnels* (pp. 106–119). Paris: Dunod.

Cyrulnik, B. (1999). *Un merveilleux malheur.* Paris: Odile Jacob.

Davidson, R., & Harrington, A. (Eds.). (2002). *Visions of compassion: Western scientists and Tibetan Buddhists examine human nature.* New York: Oxford University Press.

Davies, B., Clarke, D., Connaughty, S., Cook, K., MacKenzie, B., McCormick, J., et al. (1996). Caring for dying children: Nurses' experiences. *Pediatric Nursing, 22,* 500–507.

Davies, C., & Sharp, P. (2001). Assessment and evaluation of reflection. In S. Burns & C. Bulman (Eds.), *Reflective practice in nursing: The growth of the professional practitioner* (2nd ed., pp. 52–78). London: Blackwell Science.

Davis, C. G., & McKearney, J. M. (2003). How do people grow from their experience with trauma and loss? *Journal of Social and Clinical Psychology, 5*(22), 477–492.

De Beauvoir, S. (1964). *A very easy death* (P. O'Brian, Trans.). New York: Pantheon Books.

De Hannezel, M. (1995). *La mort intime: Ceux qui vont mourir nous apprennent à vivre.* Paris: Editions Robert Laffont.

De Montigny, J. (1993). Distress, stress and solidarity in palliative care. *Omega: Journal of Death and Dying, 27*(1), 5–15.

De M'Uzan, M. (1977). Le travail du trépas. In a *De l'art à la mort: Itinéraire psychnalytique* (pp. 182–199). Paris: Gallimard.

Dewald, P. (1982). Serious illness in the analyst: Transference, countertransference, and reality responses. *Journal of the American Psychoanalytic Association, 30,* 347–365.

Dickinson, G. E., & Field, D. (2002). Teaching end-of-life issues: Current status in United Kingdom and United States medical schools. *American Journal of Hospice & Palliative Care, 19*(3), 181–186.

Diet, E. (1996). Le thanatophore: Travail de mort et destructivité dans les institutions. In R. Kaës, J. P. Pinel, O. Kernberg, A. Correale, E. Diet, & B. Duez (Eds.), *Souffrance et psychopathology des liens institutionnels* (pp. 121–159). Paris: Dunod.

Doka, K. J. (Ed.). (1989). *Disenfranchised grief: Recognizing hidden sorrow.* Lexington, MA: Lexington Books.

Donnelly, M. M. (2006). *Critical incidents, counsellors and school communities: Professional and personal narratives.* Doctoral dissertation, University of Sydney.

Dossey, L. (1984). *Beyond illness: Discovering the experience of health* (pp. 83–93). Boulder, CO: New Science Library.

Downe-Wamboldt, B., & Tamlyn, D. (1997). An international survey of death education trends in faculties of nursing and medicine. *Death Studies, 21*(2), 177–188.

Dutton, J. E., Frost, P. J., Worline, M. C., Liliius, J. M., & Kanov, J. M. (2002). Leading in times of trauma. *Harvard Business Review, 80*(1), 54–61.

Eakes, G. G. (1984). Grief resolution in hospice nurses. *Nursing & Health Care, 11,* 243–248.

Egan, K. (1998). *Patient-family value based end-of-life care model.* Lergo: Hospice Institute of the Florida Suncoast.

Egan, K. A., & Labyak, M. J. (2001). Hospice care: A model for quality end-of-life care. In B. R. Ferrell & N. Coyle (Eds.), *Textbook of palliative nursing* (pp. 7–26). Oxford: Oxford University Press.

Eifried, S. (2003). Bearing witness to suffering: The lived experience of nursing students. *Journal of Nursing Education, 42*(3), 59–67.

Engel, G. L. (1977). The need for a new medical model: A challenge for biomedicine. *Science, 196,* 129–136.
Engel, G. L. (1980). The clinical application of the biopsychosocial model. *American Journal of Psychiatry, 137,* 535–544.
Engel, G. L. (1997). From biomedical to biopsychosocial: Being scientific in the human domain. *Psychosomatics, 38,* 521–528.
Enriquez, E. (2003). Le travail de la mort dans les institutions. In R. Kaës, J. Bleger, E. Enriquez, F. Fornari, P. Fustier, R. Roussillon et al. (Eds.), *L'institution et les institutions: Études psychanalytiques* (pp. 62–94). Paris: Dunod.
Eyetsemitan, F. (1998). Stifled grief in the workplace. *Death Studies, 22*(5), 469–479.
Farber, A., & Farber, S. (2006). The respectful death model: Difficult conversations at the end of life. In R. S. Katz & T. A. Johnson (Eds.), *When professionals weep: Emotional and countertransference responses in end-of-life care* (pp. 221–236). New York: Routledge.
Feeney, B. C., & Collins, N. L. (2004). Interpersonal safe haven and secure base caregiving processes in adulthood. In W. S. Rholes & J. A. Simpson (Eds.), *Adult attachment: Theory, research, and clinical implications* (pp. 300–338). New York: Guilford Press.
Feinsilver, D. (1998). The therapist as a person facing death: The hardest of external realities and the therapeutic action. *International Journal of Psychoanalysis, 79,* 1131.
Feldstein, M. A., & Buschman-Gemma, P. (1995). Oncology nurses and chronic compounded grief. *Cancer Nursing, 18*(3), 228–236.
Ferguson, E. D. (1989). Adler's motivational theory: An historical perspective on belonging and the fundamental human striving. *Individual Psychology, 45,* 355–361.
Ferguson, E. D. (2000). Individual Psychology ahead of its time. *Journal of Individual Psychology, 56,* 14–20.
Field, D. (1996). Awareness and modern dying. *Mortality, 1*(3), 255–266.
Figley, C. R. (1989). *Helping traumatized families.* San Francisco: Jossey-Bass.
Figley, C. R. (Ed.). (1995). *Compassion fatigue: Coping with secondary traumatic stress disorder in those who treat the traumatized.* New York: Brunner-Mazel.
Figley, C. R. (1999). Compassion fatigue: Toward a new understanding of the costs of caring. In B. H. Stamm (Ed.), *Secondary traumatic stress: Self-care issues for clinicians, researchers, and educators* (2nd ed., pp. 3–28). Baltimore, MD: Sidran Press.
Fins, J. J., Miller, F. G., Acres, C. A., Bacchett, M. D., Huzzard, L. L., & Rapkin, B. D. (1999). End-of-life decision-making in the hospital: Current practice and future prospects. *Journal of Pain and Symptom Management, 17,* 6–15.
Fowler, K., Poehling, K., Billheimer, D., Hamilton, R., Wu, H., Mulder, J., & Frangould, H. (2006). Hospice referral practices for children with cancer: A survey of pediatric oncologists. *Journal of Clinical Oncology, 24,* 1099–1104.
Foxall, J. M., Zimmerman, L., Standley, R., & Bené, B. (1990). A comparison of frequency and sources of nursing job stress perceived by intensive care, hospice and medical-surgical nurses. *Journal of Advanced Nursing, 15,* 577–584.
Fredriksson, L., & Eriksson, K. (2001). The patient's narrative of suffering: A path to health? *Scandinavian Journal of Caring Sciences, 15,* 3–11.
Freud, S. (1957). Mourning and melancholia (J. Riviere, Trans.). In J. Sutherland (Ed.), *Collected papers* (Vol. 4, pp. 152–170). London: Hogarth Press. (Original work published 1917)

Fussel, F. W., & Bonney, W. C. (1999). A comparative study of childhood experiences of psychotherapists and physicists: Implications for clinical practice. *Psychotherapy, 27*(4), 505–512.

Gabbard, G. O. (1999). An overview of countertransference: Theory and technique. In O. G. Gabbard (Ed.), *Countertransference issues in psychiatric treatment* (pp. 1–25). Washington, DC: American Psychiatric Press.

Gaylin, W. (1976). *Caring.* New York: Knopf.

Gilbert, P. (Ed.). (2005). *Compassion: Conceptualizations, research and use in psychotherapy.* London: Routledge.

Gold, J. H., & Nemiah, J. C. (Eds.). (1993). *Beyond transference: When the therapist's real life intrudes.* Washington, DC: American Psychiatric Press.

Goldman, A., Hewitt, M., Collins, G. S., Childs, M., & Hain, R. (2006). Symptoms in children/young people with progressive malignant disease: United Kingdom Children's Cancer Study Group/Paediatric Oncology Nurses Forum survey. *Pediatrics, 117,* 1179–1186.

Gosling, R. H. (1979). Another source of conservatism in groups. In G. Lawrence (Ed.), *Exploring individual and organizational boundaries: A Tavistock open systems approach* (pp. 77–151). Chichester, UK: John Wiley & Sons.

Grandley, A. A. (2000). Emotional regulation in the workplace: A new way to conceptualize emotional labor. *Journal of Occupational Health Psychology, 5,* 85–110.

Gray-Toft, P., & Anderson, J. G. (1986–1987). Sources of stress in nursing terminal patients in a hospice. *Omega: Journal on Death and Dying, 17,* 27–39.

Grossmann, K. E., Grossmann, K., & Waters, E. (2005). *Attachment from infancy to adulthood: The major longitudinal studies.* New York: Guilford Press.

Gundersen, L. (2001). Physician burnout. *Annals of Internal Medicine, 135,* 145–149.

Hafferty, F. W., & Franks, R. (1994). The hidden curriculum, ethics teaching, and the structure of medical education. *Academic Medicine, 69,* 861–871.

Haidet, P., & Stein, H. F. (2006). The role of student-teacher relationship in the formation of physicians: The hidden curriculum as process. *Journal of General Internal Medicine, 21*(Suppl. 1), 516–521.

Haley, W. E., Kasl-Godley, J., Neimeyer, R. A., & Kwilosz, D. M. (2003). Roles for psychologists in end-of-life-care: Emerging models of practice. *Professional Psychology: Research and Practice, 34*(6), 626–633.

Hall, P., & Weaver, L. (2001). Interdisciplinary education and teamwork: A long and winding road. *Medical Education, 35,* 867–875.

Halpern, J. (2001). *From detached concern to empathy: Humanizing medical practice.* New York: Oxford University Press.

Halpert, E. (1982). When the analyst is chronically ill or dying. *Psychoanalytic Quarterly, 51,* 372–389.

Halton, W. (2000). Some unconscious aspects of organizational life. In A. Obholzer & V. Z. Roberts (Eds.), *The unconscious at work: Individual and organizational stress at work* (2nd ed., pp. 11–18). London: Brunner-Routledge.

Hartocollis, P. (1983). *Time and timelessness, or The varieties of temporal experience.* New York: International Universities Press.

Hazan, C. G., & Shaver, P. (1990). Love and work: An attachment theoretical perspective. *Journal of Personality and Social Psychology, 59,* 270–280.

Heller, K. S., & Solomon, M. Z. (2005). Continuity of care and caring: What matters to parents of children with life-threatening conditions. *Journal of Pediatric Nursing, 20*, 335–346.

Heustis, R., & Jenkins, M. (2005). *Companioning at a time of perinatal loss: A guide for nurses, physicians, social workers, chaplains and other bedside caregivers.* Fort Collins, CO: Companion Press.

Hickey, M. (1990). What are the needs of critically ill patients? A review of the literature since 1976. *Heart & Lung, 19*(4), 401–415.

Hilden, J. M., Emanuel, E. J., Fairclough, D. L., Link, M. P., Foley, K. M., Carridge, B. C., et al. (2001). Attitudes and practices among pediatric oncologists regarding end-of-life care: Results of the 1998 American Society of Clinical Oncology Survey. *Journal of Clinical Oncology, 19*(1), 205–212.

Hinds, P. S., Puckett, P., Donohoe, M., Milligan, M., Payne, K., Phipps, S., et al. (1994). The impact of a grief workshop for pediatric oncology nurses on their grief and perceived stress. *Journal of Pediatric Nursing, 9*, 388–397.

Hochschild, A. R. (1983). *The managed heart: Commercialization of human feeling.* Berkeley: University of California Press.

Hogan, N. S., & Schmidt, L. A. (2002). Testing the grief to personal growth model using structural equation modeling. *Death Studies, 26*(8), 615–634.

Huggard, P. (2003). Compassion fatigue: How much can I give. *Medical Education, 37*(2), 163–164.

International Work Group on Death, Dying, and Bereavement. (1979). Assumptions and principles underlying standards for care of the terminally ill. *American Journal of Nursing, 79*, 296–297.

International Work Group on Death, Dying, and Bereavement. (1993a). Palliative care for children. *Death Studies, 17*(3), 277–280.

International Work Group on Death, Dying, and Bereavement. (1993b). A statement of assumptions and principles concerning psychosocial care of dying persons and their families. *Journal of Palliative Care, 9*(2), 29–32.

International Work Group on Death, Dying, and Bereavement. (2002). Assumptions and principles about psychosocial aspects in disasters. *Death Studies, 26*(6), 449–462.

International Work Group on Death, Dying, and Bereavement. (2006). Caregivers in death, dying and bereavement situations. *Death Studies, 30*(7), 649–664.

Janoff-Bulman, R. (1992). *Shattered assumptions.* New York: Free Press.

Jasper, M. (2003). *Beginning reflective practice: Foundations in nursing and health care.* Cheltenham, UK: Nelson Thornes.

Jellinek, M. S., Todres, I. D., Catlin, E. A., Cassem, E. H., & Salzman, A. (1993). Pediatric intensive care training: Confronting the dark side. *Critical Care Medicine, 21*(5), 775–779.

Jenkins, J. F., & Ostchega, Y. (1986). Evaluation of burnout in oncology nurses. *Cancer Nursing, 9*, 108–116.

Joinson, C. (1992). Coping with compassion fatigue. *Nursing, 22*(4), 116–122.

Jones, W. H. S. (Trans.). (1923). *Hippocrates* (Vol. 2). Cambridge, MA: Loeb Classical Library.

Kaës, R. (2003). Réalité psychique et souffrance dans les institutions. In R. Kaës, J. Bleger, E. Enriquez, F. Fornari, P. Fustier, R. Roussillon et al. (Eds.), *L'institution et les institutions: Études psychanalytiques* (pp. 1–46). Paris: Dunod.

Kahn, W. A. (1992). To be fully there: Psychological presence at work. *Human Relations, 45*(4), 321–349.

Kahn, W. A. (1995). Organization change and the provision of secure base: Lessons from the field. *Human Relations, 48*(5), 489–514.

Kahn, W. A. (2001). Holding environments at work. *Journal of Applied Behavioral Science, 37*(3), 260–279.

Kahn, W. A. (2002). Managing the paradox of self-reliance. *Organizational Dynamics, 30*(3), 239–256.

Kahn, W. A. (2005). *Holding fast: The struggle to create resilient caregiving organization.* New York: Brunner-Routledge.

Kakridis, I. T. (1986). [*Greek mythology*] (Vols. 2–3). Athens: Ekdotiki Athinon.

Kaplan, L. (2000). Toward a model of a caregiver grief: Nurses' experiences of treating dying children. *Omega: Journal of Death and Dying, 41*, 187–206.

Kastenbaum, R. (1977). *Death, society and human experience.* Saint Louis, MO: Mosby.

Katz, R. S., & Johnson, T. A. (2006a). Suffering and the caring professional. In R. S. Katz & T. A. Johnson (Eds.), *When professionals weep: Emotional countertransference responses in end-of-life care* (pp. 13–26). New York: Routledge.

Katz, R. S., & Johnson, T. A. (Eds.). (2006b). *When professionals weep: Emotional countertransference responses in end-of-life care.* New York: Routledge.

Kauffman, J. (1995). Blinkings: A thanatocentric theory of consciousness. In J. Kauffman (Ed.), *Awareness of mortality* (pp. 75–89). Amityville, NY: Baywood.

Kearney, M. (1996). *Mortally wounded: Stories of soul, pain, death and healing.* New York: Touchstone Books.

Kearney, M. (2000). *A place of healing: Working with suffering in living and dying.* Oxford: Oxford University Press.

Kember, D., Wong, F., & Young, E. (Eds.). (2001). *Reflective teaching and learning in health professions.* London: Blackwell Science.

Kern, H. (2000). *Through the labyrinth: Designs and meanings over 5,000 years.* Munich: Prestel.

Ketchum, L. D., & Trist, E. (1992). *All teams are not equal: How employee empowerment really works.* London: Sage.

Kleinman, R. E. (1992). We have the solution: Now what's the problem? *Pediatrics, 90*(1), 113–115.

Kobasa, S. C. (1979). Stressful life event, personality, and health: An inquiry into hardiness. *Journal of Personality and Social Psychology, 37*, 1–17.

Krakauer, E. L., Crenner, C., & Fox, K. (2002). Barriers to optimum end-of-life care for minority patients. *Journal of American Geriatrics Society, 50*, 182–190.

Kramer, B. J., Pacoureck, L., & Hovland-Scafe, C. (2003). Analysis of end-of-life content in social work textbooks. *Journal of Social Work Education, 39*, 299–320.

Kübler-Ross, E. (1969). *On death and dying.* New York: Macmillan.

Larson, D. G. (2000). Anticipatory mourning: Challenges for professional and volunteer caregivers. In T. A. Rando (Ed.), *Clinical dimensions of anticipatory mourning* (pp. 379–395). Champaign, IL: Research Press.

Larson, D., & Hoyt, W. (2007). What has become of grief counseling? An evaluation of the empirical foundations of the new pessimism. *Professional Psychology: Research and Practice, 38*(4), 347–355.

Lee, P. W., & Kwan, T. T. C. (2006). Providing end-of-life care: Enhancing effectiveness and resilience. In C. L. W. Chan & A. Y. M. Chow (Eds.), *Death, dying and bereavement: A Hong Kong experience* (pp. 209–224). Hong Kong: Hong Kong University Press.

Leiper, R., & Casares, P. (2000). An investigation of the attachment organization of clinical psychologists and its relationship to clinical practice. *British Journal of Medical Psychology, 73,* 449–464.

Lerea, L. E., & LiMauro, B. F. (1982). Grief among healthcare workers: A comparative study. *Journal of Gerontology, 37,* 604–608.

Lev, E. (1989). A nurse's perspective on disenfranchised grief. In K. J. Doka (Ed.), *Disenfranchized grief: Recognizing hidden sorrow* (pp. 287–299). Lexington, MA: Lexington Books.

Levi, P. (1969). *Is this is a man—The truce* (S. Woolf, Trans.). U.K: Abacus.

Levy, A. (1973). Le changement comme travail. *Connexions, 7.*

Lewis, C. S. (1961). *A grief observed.* London: Faber & Faber.

Liben, S., Papadatou, D., & Wolfe, J. (2008). Paediatric palliative care: Universal challenges and emerging ideas. *Lancet, 371,* 852–864.

Liddell, H. G., & Scott, R. (Eds.). (1994). *Liddell & Scott's Greek-English lexicon* (7th ed.). Oxford: Oxford University Press.

Lindemann, E. (1944). Symptomatology and management of acute grief. *American Journal of Psychiatry, 101,* 141–148.

Lindholm, L., & Eriksson, K. (1993). To understand and alleviate suffering in a caring culture. *Journal of Advanced Nursing, 18*(9), 1354–1361.

Luca, M. (Ed.). (2004). *The therapeutic frame in the clinical context.* New York: Brunner-Routledge.

MacLeod, R. D. (2004). Challenges for education in palliative care. *Progress in Palliative Care, 12*(3), 117–121.

MacLeod, R. D., Parkin, C., Pullon, S., & Robertson, G. (2003). Early clinical exposure to people who are dying: Learning to care at the end of life. *Medical Education, 37*(1), 51–58.

Maeve, M. K. (1998). Weaving a fabric of moral meaning: How nurses live with suffering and death. *Journal of Advanced Nursing, 27,* 1136–1142.

Maguire, P., & Pitceathly, C. (2005). Learning counseling. In D. Doyle, G. W. Hanks, & N. MacDonald (Eds.), *Oxford textbook of palliative medicine* (2nd ed., pp. 1176–1182). New York: Oxford University Press.

Main, M., & Goldwyn, R. (1984). *Adult attachment scoring and classificatory system.* Berkeley: University of California.

Malacrida, R., Betteline, C., Degratem, A., Martinez, M., Baida, F., Piazza, J., et al. (1998). Reasons for dissatisfaction: A survey of relatives of intensive care patients who die. *Critical Care Medicine, 26*(7), 1187–1193.

Mann, J. (1973). *Time-limited psychotherapy.* Cambridge, MA: Harvard University Press.

Marquis, S. (1993). Death of the nursed: Burnout of the provider. *Omega: Journal of Death and Dying, 27*(1), 17–34.

Maslach, C. (1982). *Burnout: The cost of caring.* Englewood Cliffs, NJ: Prentice Hall.

Mayer, E. L. (1994). Some implications for psychoanalytic technique drawn from analysis of a dying patient. *Psychoanalytic Quarterly, 63*(1), 1–18.

McCann, I. L., & Pearlman, L. A. (1990). Vicarious traumatization: A framework for understanding the psychological effects of working with victims. *Journal of Trauma Stress, 3*, 131–149.

McClure, D. G. (2004). Employee assistance program strategies. In J. C. Thomas & M. Hersen (Eds.), *Psychopathology in the workplace: Recognition and adaptation* (pp. 345–360). New York: Taylor & Francis.

McDermott, S., & Demmer, C. (2008). Analysis of end-of-life content in selected introductory health education textbooks. *Illness, Crisis & Loss, 16*(3), 237–257.

Meekin, S. A., Klein, J. E., Fleischman, A. R., & Fins, J. J. (2000). Development of a palliative education assessment tool for medical student education. *Academic Medicine, 75*(10), 986–992.

Menzies-Lyth, I. (1988). *Containing anxiety in institutions: Selected essays* (pp. 43–83). London: Free Association Books.

Menzies-Lyth, I. (1990). *The dynamics of the social: Selected essays* (pp. 1–18). London: Free Association Books.

Meyer, E. C., Burns, J. P., Griffith, J. L., & Truog, R. D. (2002). Parental perspectives on end-of-life care in the pediatric intensive care unit. *Critical Care Medicine, 30*(1), 226–231.

Miller, E. J., & Gwynne, G. (1972). *A life apart.* London: Tavistock.

Morasz, L. (1999). *Le soignant face à la souffrance.* Paris: Dunod.

Morgan, M. A. (1987). Learner-centered learning in an undergraduate interdisciplinary course about death. *Death Studies, 11*, 183–192.

Morris, J. A., & Feldman, D. C. (1996). The dimensions, antecedents, and consequences of emotional labor. *Academy of Management Review, 21*(4), 986–1010.

Morrison, A. L. (1997). Ten years of doing psychotherapy while living with a life-threatening illness: Self-disclosure and other ramifications. *Psychoanalytic Dialogues, 7*(2), 225–241.

Neff, K. D. (2003). Self-compassion: An alternative conceptualization of a healthy attitude toward oneself. *Self and Identity, 2*, 85–102.

Neimeyer, R. A. (1998). *Lessons of loss: A guide to coping.* New York: McGraw-Hill.

Neimeyer, R. A. (2001). Meaning reconstruction and loss. In R. A. Neimeyer (Ed.), *Meaning reconstruction and the experience of loss* (pp. 1–12). Washington DC: American Psychological Association.

Neimeyer, R. A. (2006). Re-storying loss: Fostering growth in post traumatic narrative. In L. Calhoun & R. Tedeschi (Eds.), *Handbook of posttraumtic growth: Research and practice* (pp. 68–80). Mahwah, NJ: Erlbaum.

Nolen-Hoeskema, S., & Larson, J. (1999). *Coping with loss.* Mahwah, NJ: Erlbaum.

Norton, J. (1963). Treatment of a dying patient. *The Psychoanalytic Study of the Child, 18*, 541–560.

Nuland, S. (1994). *How we die.* New York: Knopf.

Obholzer, A., & Roberts, V. Z. (Eds.). (1994). *The unconscious at work: Individual and organizational stress in the human services.* London: Routledge.

Oehler, J. M., & Davidson, M. G. (1992). Job stress and burnout in acute and non acute pediatric nurses. *American Journal of Critical Care, 2*, 81–90.

Oliviere, D. (2006). User involvement—the patient and carer as team members? In P. Speck (Ed.), *Teamwork in palliative care* (pp. 41–64). Oxford: Oxford University Press.

Olthius, G., & Dekkers, W. (2003). Medical education, palliative care and moral attitude: Some objectives and future perspectives. *Medical Education, 37*(10), 928–933.

Oneschuk, D., Hanson, J., Bruera, E. (2000). An international survey of undergraduate medical education in palliative medicine. *Journal of Pain & Symptom Management, 20*(3), 174–179.

Oppenheim, D. (2007). *Littérature et expérience-limite.* Paris: Campagne Première.

Oxford Advanced Learner's Dictionary. (2005, 7th edition). S. Wehmeier, C. McIntosh, J. Turnbull, M. Ashby (Eds.). Oxford, UK: Oxford University Press.

Papadatou, D. (1991). Working with dying children: A professional's personal journey. In D. Papadatou & C. Papadatos (Eds.), *Children and death* (pp. 285–292). Washington, DC: Hemisphere.

Papadatou, D. (1997). Training health professionals in caring for dying children and grieving families. *Death Studies, 21*(6), 575–600.

Papadatou, D. (2000). A proposed model on health professionals' grieving process. *Omega: Journal of Death and Dying, 41,* 59–77.

Papadatou, D. (2001). The grieving health care provider: Variables affecting the professional responses to a child's death. *Bereavement Care, 20*(2), 26–29.

Papadatou, D. (2006). The healthcare providers' responses to the death of a child. In A. Goldman, R. Hain, & S. Lieben (Eds.), *Oxford textbook of palliative care for children* (pp. 521–532). Oxford: Oxford University Press.

Papadatou, D., Anagnostopoulos, F., & Monos, D. (1994). Factors contributing to the development of burnout in oncology nursing. *British Journal of Medical Psychology, 67,* 187–199.

Papadatou, D., Bellali, T., Papazoglou, I., & Petraki, D. (2002). Greek physicians' and nurses' grief as a result of caring for children dying of cancer. *Pediatric Nursing, 28*(4), 345–353.

Papadatou, D., Corr, C. A., Frager, G., & Bouri, M. A. (2003). *Training curriculum in pediatric palliative care.* Alexandria, VA: National Hospice and Palliative Care Organization.

Papadatou, D., & Iossifides, M. (2004). Death and dying in the Greek culture. In J. Morgan & P. Languani (Eds.), *Death and bereavement around the world* (Vol. 3, pp. 55–68). Amityville, NY: Baywood.

Papadatou, D., Martinson, I. M., & Chung, P. M. (2001). Caring for dying children: A comparative study of nurses' experiences in Greece and Hong Kong. *Cancer Nursing, 24*(5), 402–412.

Papadatou, D., Papazoglou, I., Petraki, D., & Bellali, T. (1999). Mutual support among nurses who provide care to dying children. *Illness, Crisis & Loss,* 7(1), 37–48.

Parkes, C. M. (1971). Psychosocial transitions: A field of study. *Social Science and Medicine, 5,* 101–115.

Parkes, C. M. (1972). *Bereavement: Studies of grief in adult life.* New York: International Universities Press.

Parkes, C. M. (1988). Bereavement as a psychosocial transition: Processes of adaptations to change. *Journal of Social Issues, 44,* 53–65.

Parkes, C. M. (2006). *Love and loss: The roots of grief and its complications.* London: Routledge.

Parkes, C. M. (in press). *On the psychology of extremism.*

Parkes, C. M., Relf, M., & Couldrick, A. (1996). *Counselling in terminal care and bereavement.* Oxford: Blackwell.

Parsons, T. (1978). Death in the Western world. In T. Parson (Ed.), *Action theory and the human condition* (pp. 331–351). New York: Free Press.

Payne, M. (2000). *Teamwork in multiprofessional care.* New York: Palgrave.

Pearlman, L. A. (1999). Notes from the field: Laurie Anne Pearlman: What is vicarious traumatization? In B. H. Stamm (Ed.), *Secondary traumatic stress: Self-care issues for clinicians, researchers, and educators* (2nd ed., pp. xlv–lii). Baltimore, MD: Sidran Press.

Pearlman, L. A., & Saakvitne, K. (1995). Treating therapists with vicarious traumatization and secondary traumatic stress disorders. In C. R. Figley (Ed.), *Compassion fatigue: Coping with secondary traumatic stress disorder in those who treat the traumatized* (pp. 151–177). New York: Brunner-Mazel.

Pennebaker, J. W. (1995). *Emotion, disclosure and health.* Washington, DC: American Psychological Association.

Pennebaker, J. W. (2000). Telling stories: The health benefits of narratives. *Literature and Medicine, 19*(1), 3–18.

Pfifferling, J., & Gilley, K. (2000). Overcoming compassion fatigue. *Family Practice Management, 7,* 39–45.

Philip, C., & Stevens, E. (1992). Countertransference issues for the consultant when a colleague is critically ill (or dying). *Clinical Journal of Social Work, 4,* 411–420.

Pinel, J. P. (1996). La déliason pathologique des liens institutionnels. In R. Kaës, J. P. Pinel, O. Kernberg, A. Correale, E. Diet, & B. Duez (Eds.), *Souffrance et psychopathology des liens* (pp. 51–79). Paris: Dunod.

Pines, A. M., & Aronson, E. (1988). *Career burnout: Causes and cures.* New York: Free Press.

Plante, A., Dumas, J., & Houle, M. (1993). Les deuils à répétition. *Nursing Quebec, 13*(2), 46–51.

Potamianou, A. (2003). Reflections on the foundations and development of thinking. *Israel Psychoanalytic Journal, 1*(3), 311–330.

Randall, F., & Downie, R. S. (2006). *The philosophy of palliative care: Critique and reconstruction.* Oxford: Oxford University Press.

Rando, T. A. (1993). *Treatment of complicated mourning.* Champaign, IL: Research Press.

Rashotte, J., Fothergrill-Bourbonnais, F., & Chamberlain, M. (1997). Pediatric intensive care nurses and their grief experiences: A phenomenological study. *Heart & Lung, 26,* 372–386.

Rawlinson, F., & Finlay, I. (2002). Assessing education in palliative medicine: Development of a tool based on the Association for Palliative Medicine Core Curriculum. *Palliative Medicine, 16*(1), 51–55.

Rawnsley, M. M. (1990). Professional caregivers as survivors: An unsanctioned grief. In V. Pine, O. Margolis, K. Doka, A. Kutscher, D. Schaefer, M. Siegel, & D. J. Cherico (Eds.), *Unrecognized and unsanctioned grief: The nature and counseling of unacknowledged loss* (pp. 143–151). Springfield, IL: Charles C. Thomas.

Redding, K. K. (1999). *When death knocks on the analytic door.* Doctoral dissertation, Los Angeles Institute and Society for Psychoanalytic Studies.

Reese, D., & Sontag, M. A. (2001). Successful interprofessional collaboration on the hospice team. *Health and Social Work, 26,* 167–175.

Rehnsfeldt, A., & Eriksson, K. (2004). The progression of suffering implies alleviated suffering. *Scandinavian Journal of Caring Sciences, 18,* 264–272.

Report of the Pew-Fetzer Task Force on Advancing Psychosocial Health Education. (2000). *Health professions education and relationship-centered care.* San Fransisco, CA: Pew Health Professions Commission.

Rholes, S. W., & Simpson, J. A. (Eds.). (2004a). *Adult attachment: Theory, research, and clinical implications.* New York: Guilford Press.

Rholes, S. W., & Simpson, J. A. (2004b). Attachment theory: Basic concepts and contemporary questions. In S. W. Rholes & J. A. Simpson (Eds.), *Adult attachment: Theory, research, and clinical implications* (pp. 3–16). New York: Guilford Press.

Rice, A. K. (1963). *The enterprise and its environment.* London: Tavistock.

Roberts, V. Z. (1994). Till death us do part. In A. Obholzer, & V. Z. Roberts (Eds.), *The unconscious at work: Individual and organizational stress in the human services* (pp. 75–83). London: Routledge.

Rogers, C. (1957). The necessary and sufficient conditions of therapeutic personality change. *Journal of Consulting Psychology, 21,* 95–103.

Rogers, C. (1961). *On becoming a person.* Boston: Houghton Miffin.

Roose, L. J. (1969). The dying patient. *International Journal of Psychoanalysis, 50,* 385–432.

Rosenbaum, M. E., Lobas, J., & Ferguson, K. (2005). Using reflection activities to enhance teaching about end-of-life care. *Journal of Palliative Medicine, 8,* 1186–1195.

Rouchy, J. C., & Desroche, M. S. (2004). *Institution et changement: Processus psychique et organization.* Ramonville Saint-Agne: Editions Erès.

Rowe, H. (1996). Mutlidisciplinary teamwork: Myth or reality? *Journal of Nursing Management, 4*(2), 93–101.

Rowe, J. (2003). The suffering of the healer. *Nursing Forum, 38*(4), 16–20.

Rubin, S. (1981). A two-track model of bereavement: Theory and application in research. *American Journal of Orthopsychiatry, 51,* 101–109.

Rushton, C. H. (2004). The other side of caring: Caregiver suffering. In B. S. Carter & M. Levetown (Eds.), *Palliative care for infants, children and adolescents: A practical handbook* (pp. 220–243). Baltimore, MD: Johns Hopkins University Press.

Saakvitne, K., & Pearlman, L. (1996). *Transforming the pain: A workbook on vicarious traumatization for helping professionals who work with traumatized clients.* New York: Norton.

Sahler, O. J., Frager, G., Levetown, M., Cohn, F. G., & Lipson, M. A. (2000). Medical education about end-of-life care in the pediatric setting: Principles, challenges, and opportunities. *Pediatrics, 105*(3), 575–584.

Sanders, C. M. (1999). *The mourning after: Dealing with adult bereavement* (2nd ed.). New York: John Wiley & Sons.

Sartain, S., Clarke, C. L., & Heyman, R. (2000). Hearing the voices of children with chronic illness. *Journal of Advanced Nursing, 32*(4), 913–921.

Saunders, J. M., & Valente, S. M. (1994). Nurses' grief. *Cancer Nursing, 17,* 318–325.

Schaverien, J. (2002). *The dying patient in psychotherapy.* New York: Palgrave Macmillan.

Schofield, R. F., & Amodeo, M. (1999). Interdisciplinary teams in health care and human services settings: Are they effective? *Health and Social Work, 24,* 210–219.

Seale, C. (1996). Living alone towards the end of life. *Ageing and Society, 16,* 75–91.

Seale, C. (1998). *Constructing death: The sociology of dying and bereavement.* Cambridge: Cambridge University Press.

Shanfield, S. B. (1981). The mourning of the health care professional: An important element in education about death and loss. *Death Education, 4,* 385–395.

Shaw, R. (2003). *The embodied psychotherapist: The therapist's body story.* East Sussex: Brunner-Routledge.

Shread, T. (1984). Dealing with nurses' grief. *Nursing Forum, 21,* 43–45.

Skogstad, W. (2000). Working in a world of bodies. In R. D. Hinshelwood & W. Skogstad (Eds.), *Observing organizations: Anxiety, defence and culture in health care* (pp. 101–121). London: Routledge.

Skovholt, T. (2001). *The resilient practitioner: Burnout prevention for counselors, therapists, teachers and health professionals.* Boston: Allyn & Bacon.

Slater, J. (1988). The bereaved nurse. *Nursing Standard, 3,* 34–35.

Smith, D. H. (2005). *Partnership with the dying: Where medicine and ministry should meet.* Lanham, MD: Rowan & Littlefield.

Smith-Pickard, P. (2004). Challenging therapy: An existential perspective on the frame. In M. Luca (Ed.), *The therapeutic frame in the clinical context* (pp. 128–141). New York: Brunner-Routledge.

Solomon, M. Z., & Browning, D. (2005). Relationships matter and so does pain control. *Journal of Clinical Oncology, 23*(36), 9055–9057.

Sourkes, B. M. (1982). *The deepening shade: Psychological aspects of life threatening illness* (pp. 3–21). Pittsburgh, PA: University of Pittsburgh Press.

Speck, P. (2000). Working with dying people: On being good enough. In A. Obholzer & V. Z. Roberts (Eds.), *The unconscious at work: Individual and organizational stress in the human sciences* (2nd ed., pp. 94–100). London: Brunner-Routledge.

Speck, P. (2006a). Maintaining a healthy team. In P. Speck (Ed.), *Teamwork in palliative care* (pp. 95–115). Oxford: Oxford University Press.

Speck, P. (2006b). Team or group—spot the difference. In P. Speck (Ed.), *Teamwork in palliative care* (pp. 7–23). Oxford: Oxford University Press.

Speck, P. (2006c). Leaders and followers. In P. Speck (Ed.), *Teamwork in palliative care* (pp. 65–82). Oxford: Oxford University Press.

Spickard, A., Gabbe, S., & Christensen, J. (2002). Mid-career burnout in generalists and specialist physicians. *Journal of American Medical Association, 288,* 1447–1450.

Stamm, B. H. (1997). Measuring compassion satisfaction as well as fatigue: Developmental history of the compassion satisfaction and fatigue test. In C. F. Figley (Ed.), *Treating compassion fatigue* (pp. 107–119). Philadelphia: Brunner-Mazel.

Stamm, B. H. (Ed.). (1999). *Secondary traumatic stress: Self-care issues of clinicians, researchers, and educators* (2nd ed.). Baltimore, MD: Sidran Press.

Steinhauser, K. E., Christakis, N. A., Clipp, E. C., McNeilley, M., McIntyre, L. M., & Tulsky, J. A. (2000). Factors considered important at the end of life by patients, family, physicians and other providers. *Journal of American Medical Association, 284*(19), 2477–2482.

Steinhauser, K. E., Clipp, E. C., McNeilly, M., Christakis, N. A., McIntyre, L. M., & Tulsky, J. A. (2000). In search of a good death: Observations of patients, families and providers. *Annals of Internal Medicine, 132,* 825–832.

Stern, D. N. (2004). *The present moment in psychotherapy and everyday life.* New York: Norton. [*Le moment present en psychotherapie: Un monde dans un grain de sable* (M. Garene, Trans.). Paris: Odile Jacob.]

Stowers, S. J. (1983). Nurses cry too. *Nursing Management, 14,* 63–64.

Stroebe, M. S., & Schut, H. (1999). The dual process model of coping with bereavement: Rationale and description. *Death Studies, 23*(3), 197–224.

Stroebe, M. S., & Schut, H. (2001). Meaning making in the dual process model of coping with bereavement. In R. A. Neimeyer (Ed.), *Meaning reconstruction and the experience of loss* (pp. 55–73). Washington, DC: American Psychological Association.

Stroebe, M. S., Hansson, R. O., Stroebe, W., & Schut, H. (Eds.). (2007). *Handbook of bereavement research: Consequences, coping, and care* (5th ed.). Washington, DC: American Psychological Association.

Sullivan, A. M., Lakoma, M. D., Billings, J. A., Peters, A. S., Block, S. D., & PCEP Core Faculty. (2003). Teaching and learning end-of-life care: Evaluation of a faculty development program in palliative care. *Academic Medicine, 80*(7), 657–668.

Sullivan, A. M., Lakoma, M. D., & Block, S. D. (2003). The status of medical education in end-of-life care: A national report. *Journal of General Internal Medicine, 18*(9), 685–695.

SUPPORT Investigators. (1995). A controlled trial to improve the care of seriously ill hospitalized patients: The study to understand the prognoses and preferences for the outcomes and risks of treatment. *Journal of the American Medical Association, 274,* 1591–1598.

Taylor, S. E. (1983). Adjustment to threatening event: A theory of cognitive adaptation. *American Psychologist, 38,* 1161–1173.

Tedeschi, R. G., & Calhoun, L. G. (1995). *Trauma and transformation: Growing in the aftermath of suffering.* Thousand Oaks, CA: Sage.

Tedeschi, R. G., & Calhoun, L. G. (2004). Posttraumatic growth: Conceptual foundations and empirical evidence. *Psychological Inquiry,* 15, 1–18.

Tedeschi, R. G., Park, C. L., & Calhoun, L. G. (Eds.). (1998). *Posttraumatic growth: Positive changes in the aftermath of crisis.* Mahwah, NJ: Erlbaum.

Tessier, R. (1993). Introduction: Death, distress, and solidarity. *Omega: Journal of Death and Dying, 27*(1), 1–4.

Vachon, M. (1987). *Occupational stress in the care of the critically ill, the dying and the bereaved.* New York: Hemisphere.

Vachon, M. (1997). Recent research into staff stress in palliative care. *European Journal of Palliative Care, 4,* 99–103.

Van Servellen, G., & Leake, B. (1993). Burnout in hospital nurses: A comparison of acquired immunodeficiency syndrome, oncology, general medical, and intensive care units nurse samples. *Journal of Professional Nursing, 9,* 169–177.

Vazirani, R. M., Slavin, S. J., & Feldman, J. D. (2000). Longitudinal study of pediatric house officers' attitudes toward death and dying. *Critical Care Medicine, 28*(11), 3740–3745.

Vickers, M. H. (2005). Bounded grief at work: Working and caring for children with chronic illness. *Illness, Crisis, & Loss, 13*(3), 201–218.

Waldman, S. (1990). The health care giver: Unmasking grief. In V. Pine, O. Margolis, K. Doka, A. Kutscher, D. Schaefer, M. Siegel, & D. J. Cherico (Eds.), *Unrecognized and unsanctioned grief: The nature and counseling of unacknowledged loss* (pp. 152–157). Springfield, IL: Charles C. Thomas.

Wass, H. (2004). A perspective on the current state of death education. *Death Studies, 28*(4), 289–308.

Wear, D. (1998). On white coats and professional development: The formal and hidden curriculum. *Annals of Internal Medicine, 129*, 734–737.

Werth, J., Anderson, J., & Blevins, D. (Eds.). (2005). *Attending to psychosocial issues near the end of life.* Washington, DC: American Psychological Association.

White, M., & Epston, D. (1990). *Narrative means to therapeutic ends.* New York: Norton.

Wilson, H., & Ayers, K. M. S. (2004). Using significant event analysis in dental and medical education. *Journal of Dental Education, 68*, 446–453.

Wilson, H., Egan, A., & Friend, R. (2003). Teaching professional development in undergraduate medical education. *Medical Education, 7*, 482–483.

Wilson, J. P., & Lindy, J. D. (1994). Empathic strain and countertransference. In J. P. Wilson & J. D. Lindy (Eds.), *Countertransference in the treatment of PTSD* (pp. 5–30). New York: Haworth Press.

Winchester-Nadeau, J. (1998). *Families making sense of death.* Thousand Oaks, CA: Sage.

Winnicott, D. W. (1990). The theory of the parent-infant relationship. In *The maturational process and the facilitating environment: Studies in the theory of emotional development* (pp. 37–55). London: Karnac Books. (Originally published 1960)

Wolfe, J., Grier, H. E., Klar, N., Levin, S. B., Ellenbogenm J. M., Salem-Schatz, S., et al. (2000). Symptoms and suffering at the end of life in children with cancer. *New England Journal of Medicine, 342*(5), 326–333.

Wolfelt, A. D. (2006). *Companioning the bereaved: A soulful guide for caregivers.* Fort Collins, CO: Companion Press.

Wood, E. B., Meekin, S. A., Fins, J. J., & Fleischman, A. R. (2002). Enhancing palliative care education in medical school curricula: Implementation of the palliative education assessment tool. *Academic Medicine, 77*(4), 285–291.

Woolley, H., Stein, A., Forrest, G. C., & Baum, J. D. (1989). Staff stress and job satisfaction at a children's hospice. *Archives of Diseases in Childhood, 64*, 114–118.

Worden, J. W. (2008). *Grief counseling and grief therapy: A handbook for the mental health practitioner* (4th ed.). New York: Springer.

Working Group on Assisted Suicide and End-of-Life Decisions, American Psychological Association. (2000). *Report to the Board of Directors of the American Psychological Association from the APA Working Group on Assisted Suicide and End-of-Life-Decisions.* Washington, DC: American Psychological Association. Retrieved December 26, 2008, from http://www.apa.org/pi/aseolf.html

World Health Organization. (2002). *National cancer control programs: Policies and managerial guidelines* (2nd ed.). Geneva: Author.

Yalom, I. D. (2001). *The gift of therapy: Reflections on being a therapist.* London: Piatkus.

Yalom, I. D. (2008). *Staring at the sun: Overcoming the dread of death.* London: Piaktus.

Yasko, J. M. (1983). Variables which predict burnout experienced by oncology clinical nurse specialists. *Cancer Nursing, 6*, 109–116.

Yoder, G. (2005). *Companioning the dying: A soulful guide for caregivers.* Fort Collins, CO: Companion Press.

Index

Accompaniment/Accompanying process
  companion's role
    as container, 70
    as enabler, 70
    as facilitator, 70
    during birth, 67–68
    culture of, 105
    for dying/bereaved, 67, 68–69
    effectiveness of, 70
    midwife relating to, 67–68
  conditions for
    appropriate frame, establishment of, 70–79
    being fully present, 79–92
    being vulnerable enough, 92–103
    holding environment, 103–105
  definition of, 67
  end of, 110–111
  process of, frame relating to, 70–71
Adler, Alfred, 36
American Psychoanalytic Association, survey of, 106
American Psychological Association, as working group on assisted suicide and end-of-life decisions, 106
Ariadne, in myth, 62, 63, 65, 70–71, 79, 100
Ariès, P., 3
Assumptive world, 132
Attachment
  behaviors of
    explorative, 28–29
    to home and land of birth, 31–32
    to others, 29–30
    professional caregiving, 34–35
    proximity-seeking, 28
    to religion or deity, 30–31
    to significant goal or project, 32
  bond of, 24–25, 66
    insecure attachment, 35, 302–303
    secure attachment, 34–35, 302
  Bowlby's theory on, 24–25, 301–304
  dependency v., 27
  style of
    anxious/ambivalent, 302
    avoidant, 303
    disorganized/disoriented, 303
Ausloos, Guy, 230
Avoidance
  or suppression, of grief, 144–146
  systematic, of change, 226–227

Bauby, Jean-Dominique, 85
Being fully present, 79–92
  physical presence, 80–84
  psychological presence, 84–92
Being vulnerable enough, 92–103
  being highly vulnerable, experience of, 94–96
  being invulnerable, experience of, 96–97
Belonging
  cosmic belonging, 31, 37
  need to belong, 35–37
Benoliel, Jeanne Quint, 7, 128
Bereavement. *See also* Grief
  care, 10–11
    medicalized, 5
    personalized, 254
    socialized, 170
  education, 285–287, 290, 291
  pathological forms of, 11
  science and, 5–6
Biopsychosocial model of care, 6–9, 13
Birth
  companioning during, 67–68
  of human, end of human life v., 67–69
  land of, attachment to, 31–32
Bond. *See also* Attachment, bond of
  affirmation through belonging, 35–37

Boundaries
  leaders setting of, 277–278
  and modifications, of frame, 76–77
  for open teamwork, 253–254
  rigid, splitting and forming subgroups with, 224–226
  role, 277
  spatial, 277
  of team, 218
  time, 277
Bowlby, J., attachment theory of, 24–25, 301–304
Burnout, 122–123, 126
  caring, 122
  meaning, 122
  studies of, 123

Cancer, 10
Care. *See also* Bereavement, care; Caregiving; Health care professionals, educational challenges of; Palliative care
  medicalization of, 6
  personalization of, 261–262
  a relationship of, 21–38
    attachment behaviors, 28–32
    attachment bond, 24–25, 66
    bond affirmation through belonging, 35–37
    death situations, service requests in, 25–28
    partners in care, 22–24
    professional's caregiving behaviors, 32–35
Caregiver, altered sense of time for, 51–52
Caregiving. *See also* Partnership; Relationship-centered approach, to care
  care-giving behaviors, 35, 301–303
    safe haven, 32–34
    secure base, 32–34
  involvement in relationship of
    counseling skills and behaviors, 55–56
    detached concern, 57–59
    emotional, 54–55
    friendly professional interest, 54, 56–57
  meaning attributed to death, dying, and caregiving, 147
  motives and needs of, acknowledgment of, 179, 180–182
  organizations for
    myths and ideals of, 196–198
    primary tasks and functioning modes of, 198–202
  professional behaviors of, 32–35
  rewards of, 175–188
  wisdom of, 177–178
Care providers. *See also* Caregiver; Health care professionals
  altered sense of time for, 51–52
  aspects of suffering, 120–130
  countertransference of, 121–122
  death and mortality awareness by, 41–43
  education of, 12–13, 285–295
  good enough, 100, 274
  holding environment for, 242, 248–253
  illness or dying of, 108–110
  impact of death upon, 263
  motives and needs of, 180–182
  suffering of, 117–120
    aspects of, 120–128
  wounded healer myth, 115–117
Care seekers. *See also* Dying; Professional and individual seeking care, relationship between
  attachment behaviors of, 28–32
Care seeking behaviors, 301–302
  request for services, 25–28
  vulnerable v. resilient, 26–27
Change
  personal, 44–45
  risk taking and, 265
  systematic avoidance of, 226–227
  team, 260–261
Chaos, of team, 230, 231–233
Chiron, 115–116, 186–187
Chronic niceness, 97
Cognitive disruptions, 125
Cognitive level, of grief and loss, 141
Collaboration. *See* Interprofessional collaboration, of team functioning; Partnership
Collaborative alliance, 258–259
Collective rituals, 156–157
Collective somatization, of suffering, 228–229
Commitment
  to co-workers, 242
  to goals and tasks, 242
  facilitated by, 244
  to psychological presence, 84
  to relationship, 244
  work experience relating to, 243
Companion. *See also* Accompaniment.
  role of, 70
Companioning. *See* Accompaniment/Accompanying process

Compassion
description, 99
fatigue, secondary traumatic stress disorder, 125
satisfaction, 125
stress, secondary traumatic stress, 123–125, 127
studies of, 125
Competence, of team functioning
conditions for
commitment, 242, 243–248
holding environment, 242, 248–253
open teamwork, 253–256, 262
Connectedness, 182–183
Consultation
goals of, 280
methods of, 280–281
role of, 278–281
Containment
holding behaviors relating to, 251–252
with psychological presence, 84
Counseling skills and behaviors, engagement through, 55–56
Countertransference, of care providers, 121–122
Crisis
basic assumptions relating to, 237
risks v. benefits of, 240–242
types of
explosive, 238–239
multiple, 239–242
mutative, 236–238
Culture
of companioning, 105
myths in, 63–64
of team, 206–209

Dali, Salvadore, 85
Death
confrontation of, 11–12
denial of, 3
exposure to
by care providers, 41–43
direct and indirect, 40
good/appropriate, 8, 30, 136, 138, 159, 180, 245, 298
impact of, on care providers, 263
meanings attributed to, make sense of, 148–152, 171
medical model of care's defining of, 6
mortality awareness, 40–47
representation relating to, 4, 44
science, society, and, 3–20
system of, 3–4
terror of, 178
violence of, 48
violence v. vitalizing force of, 48–49
Western societies and, 4–5
de Beauvoir, Simone, 85
Dehumanization of care, 6
Delayed grief, 132
Denial
of death, 3
and suppression, of suffering, 178–179
Depersonalization, dysfunctional, 145
Detached concern, 58–59
Development
of holding environment, 103–105
of open teamwork, 255–256
of stages in interprofessional collaboration, 258–259
of team rules, 210
and growth, 258–259
and use, of rituals, 264–265
Diagnostic Statistical Manual of Mental Disorders, 11
Discrimination, of care providers, 117, 118, 195
Disenfranchisement, of grief, 128–129
Disorganization
of team functioning
chaos in, 230, 231–233
dysfunctional patterns in, 230–231
immobilization in, 230, 233–235
intervention in, 235–236
of narratives, 273
Distorted grief, 132
Dying
as second birth, 68
companioning for, 67, 68–69
integration of, 200
make sense of, 152–153
of care provider, 108–110
process of, making sense of, 152–153
The Dying Patient in Psychotherapy (Schaverien), 108
Dysfunctional team patters and solutions
as cause of disorganization, 230–231
favoring conditions of, 218–219
serving purposes of, 219–220
types of
collective somatization of suffering, 228–229
fragmentation of care, 221–222
idealization of care, 229–230
inhibition or disqualification, of reflection, 226

Dysfunctional team patters and solutions (*continued*)
  overinvestment and over-eroticization of relationships, 227–228
  scapegoating, 223–224
  splitting and subgrouping, 224–226
  systematic avoidance of change, 226–227
  violent acts and behaviors, 222–223
vs, functional patterns, 217–230

Education
  of care providers, 12–13
  challenges in, 285–295
  educators, leaders as, 283
  learning objectives of, 288–290
  relational learning in, 287–288
Embodiment, 59, 98, 99
Emotional involvement, 54–55
Emotional labor
  definition of, 214–215
  display rules relating to, 214
  surface v. deep acting, 214
Emotional support of coworkers, 247
Empathy, 98–99
  body, physical presence relating to, 80–81
  definition of, 98
Existential issues, addressing of, 180, 181, 185–186
Experience(s)
  of altered sense of time, 50–54
  of being vulnerable enough, 92–103
  of caregiving, 166
  containment of, 252
  of death and loss, 262–263
  of suffering, 117–120
  elaboration of, facilitation of, 252
  nadir, 184
  peak, 184
  self-understanding and, openness to, 180, 183–184
Experiencing and avoiding loss and grief, fluctuation between, 139–141, 172
Explorative behaviors, 28–29
Explosive crises, 238–239
Expression, of grief, 170–171

Facilitation
  of elaboration of experiences, 252
  of open teamwork, 253
Fragmentation, of care, 221–222
Frame
  boundaries and modifications, 76–77
  co-creation of, 72–74
  portability of, 77–79
  stability and flexibility of, 74–76
Freud, Sigmund, 43, 121, 131
Functional team patterns and solutions, 260–265
  favoring conditions of, 218–219
  serving purposes of, 261
  types of
    acknowledgment of universality v. uniqueness of caregivers' responses to loss and death, 263
    hope, instillation of, 263
    integration of services through interdisciplinary collaboration, 262
    personalization of care of, 261–262
    play patterns and humor, use of, 264
    risk taking and change, 265
    solidarity, through caring acts and behaviors, 263–264
    'working through loss' and death experiences, 262–263
Functioning modes, of caregiving organizations, 198–202

Good-enough care provider
  characteristics of, 100, 104
  parent
    Winnicott, definition of, 248
  team
    growth and evolution of, 269–270
    leaders in, 275–278, 283
    pertinent information used by, 270–271
    strengths and limitations of, 271
    supervision and consultation, methods of, 280–281
    supervisors and consultants of, 278–280
Grief
  chronic and compounded, 161–162
  in coexistence with trauma responses, 163–164
  complications of, 160–161
  delayed, 132
  disenfranchisement of, 128–129
  distorted, 132
  distress of, 129
  expression of, 170–171
  as healthy response to death situations, 128–130
  incremental, 160
  inhibited, 162–163
  leader's role relating to, 275
  losses eliciting grief, classifications of, 11

overload of, 159–160
phases of, 132
research on, 129–130
responses of, 128, 129
support for, 171–172
theories and models of, for professionals, 131–173
experience of, 161
avoidance or suppression, 144–146
work of, 131
Grief Experience Inventory, 161
Growth
of person, 65–67
personal, 164–168
proposition 6 relating to, 164–168
team, 207, 236–242, 260–261, 264, 281

Handbook of Bereavement Research: Consequences, Coping, and Care (Stroebe, Hansson, Stroebe, Schut), 133
Helping relationship, distinct features of, 39–59
altered sense of time, experience of, 50–54
caregiving relationship, involvement in, 54–59
death and mortality awareness, exposure to, 40–47
suffering v. growth potential, inevitability of, 47–50
Hercules, 115–116, 187
Hierarchical splits, 225
Hippocrates, xi
Hochschild, Arlie Russell, 214
Holding behaviors
containment, 251–252
empathic acknowledgment, 252
enabling perspective, 252
Holding environment
characteristics of
protection/order/predictability/continuity of, 249
development of, 103–105
for care seekers/care providers, 242, 248–253
holding behaviors in, 251–252
functions of, 252
containment of experiences, 252
elaboration of experiences, 252
promotion of interdependence, 252
tempering or transformation of suffering, 252
Holistic and biopsychosocial model, of care, 6–9, 13
Hope, instillation of, 263

Idealization, of care, 229–230
Ideals. *See* Myths/mythology
Identity group splits, 225
Illness or dying, of care provider, 108–110
Immobilization, of team, 230, 233–235
Incremental grief, 160
Informational support, 242, 246–248
Inhibited grief, 162–163
Inhibition or disqualification, of reflection, 226
Insecure attachments, 35
Instrumental support, of co-workers, 247
Interconnectedness and interdependence, promotion of, 252
Interdisciplinary teams, 256–257, 259–260
Internal working model, 173, 303
International Work Group on Death, Dying, and Bereavement, 104, 180, 278
Interprofessional collaboration, of team functioning
developmental stage of
coexistence, 258
collaborative alliance, 258–259
mutual acknowledgment and parallel collaboration, 258
interdisciplinary, 256–257, 259–260
multidisciplinary, 256
transdisciplinary, 257, 259–260
Intersubjective field, definition of, 17
Interventions
life-sustaining, use of, 10
of organizations, for coping with suffering, 127
psychological, of Merimna, 73, 282
in team's disorganization, 235–236
Intimacy
fear of, 179
of involvement, 55
Involvement
active engagement, 22, 122
in caregiving relationship, 54
depersonalization, 95, 145, 201, 223
detached concern, 57–59
emotional, 54–55, 122, 211
emotional detachment, 57–58
friendly professional interest, 54, 56–57
indifference relating to, 217, 223
intimacy of, 55
in partnership, 23
Invulnerable, experience of being, 96–97

Journey
of dying or bereaved, 64, 65–66
of Theseus through the labyrinth, 62, 63, 64, 65, 70–71, 79, 100

Kahlo, Frida, 85
Kern, Hermann, 63
Kollwitz, Käthe, 85
Kübler-Ross, Elisabeth, 7, 97

Labyrinth
in caregiving, 65
Christianity and, 63–64
myth of, 61–67
in reality, 62–64, 67–70
ritual relating to, 63
La competence des families: Temps, chaos, processus (Ausloos), 230
Leadership, style of, 275
Leaders, in good-enough team
boundaries set by, 277–278
competency of, 276
as educators, 283
effectiveness of, 275
environment created by, 276
as learners, 283
as parental figures, 276
responsibilities of, 277
Lessons
from clinical experience, 274, 282
of myth, 64–67
Levi, Primo, 85
Lewis, C. S., 85
Lifestyle, definition of, 168
"The Life of the Almond Tree," 89
Loss
and death experiences, working through of, 262–263
nature of, 135–139

The Managed Heart: Commercialization of Feeling (Hochschild), 214
Martinson, Ida, 7, 129
Maze, myth of, 62–64
Meaning construction, support of, 247
Meaning
burnout, 122
collective, 155–159
construction, 247
content of meanings attributed to death, dying, and caregiving, 153–155
patterns of meaning attribution, 148
personal, 21, 43, 82, 86, 134, 155, 158, 287
related to caregiving
disease-related, 153
relationship-related, 154
related to death
in light of one's life trajectory, 150
lack of, 179
multiple, 151
philosophical or spiritual, 150
religious, 150
scientific/biological, 149
Members
care providers as team members, 195, 203–204
patient and family as team members, 195
Merimna, psychological intervention of, 73
Midwife, companioning role of, 67–68
Minority ethnic people, relationship-centered approach relating to, 10
Models of care or approaches to care
biopsychosocial and holistic, 6–9, 13
case-management, 5
fluctuation relating to, 134
medical, 5–6
patient-centered/family-centered approach, 7–8
relationship-centered approach, 13–16
loss and grief
avoidance of, 134
experiencing of, 134
for professionals' grieving process, 131–173
Mortality
acceptance of, 180, 185–186
awareness of, 40–47, 138–139
confrontation of, 52
Motives and needs, acknowledgment of, 179
to address existential concerns, 181
to address personal loss or trauma, 181
to be needed, loved, appreciated by others, 181
to be unique and distinct, 181–182
to make difference in others' lives, 180–181
Mount, Balfour, 7
Multidisciplinary teams, 256
Munch, Edward, 85
Mythology. *See* Myths.
Myths
in mythology
Ariadne, 62, 63, 65, 70–71, 79, 100
Chiron (the wounded healer), 115–117
Hercules, 115–116, 187
labyrinth v. maze of, 61–67
lessons of, 64–67

Minotaur, 61–67, 70–71, 100
Pandora and Prometheus, 297–298
Theseus, 62, 63, 64, 65, 70–71, 79, 100
in organizations
as ideals, 196–198

Nadir experience, 184
Narratives
disruptions, 272–273
team/collective, 271–273
Needs. *See* Motives and needs, acknowledgment of
Norton, Janice, 54

Open teamwork. *See also* Team(s).
boundaries for, 253–254
challenges of, 254–255
competence of, 253–256, 262
facilitation of, 253
as meaningful, 254
new initiatives and developments of, 255–256
service integration, 254, 262
Organizations
for caregiving, 191–202
culture of, team functioning influenced by, 206–209
definition of, 191
functioning mode of, 198
interventions of, for coping with suffering, 127
as multinuclear system of relations, 193
myths and ideals of, 196
social defense system, 200, 209

Palliative care
approach to
care personalized by, 9
as holistic, 7–9
limitations of, 9–10
partnership in, 8–9, 21
education, 285–287
pediatric, 10
Pandora and Prometheus, myth of, 297–298
Partnership
attachment bond relating to, 24
description of, 21–24
involvement in, 23
in palliative care approach, 8–9, 21
Partners in care
advantages of, 23
complementarity in, 22–23
role in, 22
shared goals in, 22
shortcomings of, 23–24
Past unaddressed or traumatic personal losses, emergence of, 138
Pathological forms, of bereavement, 11
Patient-professional relationship, 21
Patterns. *See also* Dysfunctional coping patterns/solutions, of team; Functional team patterns and solutions
dysfunctional, as cause of disorganization, 230–231
to make sense of death-related events, 148
Peak experience, 184
Pearlman, Laurie Anne, 126
Pediatric ICU, team rules of, 211–212
Pediatric oncology, team rules for, 210–211
Pediatric palliative care, 10
Personal growth. *See also* Growth
opportunities for, 164–168
Personalization, of care, 261–262
Person-professional relationship, 21, 39
Philosophical meanings, 150
Presence
absence v., 91–92
being fully present, 79–92
physical, 80–84
psychological, 84–92
Present moments, sharing of, 87–91
Primary tasks and functioning modes, of caregiving organizations, 198–202
dying/dead/bereaved, integration of, 200
suffering, regulation of, 200–201
time management, 201–202
Principles of team functioning, 203–204
Private practice, working in, 105–108
Process. *See also* Accompanying process; Grieving process
of accompaniment, frame relating to, 70–71
of learning, evaluation of, 291–293
reflective, of psychological presence, 87
of team, 218–219
threading, myth relating to, 66
Professional-person relationship, 194–195
Professional, caregiving behaviors of
attachments relating to
insecure, 35
secure, 34–35
safe haven provided as, 32–34
secure base provided as, 33–34
Professional goals and expectations, non-realization of, 136–137
Professionals, grieving process model for. *See* Grieving process

Projects or goals, attachment to, 32
Prometheus and Pandora, myth of, 297–298
Proposition 1, of grieving process model
nature of loss relating to
assumptions about ourselves/others/life, 137–138
own mortality, awareness of, 138–139
past unaddressed or traumatic personal losses, emergence of, 138
personal bond, 135
professional goals and expectations, non-realization of, 136–137
valued relationship, 135–136
personal loss relating to, 134
Proposition 2, of grieving process model
experience of grief and loss, 141–144
experiencing and avoiding loss and grief, fluctuation between, 139–141, 172
grief, avoidance or suppression of, 144–146
Proposition 3, of grieving process model
contribution and role, making sense of, 153–155
death/dying/caregiving, meanings attributed to 146–159,179
death, making sense of, 148–152
dying process, making sense of, 152–153
Proposition 4, of grieving process model
collective/shared meanings in, 155–159
through rituals, 156–157
through talking, 156
Proposition 5, of grieving process model, grief relating to
chronic and compounded, 161–162
in coexistence with trauma responses, 163–164
complications of, 160–161
inhibited, 162–163
overload of, 159–160
Proposition 6, of grieving process model, growth relating to
associated with
our life perspective, 166–168
our view and experience of caregiving, 166
perception of others, 165–166
perception of ourselves, 165
personal, opportunities for, 164–168
Proposition 7, of grieving process model, variables relating to, 168–173
education- and profession-related, 170
personal and work-related, 168–169
situational, 169–170
sociocultural, 170–173
Providers, of care. *See* Care providers
Proximity-seeking behaviors, 28
Psychological presence, 84–92

Redding, Karen, 107
Reflection
inhibition or disqualification of, 226
as reflective practice, 87
as reflective process, working through, elaboration of experiences, 287–288
Regulation, of suffering, 200–201
Relational learning and reflective practice, promotion of, 287–288
Relationship(s). *See also* Attachment; Partnership
with body, 47
of care, 21–38
caregiving rewards relating to, 177–178
with care providers, 12–13
distant/avoidant, 54, 219, 235
with dying/bereaved/co-workers, curricula for, 288–290
enmeshed, 23, 53, 95, 161, 169, 181, 219
helping, 39–59
with oneself and one's human existence, 47–48
overinvestment and over-eroticization of, 227–228
patient-professional, 21
person-professional, 21, 39
service requests, in death situations relating to, 25–26
suffering relating to
with larger community, 195
with other professionals, 195
between professional and individual seeking care, 194–195
among team members, 195
valued, loss of, 135–136
Relationship-centered approach, to care, 9–19, 194
administrative level of, 18
basic components of, 16
basis of, 13
bereavement care relating to, 10–11
care providers in
education of, 12–13
relationships with, 12–13
role of, 5–6
educational level of, 18–19
intersubjective field relating to, 17
minority ethnic people relating to, 10
patient- and family-centered approach to, 18
personal level of, 18
reciprocal influence relating to, 13–15

satisfaction linked to, 12
skills associated with, 12–13
studies about, 14
Relationship-related meanings, 154
Religion
attachment to, 30–31
meanings related to, 150
Resilience
of dying and bereaved, 26–27, 33S
of team, 260–267
Rewards, of caregiving, 175–188
Riddle of disease, 5, 136
Rippling, 180, 184–185
Risks and benefits, of team crises, 240–242
Risk taking, change and, 265
Rituals
collective, 156–157
development and use of, 264–265
Rogers, Carl, 55
Rules
display, 214
of teams, 209–217
over-regulation, 213
in therapy, 71–72
transgression of, 212–213
under-regulation, 213

Safe haven, provision of, 32–34
Safe space, in psychological presence, 86
SARS epidemic, 237
Satisfaction. *See also* Rewards of caregiving
related to models of care, 12
Saunders, Cicely, 7, 197–198
Scapegoating, 223–224
Schaverien, J., 108
Schut, H., 133
Science, society, death, and, 3–20
Scientific meanings, 149
Secondary traumatic stress, 123–124, 127
Secure attachments, 34–35
Secure base, provision of, 33–34
Self-care strategies, for coping with suffering, 127
Self-understanding, openness to, 180, 183–184
Services in death situations
request for, 25–28
integration of, 254, 262
review and validation of, 265
Situational meanings, of death/dying/caregiving, 147
Skills
behaviors and, counseling, 55–56
in relationship-centered approach to care, 12–13
Society, science and death, 3–20
biopsychosocial and holistic model, of care, 6–9, 13
medical model, of care, 5–6
relationship-centered approach, to care, 9–19
Somatization, collective, of suffering, 228–229
Spatial boundaries, 277
Spiritual meanings, 150
Splitting, 224–226
St. Christopher's Hospice, 197–198
Stress. *See* Compassion stress, compassion fatigue and; Secondary traumatic stress
Stroebe, M. S., 133
Stroebe, W., 133
Suffering
of care providers, 49–50, 117–120
collective somatization of, 228–229
containment of, 84, 251, 253
coping with, 127
levels of, 47–48
no immunity to, 116
of professionals, 49–50
regulation of, 200–201
of relationships, 194–195
suppression and denial of, 178–179
of team, 219
tempering or transforming of, 252
transformed through
personal story sharing, 84–85
present moments sharing, 87–91
in workplace, 193–196
v. growth, 49–50
Supervision
consultation and, methods of, 280–281
goals of, 280–281
role of, 278, 280–281
Support. *See also* Commitment
through caring acts and behaviors, 263–264
types of mutual support, 171, 246–247, 263–264
Suppression
avoidance and, of grief, 144–146
denial and, of suffering, 178–179
Survey, of American Psychoanalytic Association, 106

Tasks. *See* Commitment; Primary tasks and functioning modes, of caregiving organizations
Tasma, David, 197

Team(s). *See also* Good-enough team
  boundaries of, 218
  change of, 260–261
  chaos of, 230, 231–233
  crisis of, 157–158
  disorganization of, 230–236
    chaos in, 230, 231–233
    immobilization in, 230, 233–235
  external opportunities and threats of, 281
  functional behavior patterns of, 260–265
  functioning of, in death situations
    competence of, 242–256
    crises relating to, 236–242
    dynamics of, 204–205
    functional v. dysfunctional behavior patterns, 217–230
    interprofessional collaboration of, 256–260
    organization's culture influence on, 206–209
    resilience/effectiveness/creativity of, 260–267
    understanding of, 203–204
  growth of, 207, 236–242, 260–261, 264, 281
  interdisciplinary, 256–257, 259–260
  internal strengths and weaknesses of, 281
  interventions, 235–236
  marasme and immobility of, 230, 233–235
  members of, relationship among, 195
  mesocosmos of, 277
  multidisciplinary, 256
  process of, 218–219
  rules of
    development of, 210
    display, 214
    explicit or implicit, 209
    functions of, 212
    incongruence relating to, 214, 215, 216–217
    over-regulation of, 213
    for pediatric ICU, 211–212
    for pediatric oncology, 210–211
    transgression of, 212–213
    under-regulation of, 213
  splitting relating to, 224–226
  time of, 219
  transdisciplinary, 257, 259–260
  work style of, 169
Time
  altered sense of time, 51–52
  boundaries of, 277
  lived, 52
  management of, 201–202
  organizational, 201–202
  of team, 219
Touch, with physical presence, 83–84
Training outcomes and learning process, evaluation of, 291–293
Transdisciplinary teams, 257, 259–260
Transformation
  v. growth potential, 48, 65–67
  of suffering, 252
  through personal story sharing, 84–85
  through present moments sharing, 87–91
Trauma
  achievements and, team narratives of, 271–275
    absence of, 272–273
    disorganization of, 273
    dominant, 273
  personal loss of, addressing of, 181
  responses of, grief in coexistence with, 163–164
Traumatic stress, secondary, 123–124, 127
Traumatization, vicarious, of care providers, 125–126, 127

Under-regulation, of rules, 213

Vicarious traumatization, of care providers, 127
  avoidance/prevention of, 126
  symptoms of, 125
View and experience, of caregiving, 166
Violence and vitalizing force, of death, 48–49
Violent acts and behaviors, 222–223
Virgin Mary, 31, 101
Vulnerability. *See* Being vulnerable enough

Wald, Florence, 7
Winnicot, D. W., 99, 248, 249
Work style, of team, 169
Working
  in private practice, 105–106
  through loss experiences (elaboration), 252
World Health Organization, 96
Wounded healer, myth of, 115–117